EDUCATING
PHYSICAL
THERAPISTS

EDUCATING
PHYSICAL
THERAPISTS

Gail M. Jensen, PT, PhD, FAPTA, FNAP

Elizabeth Mostrom, PT, PhD, FAPTA

Laurita M. Hack, PT, DPT, MBA, PhD, FAPTA

Terrence Nordstrom, PT, EdD, FAPTA, FNAP

Jan Gwyer, PT, PhD, FAPTA

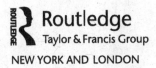

Routledge
Taylor & Francis Group

NEW YORK AND LONDON

First published 2019 by SLACK Incorporated

Published in 2024 by Routledge
605 Third Avenue, New York, NY 10158

and by Routledge
4 Park Square, Milton Park, Abingdon, Oxon, OX14 4RN

Routledge is an imprint of the Taylor & Francis Group, an informa business

Cover Artist: Justin Dalton

Library of Congress Cataloging-in-Publication Data
Names: Jensen, Gail M., author. | Mostrom, Elizabeth, author. | Hack, Laurita

Mary, author. | Nordstrom, Terrence, author. | Gwyer, Jan, author.
Title: Educating physical therapists / Gail M. Jensen, Elizabeth Mostrom,
Laurita M. Hack, Terrence Nordstrom, Jan Gwyer.
Description: Thorofare, NJ : Slack Incorporated, [2019] | Includes bibliographical references and index.
Identifiers: LCCN 2018042100
(print) | ISBN 9781630914110   (paperback)
Subjects: | MESH: Physical Therapy Specialty--education | United States
Classification: LCC RM725 (print) | NLM WB 18 | DDC
615.8/2--dc23
LC record available at https://lccn.loc.gov/2018042100

ISBN:9781630914110(pbk)
ISBN:9781003523949(ebk)

DOI: 10.4324/9781003523949

DEDICATION

Gail M. Jensen, PT PhD, FAPTA, FNAP: To Judy whose resilience is a model for all of us and her patience and support of me are never ending.

Elizabeth Mostrom, PT, PhD, FAPTA: To Herm who traveled this road by my side and whose love, humor, and patience sustains me.

Laurita M. Hack, PT, DPT, MBA, PhD, FAPTA: To Jack, Sarah, Jeff, Eleanor, and MW who make life a joy.

Terrence Nordstrom, PT, EdD, FAPTA, FNAP: To Cindy who was with me at the beginning of this journey and now is here in spirit, to Deirdre for bringing joy to our "work in progress," and my sons and grandchildren for reminding me what really matters.

Jan Gwyer, PT, PhD, FAPTA: To Marty, and all the students and clinicians who shared their wisdom, which made all the difference.

CONTENTS

Dedication V

Acknowledgments ix

About the Authors xi

Contributing Authors xiii

Foreword by Lee S. Shulman, PhD xv

Preface xvii

**Part I   Exploring Excellence in Professional Education:
              Following in Footsteps** 1

Chapter 1   Educating Physical Therapists: Context, Challenges, and Opportunities 3

Chapter 2   Excellence in the Professions: Past and Present Work of the Carnegie Foundation
             for the Advancement of Teaching 15

**Part II   Portraits of Excellence and Innovation: Model Dimensions, Elements,
              Paradigm Cases, and Recommendations** 23

Chapter 3   Research Design, Methods, and Evolving Frameworks 25

Chapter 4   The Culture of Excellence in Physical Therapist Education:
             Where Values and Vision Begin 39

Chapter 5   The Nexus: Bridging Our Academic and Clinical Worlds 59

Chapter 6   The Praxis of Learning: Opportunities Abound 75

Chapter 7   Organizational Context: Essential for Supporting Excellence 95

**Part III   Transforming Physical Therapist Education:
              Accelerating Positive Change** 111

Chapter 8   Creating a Culture of Excellence 113

Chapter 9   Advancing Learning and the Learning Sciences 125

Chapter 10   Organizational Imperatives 147

Chapter 11   Systems-Based Reform 155

Part IV   The Way Forward: Visions of What Could Be 173

Chapter 12   Understanding and Embracing the Potential of Interprofessional Education 175

             *Scott Reeves, PhD, MSc; Amber Fitzsimmons, PT, MS, DPTSc;
             and Simon Kitto, PhD*

Chapter 13   Practice-Based Education: Realizing Excellent Education for
             Future-Oriented Practice 189

             Joy Higgs, AM, BSc, MHPEd, PhD, NSW, PFHEA

Chapter 14   Directions for Education Research in Health Professions:
             Opportunities for Physical Therapy 201

             Stephen Loftus, PhD and Kathryn Huggett, PhD

Chapter 15   Educating for Professional Responsibility: Integration Across
             Habits of Head, Hand, and Heart 211

             Patricia Benner, RN, PhD, FAAN and Ruth Purtilo, PT, PhD, FAPTA

Chapter 16   Opportunities and Priorities for Physical Therapist Education:
              Perspectives From the Profession 223
              Steven B. Chesbro, PT, DPT, EdD and
              William G. Boissonnault, PT, DPT, DHSc, FAAOMPT, FAPTA

Chapter 17   Envisioning Our Future: The Way Forward 237

Appendix A 251

Appendix B 263

Financial Disclosures 273

Index 275

ACKNOWLEDGMENTS

We are grateful to all of the people who have contributed to our research and this book. First of all and most importantly, we thank those students, residents, academic and clinical faculty, and administrators across academic and clinical sites that hosted our visits, shared multiple documents, arranged logistics, and gave time for interviews, observations, and focus groups. We learned so much from all of you and have continued to share throughout our dissemination work how fortunate we have been to observe excellence and innovation in action. We have often said we wish everyone in the profession could have the experiences we had through our site visits and data collection process. We are indebted to these institutions and organizations:

- Arcadia University; Glenside, Pennsylvania
- Brooks Rehabilitation and the Institute of Higher Learning; Jacksonville, Florida
- Glendale Adventist Therapy and Wellness Center; Los Angeles, California
- Good Shepard Penn Partners; Philadelphia, Pennsylvania
- Madonna Rehabilitation Hospital; Lincoln, Nebraska
- MGH Institute of Health Professions; Charleston, Massachusetts
- Therapeutic Associates Physical Therapy; Portland, Oregon
- University of Delaware; Newark, Delaware
- University of Florida; Gainesville, Florida
- University of Southern California; Los Angeles, California
- Washington University in St. Louis; St. Louis, Missouri

Our consultants, Drs. Patricia O'Sullivan and Lee Shulman, provided us with wise counsel and guidance as we planned and implemented the study. Their critical, insightful, and supportive feedback brought us to new understandings that are part of this book. Drs. Bridget O'Brien, David Irby, and Patricia Benner shared much of their research processes and findings that were instrumental in the design of our work. We thank our Advisory Panel whose role was essential in the early phases of our work as members continually provided formative feedback for many elements of our method, selection of our sites, emerging findings, and recommendations. We had the opportunity to present our research at many conferences, and we all learned so much from our colleagues who shared their ideas and influenced our methods and findings. We are grateful to our invited authors, all experts in their fields, who provided additional insights into our findings and recommendations.

This study would not have been possible without the leadership support from the American Physical Therapy Association (APTA) and the many staff members who were instrumental in the project's success—from the time of our first consultation with Dr. Shulman at the Carnegie Foundation for the Advancement of Teaching at Stanford, California to its completion. We could not have expanded the scope of our research without the support from these funders: the APTA, the APTA's Academy of Physical Therapy Education, the APTA's Orthopedic Section, and the American Council of Academic Physical Therapy (ACAPT). We also are indebted to each of our institutions for providing us the time to conduct this study; it would not have been possible without that support.

Thanks also to Tony Schiavo, acquisitions editor at SLACK Incorporated who steadfastly supported the publication of our work, Allegra Tiver for facilitating our cover art, Phil Beagle for the creation of our figures, and Elizabeth DiPietro for her skillful, careful editing.

Finally, we had the great fortune of working together to design, conduct, and document this research. We accomplished more working as a group, using a process of listening, challenging, and collaborating, than we ever could have achieved working alone. We hope that many of our colleagues have such a rich research experience in their future. We share a deep appreciation for all of the physical therapists and other colleagues who have helped us grow and develop as physical therapists and researchers across our careers. We look forward to more opportunities to work and share with colleagues and to serve our profession.

ABOUT THE AUTHORS

Gail M. Jensen, PT, PhD, FAPTA, FNAP is Dean, Graduate School and College of Professional Studies and Vice Provost for Learning and Assessment, Professor of Physical Therapy, and Faculty Associate for Center of Health Policy and Ethics at Creighton University in Omaha, Nebraska. She holds a BS in education from the University of Minnesota, and an MA in physical therapy, and PhD in educational evaluation both from Stanford University. Dr. Jensen served as principal investigator for the research on *Physical Therapist Education for the Twenty First Century (PTE-21): Innovation and Excellence in Physical Therapist Academic and Clinical Education*, that is the focus of this text. Dr. Jensen is a qualitative researcher well-known for her scholarly publications related to expert practice, clinical reasoning, professional ethics, educational theory and interprofessional education and practice. During her career she has held faculty appointments at Stanford University, Temple University, The University of Alabama at Birmingham, Samuel Merritt University, and Creighton University. She has coauthored/edited several books, including: *Handbook of Teaching for Physical Therapists, Third Edition; Leadership in Interprofessional Health Education and Practice; Realising Exemplary Practice-Based Education; Expertise in Physical Therapy Practice, Second Edition; Educating for Moral Action: A Sourcebook in Health and Rehabilitation Ethics;* and forthcoming books *Clinical Reasoning in the Health Professions, Fourth Edition,* and *Clinical Reasoning and Decision Making in Physical Therapy.* Dr. Jensen is a Catherine Worthingham Fellow of the APTA and a fellow in the Physical Therapy Academy of the National Academies of Practice. She is a recipient of the APTA's Rothstein Golden Pen Award, Lucy Blair Service Award and was the APTA's 2011 Mary McMillan Lecturer.

Elizabeth Mostrom, PT, PhD, FAPTA is Professor Emeritus at Central Michigan University where she previously served as Professor and Director of Clinical Education for the Doctoral Program in Physical Therapy, School of Rehabilitation and Medical Sciences. She holds a BS degree in health education from West Chester State College, an MS in physical therapy from Duke University, and a PhD in educational psychology from Michigan State University. Dr. Mostrom is a qualitative and education researcher whose scholarly publications and presentations span the areas of student and professional learning and development, clinical education, and qualitative methods. She has been a contributing author to several books including the first and second editions of *Expertise in Physical Therapy Practice; Handbook of Teaching for Physical Therapists, Second Edition;* and *Realising Exemplary Practice-Based Education and Educating for Moral Action: A Sourcebook in Health and Rehabilitation Ethics.* She coauthored/edited *Handbook of Teaching for Physical Therapists, Third Edition* with Dr. Jensen. She is a co-investigator for the study described in this book, *Physical Therapist Education for the Twenty First Century (PTE-21): Innovation and Excellence in Physical Therapist Academic and Clinical Education.* Dr. Mostrom is a past editor of the *Journal of Physical Therapy Education* and is a Catherine Worthingham Fellow of the APTA. She is a recipient of the APTA's Mary McMillan Scholarship and Lucy Blair Service Award and was the APTA's Education Section Polly Cerasoli Lecturer in 2013.

Laurita M. Hack, PT, DPT, MBA, PhD, FAPTA is Professor Emeritus at Temple University. Dr. Hack holds a BA from Wilmington College; an MS as the first professional degree in physical therapy from Case Western Reserve University; an MBA from the Wharton School, University of Pennsylvania; a PhD in higher education administration from University of Pennsylvania; and a DPT from the MGH Institute of Health Professions. She is a coauthor of *Expertise in Physical Therapy Practice, Second Edition,* and several related articles, supplying the original research on development of expertise in geriatric practice for this body of work. She has also coauthored *Evidence into Practice* with Dr. Jan Gwyer. It is a text on the integration of clinical decision making, respect for patient values, and evidence from the literature into practice. She is currently a co-investigator in the grant, *Physical Therapist Education for the Twenty First Century (PTE-21): Innovation and Excellence in Physical Therapist Academic and Clinical Education.* This study has resulted in several presentations, articles, and this text. Dr. Hack has extensive clinical experience in outpatient, nursing home, and homecare practice, especially in geriatrics, and has taught in the areas of practice management, geriatrics, clinical decision making, critical inquiry, evidence-based practice, ethics, communications, and health care systems. She has served the APTA as President of the Community/Home Health Section, the Health Policy Section and the Education Section. She has also served as Vice Speaker and Secretary of the APTA. She is a Catherine Worthingham Fellow of the APTA and has received the APTA's Lucy Blair Service Award and Baethke-Carlin Award for Teaching Excellence. She is the APTA's 2018 Mary McMillan Lecturer.

Terrence Nordstrom, PT, EdD, FAPTA, FNAP is a Professor of Physical Therapy and the Vice President of Enrollment and Student Services at Samuel Merritt University. He previously served as the Director of Clinical Education and as Chair of the Department of Physical Therapy at Samuel Merritt University. He holds a Bachelor of Arts degree from the University of California Santa Cruz and a Master's degree in Physical Therapy from Stanford University in California. He received his Doctor of Education degree in Organization and Leadership from the University of San Francisco in California. Dr. Nordstrom has coauthored articles and book chapters in the areas of ethical reasoning and education research. He is currently a co-investigator in the grant, *Physical Therapist Education for the Twenty First Century (PTE-21): Innovation and Excellence in Physical Therapist Academic and Clinical Education.* This study has resulted in several presentations, articles, and this text. Dr. Nordstrom was in clinical practice for 30 years in acute care, home care and outpatient services. He held leadership positions in rehabilitation in an outpatient clinic and an academic medical center and was a co-owner of 2 independent physical therapy services. Dr. Nordstrom has held several leadership positions in the APTA, including as President and Vice President of the American Council of Academic Physical Therapy, the Ethics and Judicial Committee, and serves as an on-site reviewer for the Commission on Accreditation in Physical Therapy Education. He was named a Catherine Worthingham Fellow of the APTA in 2015.

Jan Gwyer, PT, PhD, FAPTA is Professor Emerita at Duke University. She served as a Professor of the Doctor of Physical Therapy Division, Department of Orthopaedics, School of Medicine, Duke University, Durham, North Carolina. She holds a Bachelor of Science Degree from the Medical College of Virginia and Master's and Doctor of Philosophy Degree from the University of North Carolina at Chapel Hill. Dr. Gwyer has been a practicing physical therapist for 45 years, in both inpatient and outpatient settings, with her practice focused on aspects of rehabilitation for adult patients. She has been an educator and researcher for over 30 years. Her expertise focused on higher education, clinical education, career patterns, and workforce issues in physical therapy. She is a coauthor of the first and second editions of *Expertise in Physical Therapy Practice*, and several related articles, that led to the research project that resulted in this book. She has also coauthored with Dr. Laurie Hack *Evidence into Practice*, a text on the integration of clinical decision making, respect for patient values, and evidence from the literature into practice. Dr. Gwyer has held several leadership roles in the APTA, serving on the board of the American Physical Therapy Specialists, the Clinical Instructors Education Board, and on the APTA Board of Directors. She has received APTA awards including the Lucy Blair Service Award and the Catherine Worthingham Fellow of the APTA.

CONTRIBUTING AUTHORS

Patricia Benner, RN, PhD, FAAN (Chapter 15)
Professor Emerita, Department of Social and Behavioral Sciences
University of California, San Francisco
Former Senior Scholar Carnegie Foundation for the Advancement of Teaching
San Francisco, California

William G. Boissonnault, PT, DPT, DHSc, FAAOMPT, FAPTA (Chapter 16)
Executive Vice President of Professional Affairs
American Physical Therapy Association
Alexandria, Virginia
Professor Emeritus, University of Wisconsin—Madison
Madison, Wisconsin

Steven B. Chesbro, PT, DPT, EdD (Chapter 16)
Vice President, Education
American Physical Therapy Association
Alexandria, Virginia

Amber Fitzsimmons, PT, MS, DPTSc (Chapter 12)
Associate Professor and Chair
Department of Physical Therapy and Rehabilitation Science
Department of Anatomy
University of California, San Francisco
San Francisco, California

Joy Higgs, AM, BSc, MHPEd, PhD, NSW, PFHEA (Chapter 13)
Professor in Higher Education
Charles Sturt University
Sydney, Australia

Kathryn Huggett, PhD (Chapter 14)
Director, The Teaching Academy
Robert Larner, M.D. '42 Professor in Medical Education
Assistant Dean for Medical Education
The Robert Larner, M.D. College of Medicine
University of Vermont
Burlington, Vermont

Simon Kitto, PhD (Chapter 12)
Professor, Department of Innovation in Medical Education
Faculty of Medicine
University of Ottawa
Ottawa, Canada

Stephen Loftus, PhD (*Chapter 14*)
Associate Professor of Medical Education
Oakland University William Beaumont School of Medicine
Rochester, Michigan

Ruth Purtilo, PT, PhD, FAPTA (Chapter 15)
Professor Emerita, Interdisciplinary Studies
MGH Institute of Health Professions
Boston, Massachusetts

Scott Reeves, PhD, MSc (Chapter 12)
Deceased

FOREWORD

An Office Visit

Abraham Flexner was making an office visit. In his biography of the first President of the Carnegie Foundation, Henry Pritchett, Flexner described their first meeting in 1908 as quite a surprise. Flexner was a former prep school founder and teacher from Louisville who had just published a book on the American college. His closest connection to medicine was working in a family pharmacy when he was younger and providing the funds to support his brother Simon's medical school tuition at Johns Hopkins. Hence his shock when Pritchett invited him to conduct a comprehensive study of the quality of medical education for the then-3-year-old foundation. When Flexner explained to Pritchett that he was an educator, not a physician like his brother, Pritchett affirmed that reviewing and evaluating the quality of education for physicians was a job for an astute educator, not for a physician. After reading his book on American colleges, Flexner was clearly cut out to do that job. Neither of them could have anticipated that the 1910 report would turn American medical education on its head, nor that the name *Flexner Report* would become iconic for the next century.

When she walked into my Stanford office in the mid-1980s, Gail Jensen introduced herself and explained that she was a physical therapist pursuing a doctorate in curriculum studies in the School of Education. She asked if I would become her advisor and direct her dissertation research. I wasn't surprised to have a health professional as a student, because before coming to Stanford in 1982, I held a joint appointment in educational psychology and medical education at Michigan State University. I had studied the work of physicians and nurses, and had collaborated with them, but never with a physical therapist. Indeed, I probably wasn't all that clear at the time about what physical therapists did.

Gail was interested in the most fundamental questions associated with any profession, the challenges of achieving, sustaining and judging the quality of programs. Physical therapy, like most professions, has earned the right and responsibility for holding training programs accountable to meet standards of excellence. How well do the mechanisms of review work? The heart of program quality assurance in physical therapy was a combination of self-study and a subsequent review by a peer visiting committee. Gail wanted to ask, how did visiting committees do their work? How reliable and valid was the site visit as a mode of evaluation? She designed an investigation of the site visit process in physical therapy, a splendid dissertation, and a serious contribution to the integrity of her professional field.

About 20 years later, each of our roles had changed. After several years teaching physical therapy in universities, Gail was now Dean of the Graduate School at Creighton University. I was President of the Carnegie Foundation for the Advancement of Teaching, where Flexner and Pritchett had held their earlier meeting, albeit 3000 miles further west. Gail had become a national leader in her professional field, as well as an academic administrator with broad university responsibilities. I was now leading the institution that, 100 years earlier, had conducted the *Flexner Report* of medical education. The foundation was now amid a set of studies of education in the professions of law, engineering, nursing, the clergy, medicine and business leadership. I often referred to that 12-year research program as "On the Shoulders of Flexner."

And so, once again, Gail Jensen walked into my office. This time several other leaders in the profession of physical therapy accompanied her. They wanted to discuss how they might conduct a Carnegie-like study of the education of physical therapists. The profession was in the midst of a dramatic change. The doctorate in physical therapy had become the entry-level professional degree as the standards and expectations for practice had grown in sophistication, rigor, and practice. The field needed their own *Flexner Report* and they had come to discuss how that work might unfold. My colleagues and I were at that moment working on our own revisit of the *Flexner Report*, once again studying the quality of medical education, 100 years after the original study. I felt it was a privilege to help Gail and her esteemed colleagues conduct a parallel study in their own professional field.

The volume you are about to read is the result of that initiative. It takes courage to place one's own field under a critical microscope. Like the accreditation review and site visit of an individual program, this is an evaluation of peers by peers. In accreditation, we examine one program at a time. In a study like this, peers examine the quality of education in an entire field. By studying a sample of individual programs comparatively and intensively, they test generalizations against the tough criterion of concrete instances of practice. By exploring variations in programs and visions, they appreciate the extent to which experimentation and program reforms are practically possible.

I have also come to appreciate how much has changed since my predecessor Pritchett commissioned Flexner's report. While in 1908 he had to choose between a physician and an educator to do the work, in our day we are blessed with leaders in the profession of physical therapy who are also well trained as practitioners and scholars of education. Whereas the *Flexner Report* was conducted by someone who was an outsider to the field, the present report has the virtue of an insider's perspective combined with the critical acumen of outsiders who are also sophisticated in both theory and practice in education. While Flexner did his work alone, the present report is the work of a team, a group of evaluators who bring multiple perspectives, skills, and experiences to the challenge.

When asked to describe his method, Flexner responded, "ambulando discimus, we learn by going about." The colleagues in physical therapy who conducted this study and wrote this report have also learned by going about. They have not been satisfied with broad surveys, much less with general impressions gleaned from their many years of experience. They have critically tested their ideas by juxtaposing the best ideas from clinical teaching, problem-based learning, the development of professional ethical and moral judgment and many other domains with the hard facts of observation and interaction in the field.

Physical therapists are teachers. Perhaps that's why I find it so easy to relate to the field. The work of the physical therapist is to heal the muscles and bones that need work; it is also to teach patients to manage their own lives to sustain their physical health. The work of a professional is to teach clients so well that the intervention of the professional is no longer needed. We are all educators.

I commend this volume to its readers. It takes courage to subject one's own field to this kind of critical, incisive scrutiny. Yet any field that deserves to be described as a profession must take on the highest standard of self-evaluation, both for individual practitioners and the entire professional community. They have learned by going about. We, their readers, can now profit from their journeys and use their insights to improve the work of physical therapy. I write this foreword, not as a physical therapist, but as someone whose wellbeing has been improved by the work of gifted physical therapists. You never know what will come of a visit to your office.

The authors of this volume have much to teach us, and they have taught us well. We can accept their recommendations, or we can argue with them. To ignore them is impossible.

Lee S. Shulman, PhD
Stanford, California

PREFACE

The last half-century in the United States has been characterized by constant and often dramatic change in the health care system, the nature of health care delivery, and higher education. In response, the educational preparation of professionals who deliver health care services has also evolved, albeit sometimes less rapidly, to meet new and often expanding expectations and challenges posed by these shifting sands. As a relatively recent health care profession that formally came into being approximately one century ago, physical therapy reflected these same responses, while at the same time working to build the practice, education, and research standards needed to assure it was meeting societal expectations.

By the 1960s, the need for a comprehensive nationwide study of physical therapist education was recognized and was undertaken by Catherine Worthingham. Her decade-long landmark investigation provided an overview of the current status of physical therapy education at the time and, perhaps more importantly, anticipated society's future needs and directions for physical therapy education if the profession was to continue to grow and thrive in the future. Remarkably, while the profession has experienced substantial change in the last half-century and the preparation of physical therapists has moved from apprenticeship and certificate models of education to doctoral preparation, to date there has been no comprehensive, systematic, nationwide study of physical therapy education since that of Worthingham more than 5 decades ago.

The study described in this book grew out of our recognition of the need for another comprehensive and nationwide investigation given the substantial changes in physical therapy practice and education over the past 5 decades. Our vision of the nature and scope of the project was shaped, in large part, by investigations of professional education undertaken by the Carnegie Foundation for the Advancement of Teaching in the 2000s. The Foundation's Preparation for the Professions Program (PPP) initiated under the leadership of then President, Dr. Lee Shulman, resulted in 5 far-reaching and noteworthy studies of preparation for the professions of the clergy, law, engineering, nursing, and medicine. Importantly, they also afforded the opportunity for a cross-professions examination of professional education in those fields and others.

The Carnegie studies, and the findings and recommendations that emanated from them, provided a source of inspiration and perseverance as we sought funding and began our investigative journey that spanned several years. Like the PPP studies, we chose to closely examine exemplars of excellence in professional education; in our case, across the continuum from the initial preparation for entry into the profession through post-professional residency education in both academic and clinical settings. Collectively, we brought to the endeavor more than 150 years of experience in physical therapist education, expertise in educational research and qualitative inquiry, and a deep belief in the need for and the purpose of our study. Finally, we brought an abiding hope that the findings from our study would engender the kinds of deliberative reflection, rich conversation, and thoughtful reform that had resulted from the PPP studies, and that would promise a bright future for physical therapist education well into the 21st century. While we anticipate discussion of our findings and recommendations among physical therapy academic and clinical educators and professional leaders world-wide, we also believe they are relevant to all who are interested and invested in professional education.

The are several purposes for this book. The first is to share the findings from our study, *Physical Therapist Education for the Twenty First Century (PTE-21): Innovation and Excellence in Physical Therapist Academic and Clinical Education*, and place those findings in the historical and current context for health professions education, physical therapist education, and physical therapy practice in the United States. In sharing our findings, and because of the nature of our multi-year qualitative investigation, we provide a great deal of grounded data, detailed narratives, and paradigm cases to bring readers as close as possible to what we had the good fortune to directly observe and hear as we visited sites that were exemplars of excellence in physical therapist education; in essence, we seek to paint portraits of excellence for our readers. Readers will also hear a multiplicity of voices and perspectives in this volume—ranging from those of students and residents, to academic and clinical faculty, to clinic and university administrators. A second purpose is to present the Conceptual Model of Excellence in Physical Therapist Education that emerged from ongoing and iterative analysis of our extensive data repository and to reflect on the meaning and implications of that model for future directions in educational research and practice in physical therapist education. Finally, moving forward from our findings and drawing on literature from other health professions and disciplines, we offer recommendations for consideration and action that we believe could advance and transform physical therapist education in the future. The latter purpose is fully realized and enhanced by contributions from a distinguished group of nationally and internationally known invited authors who bring key insights on our work from a variety of perspectives and disciplines.

This volume is organized into 4 main parts related to the study purposes described above. Each of the parts begins with a preface that sets the stage for what is to come in the chapters that follow. Part I provides an overview of the historical context for our study with a primary focus on (1) physical therapist education in the United States over the last century and (2) the Carnegie Foundation for the Advancement of Teaching studies of professional education during that same time. Part II provides detailed descriptions of our study design, methods and findings, and introduces the Conceptual Model of Excellence in Physical Therapist Education that arose from our analysis and that serves as a framework for the remaining chapters and parts of the book. In Part III, working from our findings and model and drawing on evidence and literature from a variety of professions and disciplines, we put forth 30 recommendations that we believe have the potential to produce transformation and positive change in physical therapist education. Finally, in Part IV, we combine our voices and visions with those of other outstanding invited authors, to consider the question of "Where do we go from here?" and to envisage the way forward with imagination and renewed purpose and energy.

Our investigative and reflective journey during the completion of this study was one of constant learning and development over the years enriched by the experiences and insights shared by our study participants, consultants, and the audiences who asked thought provoking questions as we presented emerging findings as the study unfolded. Now we invite readers to join us on that journey.

Exploring Excellence in Professional Education
Following in Footsteps

Our aim in Part I of this volume is to set the scene for what is to come. We place the description of our national study of physical therapist education, and the findings and recommendations that ensued, in the context of physical therapy's emergence as a health care profession in the 20th century and the recent comprehensive studies of professional education conducted by the Carnegie Foundation for the Advancement of Teaching.

In Chapter 1, we provide a brief overview of the history of the profession of physical therapy and physical therapist education in the United States over the last century—from birth to adulthood. In doing so, we highlight a landmark study completed by Catherine Worthingham in the 1960s—our adolescence, if you will—that set a course for future directions in physical therapist education influenced by signposts she erected. We describe key events and trends that shaped physical therapist education since that midpoint in our development as a profession and conclude the chapter with a snapshot of physical therapist education today, identifying current issues facing the profession, and anticipating future challenges and opportunities as physical therapist education moves forward in the 21st century.

In Chapter 2, we introduce the Carnegie Foundation Preparation for the Professions Program (PPP), a series of studies that investigated education in 5 professions (ie, clergy, law, engineering, nursing, medicine) during the first decade of the 21st century. The PPP studies were undertaken almost 100 years after a pioneering study of medical education, also supported by the Carnegie Foundation, that resulted in the *1910 Flexner Report* that shaped medical education for the 20th century. Like the Flexner study before them, the PPP studies have had a significant impact on professional education and research in the fields studied and promise to continue to do so. The design of the PPP studies served as a model for our study of physical therapist education, and several of their findings and recommendations for reform resonate with and inform our own findings and recommendations. We are fortunate to have been able to follow in the footsteps of the Carnegie

Foundation investigators and leadership and hope others agree, as Dr. Lee Shulman suggested in his foreword, that our readers can learn and profit from the insights we gained on our journey.

1

Educating Physical Therapists
Context, Challenges, and Opportunities

CONTEXT: THE FIRST 50 YEARS

Physical therapy as a health care practice in the United States had its beginnings in the late 19th century as unlicensed personnel with backgrounds in exercise and other forms of physical agents, joined with teams of physicians and nurses to treat people affected by the polio epidemics of that era. Then, in 1918 the Office of the US Surgeon General of the Army authorized formation of Reconstruction Aides who entered 3-month training programs to meet the therapeutic needs of soldiers serving in World War I.[1,2]

The timing of physical therapy's emergence benefited from reforms in medicine and nursing that just preceded the origins of physical therapy. At the beginning of the 1900s, medicine and nursing were both characterized by a great variability in practice that many leaders in the field considered to be dangerous to public health. The *1910 Flexner Report*,[3] commissioned by the Carnegie Foundation, coupled with formation of the Council of Medical Education of the American Medical Association, led to a structure with the scientific basis of medical education occurring within institutions of higher education, and clinical training occurring in academic medical centers and hospitals. By 1927, this structure was truly standardized with universal licensure of physicians.[4-8] The nursing profession followed a similar, but later, trajectory than medicine. *The Goldmark Report of 1923*,[9] commissioned by the Rockefeller Foundation, set criteria for both the practice of nursing in various settings, and the education of nurses, placing nursing education on a path out of hospital-based training and into institutions of higher education. Universal mandatory nursing licensure with an education requirement occurred in the 1940s.[10-12]

Physical therapy began as a profession in the United States just as medicine and nursing were turning their attention to standardizing education and practice, thereby benefiting from the work done in those fields. Mary McMillan led the development of educational programs to prepare

Jensen GM, Mostrom E, Hack LM, Nordstrom T, Gwyer J.
Educating Physical Therapists (pp 3-13).
© 2019 Taylor & Francis Group.

Reconstruction Aides for their service, and by 1928, within 10 years of the development of those programs, there were 12 programs in the United States, and the professional association of the time, the American Physiotherapy Association, had published standards for these programs.[1] The programs were grounded in practical, apprenticeship models with preparatory classroom and laboratory learning where the emphasis was on applied physical therapeutics.[1,2]

Licensure was initiated in Pennsylvania in 1911,[13] but, unlike the widespread rapid adoption seen in medicine and nursing, physical therapists were not licensed in all 50 states until the 1970s.[1,14] Much like medicine and nursing, physical therapy transitioned from apprenticeship and hospital-based training into higher education. Even so, of the 42 programs in existence in 1968, 13 were in hospitals and 1 was in a physical education school, with 28 in colleges, universities, or medical schools, and it was possible to become licensed without a bachelor's degree.[1,15]

The Worthingham Study

By the 1960s, the need for a comprehensive, national study of physical therapy education was apparent in the profession. Supported by funding from the US Social and Rehabilitation Services Administration and the American Physical Therapy Association (APTA), Catherine Worthingham embarked on a comprehensive study of physical therapy education that included other aspects of the profession, such as patterns of patient care, the clinical environment, referral patterns, and graduate outcomes. Unlike the Flexner and Goldmark studies with their detailed on-site examination of individual programs, Worthingham's study relied on survey data, as well as careful review of the educational and health care environment of the time, including referral practices and patient characteristics in physical therapy. Hislop[16], introducing the series of articles presenting the findings of the study, wrote:

> For years it has been lamented in many circles that physical therapy needs a thorough objective investigation of its entire educational system—a study which, like the *1910 Flexner Report* in medicine, would show to all the world the glowing strengths and glaring weaknesses of our schools, a report, however, which would pave the way for innovation and progress.[(p5)]

That introductory editorial recognized the thoroughness of the study and substantial contribution Worthingham's work could play for the profession, concluding that "the momentum provided by this study should carry us a long way."[16(p5)]

The Worthingham Study included all the physical therapy education programs in existence at the time (n = 42), all the associated clinical sites (n = 441), the clinical staff at those sites (n = 2402), and a survey of 1961 and 1965 graduates of those programs. Worthingham also gathered clinical data from physician referrals in physical therapy at the participating clinical sites to better understand clinical practice patterns. The findings of this comprehensive study were published in 5 parts from 1968 to 1970.[15,17-21] The first 2 parts focused on physical therapy education; the third part focused on clinical education (CE) sites, such as monetary factors, administrative structure, activities expected of students, and characteristics of the clinical staff; the fourth part focused on graduates and described geographic distribution, clinical and teaching experiences, salaries, professional development, and perceptions of their entry-level education; and the fifth part addressed clinical practice patterns, including the specialties of referring physicians, patient diagnoses, and the physical therapy services provided. Worthingham's final article[22] summarized the findings from the first 5 articles and made recommendations for the future of physical therapist education and practice that fell into the following 5 broad categories:

1. *Professional Identity*: Physical therapists need a closer approach to peer equivalence, mutual respect, and recognition of responsibility is essential.[(p1321)]
2. *Workforce*: The public is demanding that health care be available, accessible, and acceptable, yet there are not enough physical therapists to fill budgeted positions.[(p1321)]

3. *Societal Needs*: Educators in physical therapy can no longer shirk the responsibility of meeting community health needs on a local, regional, or national scale.(p1322)

4. *Bridge Between Academic and Clinical Envionments*: The fact that 73% of staff of the CE facilities in the years from 1965 to 1966 had responsibility for supervising physical therapy students, coordinating clinical supervision, or both, but only 6% participated in the development of curricula of the schools indicates the need for further contributions from this group.(p1326)

5. *Interprofessional Education*: The expanding role of the physical therapist requires an educational program which will prepare the graduate to participate with medical and other health professionals in designing and carrying out systems of health care that will meet the needs of an awakened public.(p1330)

The Worthingham Study stands as a landmark for the physical therapy profession. Worthingham collected an extraordinary amount of data from participants, representing the universe or near universe of all major stakeholders in physical therapist education. Dr. Worthingham was an extraordinary leader and systems thinker for the profession, as demonstrated by the innovative data collection mechanisms she employed in looking across all aspects of physical therapist education, as well as an assessment of the expectations of the health care system of the time for physical therapists. The real stroke of genius in her work was to place her results in the larger context of the health care and education systems.

CONTEXT: PHYSICAL THERAPIST EDUCATION 1970S TO PRESENT

In this section, we summarize key activities and changes that were occurring in the years between 1970 and today in the professional preparation of physical therapists in the United States in the context of concurrent change in health care and higher education. A timeline and summary of key activities and initiatives that influenced physical therapist education over these 5 decades are provided in Appendix A, Table A-1.

Following the Worthingham Study, another large-scale initiative, the *Project on Clinical Education in Physical Therapy*, was undertaken in the 1970s by Moore and Perry.[23] This project was developed in response to a charge from the APTA Section for Education and was federally funded by the US Department of Health, Education, and Welfare. The primary aim was to gather data about the status of CE and to anticipate future needs, especially related to clinical site and faculty development and the assessment of the quality of CE experiences. The final project report provided detailed descriptions of CE sites and faculty, the educational and evaluation processes used, and concluded with 27 focal points for further work in understanding and improving the social, education, evaluation, and organization contexts and practices for physical therapist CE in the United States.[23] The findings from this project were widely disseminated in the physical therapist education community and fueled new initiatives to investigate and improve CE. Paired with a 1979 APTA House of Delegates (HOD) adoption of a policy to move physical therapist education from baccalaureate degree preparation to a graduate degree level (HOD 06-79-08-15), such efforts were timely and important.

Building on Moore and Perry's work, Barr and colleagues[24] developed a manual with recommended standards and forms for evaluation and selection of CE sites. In a subsequent study, these authors found the standards to be valued, reliable, and valid by a large sample of academic coordinators of CE, clinical faculty, and students.[25] These standards were the basis for many of the activities that ensued during the 1980s and 1990s directed toward the improvement and standardization of CE. The standards served as a starting point for identifying potential changes and alternative models for CE as the profession moved toward post-baccalaureate preparation for physical therapists.

Following the Moore and Perry project[23] to examine and advance physical therapist education, there was a substantial acceleration in the level of activity in this realm between 1980 and today (see Appendix A). Several advances and factors within the profession itself, physical therapist and higher education, and the health care system propelled many of these activities.

In response to changing demographics and health care needs in society, widespread changes in delivery patterns, and changes within the profession, the scope of practice for physical therapists was expanding during the 1980s to 1990s. This included the delivery of therapy services to a wider variety of patient populations across diverse settings, and a focus that was moving beyond the provision of rehabilitation services to incorporate preventive, and health promotion activities. Concurrently, practice acts across the nation were gradually changing to allow for direct consumer access to physical therapists for care in contrast to previous requirements in most states for physician referral for services. This change meant there was a need for expanded knowledge and skills for physical therapists for screening for medical disease and clinical disorders that might fall outside of their scope of practice. The increasing variability in the types and complexity of patients seen by physical therapists was also creating a greater demand for specialization in the field and board certification and post-professional residencies and fellowships in several specialty areas became a reality during this time. These shifts in practice demands and health care system changes meant changes in responsibilities and expectations for physical therapists and, in combination with the exponential growth in the foundational knowledge and skills needed for practice, demanded curricular expansion in educational programs.

These changes in physical therapy meant that accreditation criteria and standards needed to be altered to reflect new practice expectations for physical therapist graduates and to ensure that professional preparation programs were accountable for assessing and meeting desired educational outcomes in both the didactic and clinical components of the program. During the mid-19th century, accreditation for physical therapist education was controlled by the American Medical Association. After many years of inability to improve educational standards, the APTA determined to take control over accreditation of physical therapy education. In 1977, the accreditation structure and processes for physical therapy put in place by the APTA were recognized by the US Department of Education. This move for the profession to finally have control over the setting of accreditation standards was a watershed change for physical therapist education.[26] Accreditation processes and criteria continued to evolve with 5 standard changes between 1977 and 2003[26] with the latest set of standards becoming effective in 2016.[27]

As professional program length, credit hours, curricular requirements, and density increased, there were changes in the degree awarded for entry into the profession. In the 1970s the great majority of physical therapist programs awarded a baccalaureate degree as the first professional degree, rather than in post-baccalaureate certificate programs. This move was not without controversy. It occurred primarily because of the availability of federal support to create schools of allied health professions and for baccalaureate degree programs. At the same time, some leaders thought a better path was to move to graduate education. They led the way in developing 6 entry-level master's degree programs.[28] The program directors responsible for these innovative programs were vibrant and risk-taking leaders, all with a strong vision of physical therapy as a profession and the need for development of graduates who would serve as change agents in the profession.

Beginning in the early 1980s, this movement toward post-baccalaureate (graduate level) preparation gained strong support as demonstrated by a 1979 HOD motion (HOD 06-79-08-15) supporting education at a postgraduate level, and by 2002 the Commission on Accreditation in Physical Therapy Education (CAPTE) was no longer accrediting programs that did not award a post-baccalaureate degree.[26] As early as the late 1980s, discussion around the need for a clinical doctoral degree had begun in the physical therapist education community[29,30] and by 1996, Creighton University awarded the first Doctor of Physical Therapy (DPT) degree to entry-level graduates.[31] The trend of increasing degree level to a clinical doctorate continued in the late 1990s and 2000s, and as of 2015 the only professional degree being awarded by accredited programs in the United States was the DPT.

The changes in practice and education described previously and the advancement of the first professional degree to the doctoral level were reflected in the APTA's *Vision 2020* sentence adopted by the HOD in 2000 that stated:[32]

> By 2020, physical therapy will be provided by physical therapists who are doctors of physical therapy, recognized by consumers and other health care professionals as the practitioners of choice to whom consumers have direct access for the diagnosis of, interventions for, and prevention of impairments, activity limitations, participation restrictions, and environmental barriers related to movement, function and health.

The elements and values embedded in *Vision 2020*, including the *International Classifciation of Functioning, Disability and Health* framework,[33] continue to influence physical therapist practice and education today but are augmented by a more recent vision statement for the physical therapy profession and the related guiding principles adopted by the HOD in 2013: "Transforming society by optimizing movement to improve the human experience."[34,35] This bold vision for the profession is currently shaping practice and physical therapist education today and promises to continue to do so in the future. A comparison of these 2 vision statements also highlights a notable shift from one that is primarily focused inward on the profession itself to one that focuses attention outward on what the profession can contribute to society.

Physical Therapist Education Today

Physical therapy programs are housed across a variety of colleges and universities with 41% at master's colleges and universities of various sizes, 36% at research universities, 17% at medical schools and other specialized health professional schools, and 6% at bachelor's colleges and universities; 51% percent of programs are at private institutions.[36] There is no common curricular model in use among the physical therapist education programs in the United States, with 75% reporting using a hybrid model, meaning some combination of systems-based, problem-based, traditional (basic science followed by clinical science, followed by physical therapy science), or other description.[36] There is a great deal of variability in the number of weeks of didactic and CE among physical therapist education programs, but the average total length of programs is 123 weeks.[36]

The CE components of professional preparation are typically comprised of short term clinical experiences, often referred to as *integrated clinical education* (ICE) experiences, that may be part-time or full-time, days or a few weeks, learning experiences with real or simulated patients that are embedded within the didactic curriculum most often during years 1 and 2 of the professional curriculum. These ICE experiences are usually followed by longer term full-time intermediate experiences in affiliated clinical sites that vary in length, weeks to months, followed by final or terminal clinical experiences that may last months to 1 year. For the CAPTE-accredited physical therapist programs in 2017, the average number of weeks students spent in full-time experiences, intermediate and final, was 37.8 weeks, representing roughly 33% of the average total number of weeks in the professional program.[36]

Physical therapy CE most commonly uses a voluntary, preceptor model of supervision/instruction with clinical affiliation agreements between the clinical agencies and the academic programs establishing the legal obligations of the parties. Preparation of clinical instructors (CIs) for clinical teaching roles is variable, although the latest CAPTE data indicate that, on average, slightly more than half of CIs supervising students have completed the APTA's CI credentialing program[36] (see Appendix A). Clinical experiences can take place in a range of settings with a wide range of patient populations across the life span, but typically programs require that students experience the delivery of care in 3 broad areas: acute and/or subacute care, ambulatory care, and rehabilitation services for individuals with long-term or chronic disabilities that require interprofessional interaction and care.

CHALLENGES AND OPPORTUNITIES

Despite the wisdom of Worthingham's work, the profession has been unable to fully meet the challenges and completely fulfill the recommendations she identified, and several of these recommendation areas remain relevant today. While the terrains of education and health care in which physical therapy education and practice occur have shifted dramatically in 50 years, we can align the challenges and opportunities for physical therapy education today within Worthingham's 5 broad areas.

A full description of physical therapist practice today is beyond the scope of this text, but we have highlighted some of the many changes in practice that are entwined with changes in education as we discuss the challenges ahead. For a longer description of practice see *Today's Physical Therapist* (http://www.apta.org/TodaysPT) or one of the many texts designed as introductions to the profession.[37]

Professional Identity

Achieving the DPT degree as the standard for entry to practice, consumer direct access to physical therapy throughout the United States, and public recognition of the profession's role in health care are all important accomplishments of the last 50 years. At this juncture in our profession's history it is important to shed the insistence on our professional autonomy that was arguably helpful in achieving these goals, and in its place cultivate a sense of both humility and agency as members of interprofessional, collaborative teams whose focus is on improving the health of patients and communities. We are also confronted with the need to have the profession's expertise in understanding and improving movement for patients and clients as the clearly identified, unique, and valued contribution of physical therapists in the health care system. There is also a challenge in framing the profession's expertise in movement in the concept of the movement system, a concept and a system that does not have a common understanding within health and medical care.[38,39] Coming to such an understanding is made more difficult by the broad range and complexity of internal and external factors that influence movement and its contribution to human experience.

Workforce

The racial and ethnic diversity of the US population will continue to increase, and despite periodic shifts in US policy regarding immigration, this will not change. Census data indicates that people who identify as multi-racial or multi-ethnic are the fastest growing demographic group.[40] Current trends suggest that the emergence of other identities, such as disability, gender, and sexual orientation, will continue to receive attention in public discourse and in policy, leading to the prominence of intersectionality as a way to understand issues of discrimination and identity.[41] As described in this social perspective, physical therapy is an overwhelmingly White profession.[42] The profession must understand how young people from communities of color, from varying economic levels, and with varying identities see the profession and make choices about whether or not to enter the profession if we are to have a workforce of necessary size and, more importantly, the fluency to address the needs of our diverse communities. We are also challenged to meet the needs of people in rural, underserved areas and in cities, suburbs, and exurbs where transportation systems, income inequality, and cost of living can be challenges to the members of the community and to the physical therapists and physical therapist assistants who comprise that workforce. The aging of the US population is another demographic trend that will present both challenges and opportunities for the profession. Meeting the needs of older people, with their multi-system, complex health problems will challenge the profession, as these needs run counter to the growing practice specialization focused on discrete systems. On the other hand, continued growth of specialties and residences in areas such as geriatrics and acute care, with a focus on management of patients with multiple system involvement, offer opportunities. This situation is very similar for medicine, as it struggles to address the primary care needs of society.

Societal Needs

While the challenges and opportunities discussed previously are vital to address if we are to meet society's needs, there are many others. The increasing incidence and prevalence of non-communicable diseases, such as heart disease, stroke, cancer, and drug addiction, coupled with the way in which social, political, economic, and cultural factors affect those diseases are a challenge for the entirety of the health care and political systems. Achieving health equity is crucial for communities across the United States if all the members of those communities are to live healthy, fulfilling lives. As the National Academies of Sciences, Engineering, and Medicine states on its website, Pathways to Health Equity:[43]

> While many communities have the resources they need to fully thrive, there are communities across the United States without sufficient access to jobs, adequate transit, safe and affordable housing, parks and open space, healthy food options, or quality education. These differences in opportunity mean that a person's health can depend on his or her zip code. In fact, life expectancy can vary by as many as 15 years depending on income level, education, and where you live.

The challenge and opportunity for physical therapy education and curricula is to place a priority on including learning experiences that prepare practitioners with the knowledge and skills as well as the cultural sensitivity, professional humility, and moral courage to participate in community-centered efforts and political and social advocacy to achieve health equity in every community.

Bridge Between Academic and Clinical Environments

One of the potential benefits of the diversity of curricular and CE models in physical therapy is the flexibility that programs could have to respond to the local environment of their community. The downside, however, is that physical therapy lacks the structural affordances and imperatives for creation of the sound clinical-academic partnerships that are common in medicine with the relationship between academic medical centers and medical schools. Though the funding for clerkship and residency training models in medicine has been under scrutiny for decades, how medical education is financed lends additional stability to that model. Now, ironically, medicine is faced with the challenge of designing more flexibility into medical education,[44] whereas physical therapy's challenge proceeds in the other direction—from variability, flexibility, and diversity to arriving at sound structural and financial partnerships between the academic and clinical environments that would enhance the potential for creating robust learning partnerships. In such partnerships, academic and clinical entities and faculty would be equally respected and valued for what they contribute to the educational endeavor and would collaborate to identify and support mutually beneficial educational outcomes.

Beyond establishing a solid infrastructure for developing these partnerships, there is another challenge but also great opportunity. If all physical therapists had a deeper understanding of learning and the learning sciences and were equally invested in an expanded professional identity from that of clinician to that of clinician-educator, the possibilities for coordination, connection, and continuity between what is learned in classrooms and what is learned through practice would be dramatically increased for all participants. Currently, in the context of reimbursement-driven productivity expectations placed on therapists, there are increasing concerns expressed by the clinical community about the cost of CE in physical therapy with little focus on potential long-term benefits. This concern has led to some agencies requiring that academic institutions pay clinical sites for the clinical experiences they provide. These concerns, and structural and financial challenges are compounded by a lack of collaboration and commitment to cooperation between academic and clinical learning environments and are often driven by perceived or real hierarchical relationships between academic institutions and clinical organizations, limited shared understandings of the importance and complexity of coherent curricular design, and insufficient mutual regard for the power and promise of practice-based workplace teaching and learning. We believe this challenge can be overcome.

Interprofessional Education

While efforts to advance interprofessional collaborative practice in health care have been evident for 3 to 4 decades,[45,46] those efforts have received significantly more attention in the last 20 years when it was apparent that failures in interprofessional collaborative practice and communication were the source of many errors in health care.[47,48] The Interprofessional Education Collaborative published core competences for interprofessional collaborative practice in 2011, subsequently revised in 2016. While the APTA was not one of the founding participating organizations of the Interprofessional Education Collaborative, they became a member in 2016. The most recent CAPTE accreditation criteria include elements that address interprofessional education in the classroom and clinical learning environments, and the CAPTE is represented as several accreditation agencies are working to develop common standards for interprofessional education and collaborative practice.[49-52] In addition to preparing physical therapists for interprofessional collaborative practice, an important corollary learning outcome is for practitioners to have the ability to improve safety and quality of care from a systems perspective.[53-55] In the current CAPTE Standards there are 2 curricular elements that specifically include quality improvement; these elements require that there are courses within the curriculum with content designed to prepare students to: (1) participate in activities for ongoing assessment and improvement of quality services; and (2) participate in practice management, including marketing, public relations, regulatory and legal requirements, risk management, staffing, and continuous quality improvement.[27] However, these criteria do not explicitly address the importance of a systems perspective and the collaborative nature of system-wide interprofessional work necessary to achieve durable quality improvement. Medical education, particularly in post-graduate residency education, provides optimal, mentored experiences for residents to have longitudinal learning experiences with quality improvement in the clinical environment. Physical therapy's challenge will be to provide the necessary knowledge in the academic learning environment, coupled with clinical experiences that are purposeful and of sufficient length to help students learn how to engage in effective systems level analysis and improvement of health care and physical therapy services.

Education Research

While Worthingham did not include education research as one of the 5 recommendations for physical therapy education, she did emphasize the need for and importance of research to provide direction for future action by the profession in each of the areas she identified for reform.[15,17-22] We are including the absolute necessity of education research as a sixth challenge and opportunity because the profession's ability to advance excellence throughout the education enterprise is dependent upon sound evidence and insights that can only come from an intentional research effort. Basic science, clinical, and health policy research are now well represented in the physical therapy literature. Major initiatives from throughout the profession, particularly from the Foundation for Physical Therapy, provided reliable sources of funding, mentorship, and a framework for guiding the focus of research in those areas. Education research has not had the same recognition, nor this level of systematic attention or commitment of financial resources. There are, however, positive signals from within the profession that might bode well for advancing education research. The Education Leadership Partnership (composed of the APTA, the American Council on Academic Physical Therapy, and the Academy of Physical Therapy Education) has convened a diverse group of education researchers to create mentorship networks and develop resources for future researchers, identify and build stable and substantive sources of funding, and establish a framework for an education research agenda that may be derived from the findings of the national study of physical therapist education described in this book.

The challenges and opportunities discussed here have been presented in the framework from Worthingham's original research and recommendations; however, her findings did not serve as an explicit, *a priori,* framework for the study of physical therapist education described in this volume. Even so, as our work proceeded, we realized that her recommendations put forth almost 50 years ago have real resonance and relevance even today. These challenges are set against the backdrop of several current questions or concerns about physical therapist education:

- Whether there are structures and models that can better serve society, including moving CE to a post-licensure experience and staged licensure
- The increasing number of new programs and enrollment growth in current programs combined with shortages of faculty and program directors
- Concerns related to escalating student indebtedness
- Questions about whether hybrid learning models can be as effective or more effective than traditional education delivery models
- Whether CE places a burden on clinical agencies that warrants a financial arrangement between academic and clinical programs

At the outset, our intention in this study was to carefully examine and shine a light on clinical and academic programs identified as exemplars of excellence and innovation in physical therapist education. In doing so, we anticipated that we would find educational practices worth celebrating and emulating, but also gaps or areas for improvement as physical therapist education moves forward in the 21st century. Where one shines a light, sometimes cobwebs appear. Our hope is that the entire profession can learn, as we did, from the excellent programs we describe and acknowledge where we can do better in envisioning and crafting learning experiences and environments that will ensure that physical therapists and physical therapy as a profession will thrive and meet our obligations to society today and in the future.

CONCLUSION

The Worthingham Study provided an excellent analysis of physical therapist education in the 1960s, and Moore and Perry provided a thorough review of CE in the 1970s. But there have been no major comprehensive, rigorous, nationwide investigations done to provide a broad-based assessment of physical therapist education in more than 40 years. The work of the Carnegie Foundation for the Advancement of Teaching's Preparation for the Professions Program looked deeply at professional education in 5 professions in the first decade of the 21st century and provided a model for our investigation and assessment of physical therapist education. The findings of the Preparation for the Professions Program are summarized in Chapter 2. Part II of this book presents an overview of our qualitative research design and the findings from our national study of physical therapist education in the second decade of the 21st century. In Part III, we make recommendations and identify specific actions that can be taken by individuals and organizations, and collectively by the stakeholders in the profession, that could result in making real changes that allow us to meet and creatively address current and future challenges in physical therapist education and practice. Part IV presents visions of what might be—of a way forward—with chapters devoted to interprofessional education and collaborative practice, an international perspective on practice-based learning, the future of education research in the profession, the importance of professional formation and the profession's social contract, and on the future of physical therapy practice and education. Collectively, we hope these pages offer a roadmap for the future—one that provides several routes for our journey to excellence.

REFERENCES

1. Pinkston D. Evolution of the practice of physical therapy in the United States. In: Barnes M, Scully R., eds. *Physical Therapy*. Philadelphia, PA: JB Lippincott; 1989:2-20.
2. Littell EH, Johnson G. Professional entry education in physical therapy during the 20th century. *J Phys Ther Educ*. 2003;17(3):3-14.
3. Flexner A. Medical education in the United States and Canada: a report to the Carnegie Foundation for the Advancement of Teaching. *Bulletin No. 4*. New York, NY: The Carnegie Foundation for the Advancement of Teaching; 1910.
4. Beck A. The Flexner Report and the standardization of American medical education. *JAMA*. 2004;291(17):2139-2140.
5. Hiatt MD, Stockton CG. Impact of the Flexner Report on the fate of medical schools in North America after 1909. *J Am Phys Surg*. 2003;8(2):37-40.
6. Hamowy R. Early development of medical licensing laws in the United States, 1875-1900. *J Libert Stud*. 1979;3(1):73-119.
7. Doukas DJ, McCullough LB, Wear S. Reforming medical education in ethics and humanities by finding common ground with Abraham Flexner. *Acad Med*. 2010;85:318-323.
8. Cooke M, Irby DM, Sullivan W, Ludmerer KM. American medical education 100 years after the Flexner Report. *N Engl J Med*. 2006;355:1339-1344.
9. Goldmark J. *Nursing and Nursing Education in the United States*. New York, NY: Macmillan Publishers; 1923.
10. Benefiel D. The story of nurse licensure. *Nurse Educ*. 2011;36(1):16-20.
11. Anderson N. Historical development of American nursing education. *J Nurs Educ*. 1981;20(1):18-36.
12. Egenes K. History of nursing. In: Roux G, Halstead JA, eds, *Issues and Trends in Nursing: Essential Knowledge for Today and Tomorrow*. Sudbury, MA: Jones and Bartlett; 2008.
13. Carlin EJ. The Pennsylvania chapter: historical highlights. *Phys Ther*. 1962;42(4):246-250.
14. Pennell MY, Stewart FA. *State Licensing of Health Occupations*. Washington, DC: US Department of Health, Education, and Welfare; 1968.
15. Worthingham C. Study of physical therapy I: curriculum patterns for basic physical therapy education. *Phys Ther*. 1968;48(1):7-20.
16. Hislop HJ. Where do we go from here? *Phys Ther*. 1968;48(1):5.
17. Worthingham C. Study of physical therapy II: the environment for basic physical therapy education:1965-1966. *Phys Ther*. 1968;48(9):935-962.
18. Worthingham C. Study of physical therapy III: the clinical environment for basic physical therapy education, part 1: facilities. *Phys Ther*. 1968;48(11):1195-1215.
19. Worthingham C. Study of physical therapy III: the clinical environment for basic physical therapy education, part 2: staff. *Phys Ther*. 1968;48(12):1353-1382.
20. Worthingham C. Study of physical therapy IV: the 1961 and 1965 graduates of the physical therapy schools. *Phys Ther*. 1969;49(5):476-499.
21. Worthingham C. Study of physical therapy V: request for physical therapy. *Phys Ther*. 1970;70(7):989-1031.
22. Worthingham C. Study of physical therapy VI: findings of the study in relation to trends in patient care and education. *Phys Ther*. 1970;70(9):1315-1332.
23. Moore ML, Perry JF: *Clinical Education in Physical Therapy: Current Status/Future Needs*. Washington, DC: American Physical Therapy Association; 1976.
24. Barr JS, Gwyer J, Talmor Z, et al. *Standards for Clinical Education in Physical Therapy: A Manual for Evaluation and Selection of Clinical Education Centers*. Washington, DC: American Physical Therapy Association; 1980.
25. Barr JS, Gwyer J, Talmor Z. Evaluation of clinical education centers in physical therapy. *Phys Ther*. 1982;62(6):850-861.
26. Nieland VM, Harris MJ. History of accreditation in physical therapy education. *J Phys Ther Educ*. 2003;17(3):52-61.

27. Commission on Accreditation in Physical Therapy Education. Standards and required elements for accreditation of physical therapist education programs. http://www.capteonline.org/uploadedFiles/CAPTEorg/About_CAPTE/Resources/Accreditation_Handbook/CAPTE_PTStandardsEvidence.pdf. Accessed February 19, 2018.

28. Daniels L. Ninth Mary McMillan Lecture: tomorrow: the master's degree for physical therapy education. *Phys Ther.* 1974;54(5):463-473.

29. Johnson G. Twentieth Mary McMillan Lecture: great expectations–a force in growth and change. *Phys Ther.* 1985;65(11):1690-1695.

30. Soderberg GL. The future of physical therapy doctoral education. *J Phys Ther Educ.* 1989;3(1):15-19.

31. Stohs SJ, Jensen GM, Paschal KA. Initiating clinical doctoral education in physical therapy: the case of Creighton University. *J Phys Ther Educ.* 2003;17(3):44-51.

32. American Physical Therapy Association. *Vision 2020.* http://www.apta.org/Vision2020/. Updated July 13, 2015. Accessed February 19, 2018.

33. World Health Organization. International classification of functioning, disability and health (ICF). http://www.who.int/classifications/icf/en/. Updated March 2, 2018. Accessed February 19, 2018.

34. American Physical Therapy Association. Vision statement for the physical therapy profession. http://www.apta.org/Vision/. Updated March 20, 2018. Accessed February 19, 2018.

35. Hayhurst C. A vision to transform society. *PT in Motion.* 2014;6(2):20-25.

36. Commission on Accreditation of Physical Therapy Education. Aggregate Program Data, 2016–2017 CAPTE. http://www.capteonline.org/uploadedFiles/CAPTEorg/About_CAPTE/Resources/Aggregate_Program_Data/AggregateProgramData_PTPrograms.pdf. Published 2017. Accessed February 1, 2018.

37. Pagliarulo M. *Introduction to Physical Therapy.* 5th ed. St. Louis, MO: Elsevier; 2016.

38. American Physical Therapy Association. *Physical Therapist Practice and the Human Movement System. An APTA White Paper.* Alexandria, VA: American Physical Therapy Association; 2015.

39. American Physical Therapy Association. The movement system brings it all together. *PT in Motion.* 2016;8(4):14-21.

40. US Census Bureau. 2010 Census Briefs. https://www.census.gov/prod/cen2010/briefs/c2010br-02.pdf. Accessed February 15, 2018.

41. Eckstrand KL, Eliason J, St. Cloud T, Potter J. The priority of intersectionality in academic medicine. *Acad Med.* 2016;91(7):907-907: doi:10.1097/ACM.0000000000001231.

42. Diversity Task Force. Report to the American Council of Academic Physical Therapy. https://www.acapt.org/docs/default-source/reports/diversity-task-force-final-report.pdf?sfvrsn=2. Published January 4, 2016. Accessed February 18, 2018.

43. National Academies of Sciences, Engineering and Medicine. Pathways to health equity. http://resources.nationalacademies.org/infographics/healthequity/healthequity.html. Accessed February 18, 2018.

44. Cooke M, Irby DM, O'Brien BC. *Educating Physicians: A Call for Reform of Medical School and Residency.* San Francisco, CA: Jossey-Bass; 2010.

45. World Health Organization. *Framework for action on interprofessional education and collaborative practice.* Geneva, Switzerland: World Health Organization; 2010.

46. Institute of Medicine. *Interprofessional Education for Collaboration: Learning How to Improve Health From Interprofessional Models Across the Continuum of Education to Practice: Workshop Summary.* Washington, DC: The National Academies Press; 2013.

47. Wachter R. *The Digital Doctor: Hope, Hype, and Harm at the Dawn of Medicine's Computer Age.* New York, NY: McGraw-Hill; 2015.

48. Dow A, Reeves S. How health professional training will and should change. In: Hoff T, Sutcliffe K, Young G, eds. *The Healthcare Professional Workforce: Understanding Human Capital in a Changing Industry.* Oxford, UK: Oxford University Press; 2017:147-172.

49. Commission on Accreditation in Physical Therapy Education. *Rules of Practice and Procedure Parts 1-16.* American Physical Therapy Association; 2017.

50. Interprofessional Education Collaborative. https://www.ipecollaborative.org/membership.html. Accessed February 26, 2018.

51. National Academies of Science, Engineering, and Medcine. *Exploring the Role of Accreditation Enhancing Quality and Innovation in Health Professions Education.* Washington, DC: National Academies Press; 2017.

52. Cox M, Blouin A, Cuff P, Paniaggua M, Phillips S, Vlasses P. The role of accreditation in achieving the quadruple aim. *National Academy of Medicine.* https://nam.edu/the-role-of-accreditation-in-achieving-the-quadruple-aim/. Published October 2, 2017. Accessed September 4, 2018.

53. Berwick D, Nolan T, Whittington, J. The Triple Aim: care, health, and cost. *Health Aff.* 2008;27:759-769.

54. Brandt B, Lutfiyya M, King J. A scoping review of interprofessional collaborative practice and education using the lens of the Triple Aim. *J Interprof Care.* 2014;28(5):393-399.

55. Kigin C, Rodgers M, Wolf S. The Physical Therapy and Society Summit (PASS) meeting: observations and opportunities. *Phys Ther.* 2010;90:1555-1567.

2

Excellence in the Professions
Past and Present Work
of the Carnegie Foundation
for the Advancement of Teaching

In the Carnegie Foundation's studies of education in the professions we intend to demonstrate how the professionals, on whom we all depend for so much of the quality of our lives, can learn to balance those technical, intellectual, and moral equations. That's what professions do.[1(pxv)]

FLEXNER STUDY OF MEDICAL EDUCATION

Since 1910, when then President of the Carnegie Foundation for the Advancement of Teaching, Henry S. Pritchett, wrote about Flexner's famous report on medical education, "The present report on medical education forms the first of a series of papers on professional schools to be issued by the Carnegie Foundation,"[2] the Carnegie Foundation has engaged in research focused on professional education. Over the next several decades, Carnegie performed a series of studies on higher education and professional education through the Carnegie Commission on Higher Education sponsored research studies.[2]

The most famous Carnegie study, the *1910 Flexner Report*, led to transformative changes in medical education. An important element in the Flexner report was the concept of *ambulando discimus*—we learn by going about. This assessment of medical education was fueled by a concern for the mediocre quality, profit motive of many schools, inadequate curricula and facilities, and a non-scientific approach to medical education.[3] Flexner visited 155 medical schools in the United States and Canada. Part of his preparation for these visits was a visit to Johns Hopkins Medical School and that became a model of comparison for his study. Flexner saw medicine as a science-based practice and argued that schools should be housed in universities, have teaching hospitals, require a clinical phase of education in academically oriented hospitals, and have thoughtful clinicians engaged in clinical research as well as patient care. Flexner identified challenges along with recommendations for change in medical education (Table 2-1).[4] Following the 1910 report, medical education changed rapidly, accreditation and licensure procedures were put in place, and the proprietary schools closed.[3-6]

Jensen GM, Mostrom E, Hack LM, Nordstrom T, Gwyer J.
Educating Physical Therapists (pp 15-22).
© 2019 Taylor & Francis Group.

TABLE 2-1

EXAMPLES OF FLEXNER'S FINDINGS, RECOMMENDATIONS FOR MEDICAL EDUCATION[3,4,6]

FINDINGS	RECOMMENDATIONS
Lack of standard curricula	Require 4 years of college, specific science courses
Too much variation in student achievement	Establish accreditation process
Limited science and laboratory experience	Integrate laboratory learning into curriculum
Limited interaction with patients	Provide clinical training at university teaching hospitals
Emphasis on memorization	
Tradition-bound curricula and faculty	Facilitate thinking like scientists; use scientific inquiry
Teaching by unqualified faculty	Faculty who are scientifically educated
Role modelling by for-profit institutions with variable quality faculty	Medical education integrated into university culture
	Scientifically based faculty role models

CARNEGIE PREPARATION FOR THE PROFESSIONS PROGRAM

The most recent Carnegie initiative in the study of professions was led by then-Carnegie President Lee S. Shulman in the Preparation for Professions Program (PPP), a study of 5 professions (clergy, law, engineering, nursing, and medicine).[1,5,7-10] The program was designed to be an integrated, comparative study of education for professional understanding, integrity, and practice in these 5 professional fields.[11]

Shulman had a long-standing interest in the education of professionals and has consistently challenged us to see what is common as well as unique across the professions. His conceptualization of what it means to prepare professionals based on the previous work of many[12-15] provides us with insight into the formulation of the PPP program. Shulman put forward 6 characteristics or features that he considers common to professions:[16]

1. *Service*: A commitment to important social ends, including a moral understanding to aim and guide practice.

2. *Understanding*: Practice that is grounded in bodies of knowledge that are created, examined and re-examined, refuted, and transformed. An important element is that professions change not only because of policy or practice, but most importantly, as the knowledge is developed, challenged, and shaped through new understandings.

3. *Practice*: Knowledge must be connected to and tested in practice, as that is where professionals do their work. The importance of connecting theory and practice, although often troubling, is essential. Consistent with Dewey's position, this theoretical learning needs to be situated in practice to be meaningful.

4. *Judgment*: Professionals do not merely apply knowledge as that is too simple and practice is complex. There is a critical process of judgment that is between knowledge and application and professionals must make judgments in uncertain conditions.

5. *Learning*: This is the most essential element of professions, as learning from experience is non-negotiable and must occur both in the academy and in the community of practice. The professional must learn how to manage change or uncertainty and reflect and learn from that experience.

6. *Community*: Being a professional requires being a member of a professional community that has public obligations and accountability to broader society.

A centerpiece of the PPP studies was the foundational importance of learning in professional education. Contrary to the Flexner study, where he went about describing the conditions in all the medical schools and exposing the variability and lack of quality in the academic environment, particularly in the proprietary schools, the PPP project centered on studying programs that were known for excellence and innovation. This positive focus allows one to also uncover areas that need improvement without emphasizing the negative aspects. Dr. William Sullivan[17], a philosopher and senior scholar at the Carnegie Foundation for the PPP studies, published a second edition of *Work and Integrity: The Crisis and Promise of Professionalism in America*, in which he put forth an indictment of professions but also set out a visionary challenge for the future. His critique of professions was that the lack of integration between cognitive training and practical skills is coupled with weak abilities to think responsibly about important social and political dimensions of their practice.[11] Work and integrity, while an inherent tension in professional work, Sullivan asserts must be a quest for all professions. "Integrity is never a given, but always a quest that must be renewed and reshaped over time. It demands considerable self-awareness and self-command."[17(pxiii)]

Sullivan argues that "All professional schools face the challenge of shaping their students' modes of thinking so as to enable their becoming contributing members of the professional context and, ultimately, the larger society."[17(p207)] He envisions that professional education has 3 major areas of development, which he calls *apprenticeships*:

1. *Cognitive or intellectual apprenticeship*: Intellectual focus and knowledge base of the profession—*habits of mind*
2. *Practice-based or skill apprenticeship*: Skills-based learning through practice; use of a variety of pedagogies from simulation to actual practice settings—*habits of hand*
3. *Professional identity apprenticeship*: Development of the student's professional self through introduction to the values, attitudes, social roles, and responsibilities of the profession—*habits of heart*

These 3 apprenticeships or *habits* (ie, head, hand, heart) served as a working model or framework that allowed a point of comparison across the 5 professions.

The term *apprenticeship* was used as a metaphor and analytic lens for exploring the "embodiment of skillful, cognitive, and ethical experiential learning required in practice disciplines."[18(p346)]

Each of the 5 PPP studies had an overarching question: How do professional schools prepare their students for their professional roles and responsibilities? Additional questions were generated for each profession but always with specific attention to processes of teaching, learning, assessment, and curriculum. In addition, all 5 studies posed the question, **Does this profession have a signature pedagogy distinctive to it among the professions?**

The research design used in the PPP studies was a qualitative case study design with some studies being supplemented with additional descriptive surveys. An interdisciplinary research team that included education researchers, psychologists, philosophers, and members of the profession being studied engaged in 2- to 3-day intensive site visits and gathered qualitative data through individual interviews, focus group sessions, review of curricular and teaching materials, and field observations of teaching and learning. The goal of the data collection and analysis process was to find exemplars of excellence or good pedagogy. Each of the 5 studies also chose their sample to represent geographic and institutional diversity. The larger cross professions sample also provided the opportunity to develop a common framework for understanding and comparing education in the professions.[5,7-10]

Selected Findings From Carnegie Studies

The Carnegie's PPP study led to the publication of 5 books, *Educating Clergy*,[7] *Educating Lawyers*,[10] *Educating Engineers*,[8] *Educating Nurses*,[9] and *Educating Physicians*,[5] along with various forms of dissemination through presentations and papers.[19-23] While the focus was on excellence, analysis of the findings led to important observations, recommendations, and action steps for education reform in each of the professions. Of particular relevance to our research in physical therapy are the key observations and recommendations generated for the studies of nursing and medicine (Table 2-2).

In the comparison across professions, the Carnegie PPP studies found that the third apprenticeship, professional formation, was the weakest and, in some fields, marginalized. Most professions focus more on expert knowledge, theory and skill development than a full understanding of the critical importance and integrative goal of professional formation and understanding of professionals' moral responsibilities to society. While medicine and nursing were more likely than law and engineering to develop the third apprenticeship of professional formation, the need for further development of habits of heart that facilitate a sustained commitment to the profession's core aims was noted. As Colby and Sullivan argue:[20]

> Professional work is inherently complex, requiring wise judgment under conditions of uncertainty, and its knowledge base is always evolving. It is this third apprenticeship that draws together and grounds the 2 most essential features of high quality work, deep expertise, and ethical commitment.[(p411)]

Lifelong professional competence and commitment for professionals requires 5 key qualities.

---

5 KEY QUALITIES FOR THE DEVELOPMENT OF SUSTAINABLE PROFESSIONALISM

1. Deep engagement with the profession's public purposes
2. Strong professional identity
3. Development of habits of salience where complex situations are understood and framed in moral terms
4. Ability to adhere to the profession's standards and ideals rather than over-riding self interest
5. Sense of moral agency

SIGNATURE PEDAGOGY

An essential component in all the Carnegie PPP studies was the identification of a signature pedagogy. Shulman defines his concept of signature pedagogy building on the observation of Erik Erikson[24] who advised that to understand a culture, one should study its nurseries:

> If you wish to understand why professions develop as they do, study their nurseries, their forms of professional preparation. When you do, you will generally detect the characteristic forms of teaching and learning that I have come to call signature pedagogies.[25(p52)]

These signature pedagogies include the 3 dimensions or apprenticeships of professional education that prepare graduates for professional work (Figure 2-1). At first glance, one might think these 3 apprenticeships (ie, habits of head, hand, heart) merely represent the 3 domains of learning—cognitive, affective, and psychomotor. As discussed earlier in this chapter, this is not the case because professional education must aim toward an integrated whole, the development and embodiment of all 3 of these apprenticeships that are required for professional practice. Shulman proposes that exploration and identification of signature pedagogies helps us gain a deeper understanding of professions.

Signature pedagogies are important because they are pervasive, they define what counts as knowledge in a field and how things become known, as well as define how knowledge is analyzed, criticized, accepted, or discarded. They almost always include public student performance and are both active and interactive. Signature pedagogies have 3 dimensions:

TABLE 2-2

KEY OBSERVATIONS AND RECOMMENDATIONS FROM THE MEDICAL AND NURSING EDUCATION CARNEGIE STUDIES

MEDICAL EDUCATION[5,6]	NURSING EDUCATION[9]
Observations:	*Observations:*
1. Curriculum content educators must distinguish more clearly between CORE material and everything else. 2. Failure to assess, acknowledge, and advance professional behaviors. 3. Inadequate attention to the skills required for effective team care in a complex health system. 4. Poor connections between formal knowledge and experiential learning. 5. Clinical education overuses inpatient experiences. 6. Commercial nature is a threat to professional identity.	1. US nursing programs are very effective in forming professional identity and ethical comportment. 2. Clinical practice assignments provide powerful learning experiences, especially in programs where educators integrate clinical and classroom teaching. 3. US nursing programs are not effective in teaching nursing science, natural sciences, social sciences, technology, and the humanities.
Recommendations:	*Recommendations:*
1. Standardization: Need for standard learning outcomes/individualization of the learning process. a. At medical school and residency levels, medical education must ensure, through assessment, learners achieve predetermined standards of competence with knowledge and performance in core domains. 2. Integration: Connect formal knowledge to clinical experience; Integration of basic, 3. clinical, and social sciences; Need for interprofessional education/teamwork. 4. Habits of inquiry and improvement: Prepare learners for routine and adaptive expertise; Learner engagement in innovation/improvement of care, exposure to population health, quality improvement, and patient safety; Move clinical education beyond university teaching hospital. 5. Identify formation: Provide formal ethics instruction, rituals that symbolize being a professional, assessment on professionalism (in the context of longitudinal mentoring); create collaborative learning environments.	1. Teach for salience: From a focus on covering decontextualized knowledge to an emphasis on teaching for a sense of salience, situated cognition, and action in situations. 2. Integration across academic and clinical: From a sharp separation of clinical and classroom teaching to an integration of the 2. 3. Clinical reasoning: From an emphasis on critical thinking to an emphasis on clinical reasoning and multiple ways of thinking. 4. Formation not socialization: From an emphasis on socialization and role-taking to an emphasis on formation. 5. Consensus on degree: Require the Bachelor of Science of Nursing entry into practice.

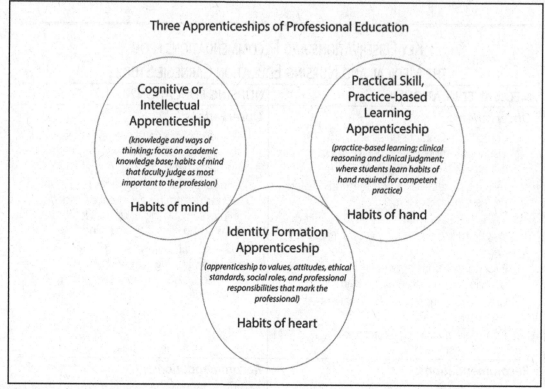

Figure 2-1. The 3 apprenticeships of professional education.

1. *Surface structure*: the concrete, operational acts of teaching and learning
2. *Deep structure*: a set of assumptions about how best to impart a body of knowledge and know-how
3. *Implicit structure*: a moral dimension that comprises a set of beliefs about professional attitudes, values and dispositions

The signature pedagogies identified in the Carnegie PPP studies are shown in Table 2-3.[5,7-10]

Why are these pedagogies important? Remember they are both pervasive and routine so they would cut across learning environments, programs, and institutions. They are important as a pedagogy that bridges theory and practice. Signature pedagogies make students feel deeply engaged, highly visible, and at times vulnerable.[26] Learning to engage in complex performances can change depending on the situation, but because the messages from these signature pedagogies become learned and internalized, you do not have to think about them. These signature pedagogies become routine and allow the learner and professional to perform complex activities without thinking about them, which frees up their attention to more challenging situations as they arise.[25]

As Shulman reminds us:[25]

Signature pedagogies make a difference. They form habits of the mind, habits of the heart, and habits of the hand the way we teach will shape how professionals behave—and in a society so dependent on the quality of its professionals, that is no small matter.(p59)

Shulman also proposes a fourth structure, or shadow dimension, of signature pedagogies; this is what may be more hidden or weakly developed in the profession's pedagogy. This shadow side can become sources of rigidity and preservation. We propose that the signature pedagogy for physical therapy is the human body as teacher. We present and explore our evidence and analysis of all 4 dimensions of physical therapy's signature pedagogy in more detail in Chapters 6 and 9.

TABLE 2-3
SIGNATURE PEDAGOGIES IDENTIFIED IN CARNEGIE'S PREPARATION FOR PROFESSIONS PROGRAM[5,7-10]

PROFESSION	SIGNATURE PEDAGOGY
Clergy	Formation: Foster professional identity and integrity Emphasis on forming in students the dispositions, habits, knowledge, and skills in professional identity and practice, commitments, and integrity
Engineering	Practice of problem solving: Knowing that (fundamental concepts) in mathematical terms and knowing how (learning to analyze problems), generating models, and using deep knowledge through intuition
Law	Thinking like a lawyer: Discern facts and principles, use processes of analytical reasoning
Nursing	Teaching for a sense of salience by guiding students through coaching
Medicine	Teaching at the bedside, develop habits of hand, practice, and performance

NEEDED: AN ARC OF PROFESSIONAL DEVELOPMENT

A final observation across the 5 professions studied in the Carnegie PPP was a critique of the well-known claim across professions about preparation of lifelong learners. The studies uncovered little evidence of educational practices across curriculum, pedagogy, and assessment that explicitly focused on developing lifelong learners. This does not merely mean gaining additional knowledge and clinical skills as one's professional career unfolds. It means much more—that there is a fundamental commitment to the profession's public purpose. This in turn, drives the critical progressive learning process that is essential in the development of expertise.[20,27-29] Bereiter and Scardamalia[30] found that many professionals fail to become lifelong learners, but instead fall into a routine level of practice and competence as they become experienced non-experts. The characteristics that counter this kind of routine level of practice are intense engagement in one's work, curiosity, and a deep commitment to the profession's aims and public purpose; it is these critical factors that result in continuous advancement of knowledge and self-directed improvement.[20]

Professional schools serve as critical gateways to the profession. Colby and Sullivan[20] argue that professional schools need to aspire to be trustee institutions and must do more to prepare students to do good work and challenge questionable, unethical work. Educators must not only focus on the knowledge and skill development of students but also must find ways to create professionals who take responsibility to influence the context of their work beyond the patient-provider relationship. The Carnegie studies found very few examples of faculty or students' deep understanding of and concern for social justice or the development of students as citizens of their professional communities with an eye toward the public purposes of professions.

Our graduates will be working in a world where the conditions of practice will continue to become increasingly complex. The structures, concepts, and findings from the Carnegie studies provide an exceptional roadmap and solid foundation for an in-depth investigation of the professional preparation of physical therapists. The chapters in Part II share the methods and evidence from our Carnegie-like study of excellence and innovation in physical therapist education.

REFERENCES

1. Shulman L. Preface. In: Sullivan WM. *Work and Integrity: The Crisis and Promise of Professionalism in America.* 2nd ed. San Francisco, CA: Jossey-Bass; 2005:xv.

2. Shulman L. Foreword. In: Cooke M, Irby D, O'Brien B. eds. *Educating Physicians: A Call for Reform of Medical School and Residency.* San Francisco, CA: Jossey-Bass; 2010:v.

3. Cooke M, Irby D, Sullivan W, Ludmerer K. American medical education 100 years after the Flexner Report. *N Engl J Med.*2010;355:1339-1343.

4. Flexner A. Medical education in the United States and Canada: a report to the Carnegie Foundation for the Advancement of Teaching. *Bulletin No. 4.* Boston, MA. http://archive.carnegiefoundation.org/pdfs/elibrary/Carnegie_Flexner_Report.pdf. Reproduced 1972. Accessed December 10, 2017.

5. Cooke M, Irby D, O'Brien B. *Educating Physicians: A Call for Reform of Medical School and Residency.* San Francisco, CA: Jossey-Bass; 2010.

6. Irby D, Cooke M, O'Brien B. Calls for reform of medical education by the Carnegie Foundation for the Advancement of Teaching. 1910-2010. *Acad Med.* 2010;85(2):220-227.

7. Foster C, Dahill L, Goleman L, Tolentino BW. *Educating Clergy: Teaching Practices and Pastoral Imagination.* San Francisco, CA: Jossey-Bass; 2006.

8. Sheppard S, Macatangay K, Colby A, Sullivan W. *Educating Engineers: Designing the Future of the Field.* San Francisco, CA: Jossey-Bass; 2009.

9. Benner P, Sutphen M, Leonard C, Day L. *Educating Nurses: A Call for Radical Transformation.* San Francisco, CA: Jossey-Bass; 2010.

10. Sullivan W, Colby A, Wegner JW, Bond L, Shulman LS. *Educating Lawyers: Preparation for the Profession of Law.* San Francisco, CA: Jossey Bass; 2007.

11. Benner P, Sullivan W. Current controversies in clinical care: challenges to professionalism—work integrity and the call to renew and strengthen the social contract. *Am J Crit Care.* 2005;14:78-80.

12. Dewey J. The relation of theory to practice in education. In: *Third Yearbook of National Society for the Scientific Study of Education: Part 1: The Relation of Theory to Practice in Education of Teachers.* Chicago, Il.: University of Chicacgo Press; 1904:9-30.

13. Brint S. *In an Age of Experts: The Changing Role of Professionals in Politics and Public Life.* Chicago, IL: University of Chicago Press; 1994.

14. Schon D. *Educating the Reflective Practitioner.* San Francisco, CA: Jossey-Bass; 1987.

15. Abbott A. *The System of Professions: An Essay on the Division of Expert Labor.* Chicago, IL: University of Chicago Press; 1988.

16. Shulman L. *Teaching as Community Property: Essays on Higher Education.* San Francisco, CA: Jossey-Bass; 2004.

17. Sullivan W. *Work and Integrity: The Crisis and Promise of Professionalism in America.* 2nd ed. San Francisco, CA: Jossey-Bass; 2005.

18. Benner P. Formation in professional education: an examination of the relationship between theories of meaning and theories of self. *J Med Philos.* 2011;36:342-353.

19. O'Brien B, Irby D. Enacting the Carnegie Foundation call for reform of medical school and residency. *Teach Learn Med.* 2013;25:S1-S8.

20. Colby A, Sullivan W. Formation of professionalism and purpose: perspectives from the preparation for the professions program. *University of St. Thomas Law Journal.* 2008;5:404-426.

21. Wegner J. The Carnegie Foundation's Educating Lawyers: 4 questions for bar examiners. *The Bar Examiner.* 2011:11-24

22. Noone J. Teaching to the 3 apprenticeships: designing learning activities for professional practice in an undergraduate curriculum. *J Nurs Educ.* 2008; 48(8):468-472.

23. Cronenwett L, ed. The future of nursing education. In: *Institute of Medicine. The Future of Nursing Education: Leading Change, Advancing Health.* Washington, DC: National Academies Press; 2011;477-483.

24. Erikson E. *Childhood and Society.* New York, NY: WW Norton and Co.; 1963.

25. Shulman LS. Signature pedagogies in the professions. *Daedelus.* 2005;134:52-59.

26. Shulman LS. Pedagogies of uncertainty. *Liberal Education.* 2005;Spring:18-25.

27. Dreyfus H, Dreyfus S, Benner P. Implications of the phenomenology of expertise for teaching and learning everyday skillful ethical comportment. In: Benner P, Tanner C, eds. *Expertise in Nursing Practice: Caring, Clinical Judgment and Ethics.* 2nd ed. New York, NY: Springer; 2009:309-333.

28. Ericsson KA, Charness N, Feltovich P, Hoffman R. *The Cambridge Handbook of Expertise and Expert Performance.* New York, NY: Cambridge Press; 2006.

29. Jensen GM, Gwyer J, Hack L, Shepard K. *Expertise in Physical Therapy Practice.* 2nd ed. St. Louis MO: Saunders, Elsevier; 2007.

30. Bereiter C, Scardamalia M. *Surpassing Ourselves: An Inquiry into the Nature and Implications of Expertise.* Chicago, IL: Open Court Press; 1993.

Portraits of
Excellence and Innovation
Model Dimensions, Elements, Paradigm Cases, and Recommendations

Our research team, following in the methodological footsteps of the Carnegie Preparation for Professions Program, presents a fascinating set of findings that paint a portrait of excellence in physical therapist education in this section of the book. This section provides the reader with detailed descriptions of many observations of excellence in teaching and learning, of leadership, and of educational structures and resources. These findings led the researchers to propose a conceptual model of excellence in physical therapist education that is at the core of this part of the book.

In Part II, we will first provide the reader with a glimpse of our investigative journey toward the iterative development of our conceptual framework of excellence in physical therapist education. Across 4 years of data collection and analysis, we reflexively refined and recontextualized our research and theory-based model of excellence in physical therapist education. The conceptual model is comprised of several dimensions, and each dimension is described in the following chapters.

In Chapter 3, we describe in detail the design and methods used in our study exploring excellence and innovation in physical therapist education in the United States. We also provide the reader with an overview of our sampling procedures and a snapshot of the academic and clinical sites that comprised our sample. Our final Conceptual Model of Excellence in Physical Therapist Education was derived from the findings of this study and represents our understanding of the attributes of excellence in physical therapist education. In our model, we refer simply to physical therapist education, as opposed to referring separately to the academic or clinical components of the educational process, because we found that the attributes identified in our model were present in both domains as we visited sites around the country.

In Chapter 4, the dimension Culture of Excellence and the 4 elements that comprise it will be described. Each of the 4 elements were found to be important to support and achieve excellence in physical therapist education. In Chapter 5, the centerpiece of the model is identified as a Nexus of linked and highly valued aims that focus the educational endeavor on patient-centered care combined with learner-centered teaching. This Nexus is essential for the realization of excellence and provides a foundation for linkages between clinical and academic learning environments. Furthermore, it serves as a conduit for the translation and transformation of the first dimension, culture of excellence, into the second dimension, Praxis of Learning. Chapter 6 delves into the Praxis of Learning dimension, with an in-depth discussion of 4 elements that focus on a variety of features of teaching and learning in the classroom and clinical setting that are markers of excellence. Chapter 7 discusses the important organizational structures and resources that we found to support excellence in both academic and clinical settings.

Collectively, Chapters 4 to 7 present an in-depth description of each component of the Conceptual Model of Excellence in Physical Therapist Education, based on our research findings. The general structure of each chapter will be as follows: First, each dimension of the model and its elements will be described in detail. Secondly, evidence supporting each element will be presented in the form of interview or observational data from the academic and clinical sites. Following these descriptions and a review of evidence, one or more paradigm cases will be presented.[1] A paradigm case is defined as "a strong instance of a pattern or style that embodies skilled know-how and understandings and multiple key meanings of a social practice."[2(p90)] We present these cases as illustrative vignettes that seek to capture what we heard and observed in classroom or clinical settings in a way that creates a vision for the reader of what the elements look like in action. Finally, an envisioned future narrative related to each dimension or element will anticipate what physical therapist education could look like in the future if the attributes we identify in our model were universally present in academic and clinical sites that provide professional and post-professional preparation for physical therapists.

The findings from our study led to the development of 30 recommendations to enhance physical therapist education in the future. While many of the recommendations are derived from our direct observations of excellence and innovation in academic and clinical education and practice, some recommendations emanate from non-observations—things that we weren't seeing or hearing—that we feel have the potential to further advance physical therapist education. The recommendations that emerged from the findings presented in this section of the book will be discussed in detail in Part III and are paired with reflective questions that arise for educators to consider related to those recommendations.

REFERENCES

1. Benner P. The role of articulation in understanding practice and experience as sources of knowledge in clinical nursing. In: Tully J, ed. *Philosophy in an Age of Pluralism: The Philosophy of Charles Taylor in Question.* New York, NY: Cambridge University Press; 1994:136-155.
2. Benner P, Sutphen M, Leonard V, Day L. *Educating Nurses: A Call for Radical Transformation.* San Francisco, CA: Jossey-Bass; 2010.

3

Research Design, Methods, and Evolving Frameworks

In Chapter 2, we shared both the past, Flexner study of medical education, and present work, Preparation for the Professions Program (PPP), from the Carnegie Foundation for the Advancement of Teaching. The books from the PPP initiative, *Educating Clergy, Educating Lawyers, Educating Engineers, Educating Nurses,* and *Educating Physicians*,[1-5] all shared study findings and recommendations for existing or envisioned innovation for professional education. In addition, publications continue to share changes occurring in these professions as many of the recommendations have been enacted.[6-11]

In this chapter, we take a closer look at our qualitative research methods, which were like the methods used in the Carnegie PPP studies but were tailored to our research purpose and questions. A central component of our research was the continued development and evolution of our conceptual framework and grounded theory development about excellence and innovation in physical therapist education.

Our study of physical therapist education was modeled after the Carnegie Foundation for the Advancement of Teaching studies of the 5 professions (clergy, law, engineering, nursing, and medicine) with the following considerations:

- To examine physical therapist professional education considering the theoretic models and findings from those studies
- To expand the findings to include a profession that had recently transitioned to doctoral-level professional education
- To conduct the first comprehensive study of physical therapy education since Worthingham's studies in the 1960s[12-17] (see Chapter 1)

Jensen GM, Mostrom E, Hack LM, Nordstrom T, Gwyer J.
Educating Physical Therapists (pp 25-38).
© 2019 Taylor & Francis Group.

Because we had the same overarching purpose as the other Carnegie studies, the team knew that we needed a research design that would generate data from multiple exemplary sites. Additionally, because of the profession's rapidly growing post-professional residency and fellowship programs, and the goal of making such programs universally accessible, it was important to represent the continuum from professional education into residency and fellowship education. This expanded focus required us to investigate learners and learning in academic and clinical learning settings in both the professional preparation and post-professional phases of physical therapist education.

The Carnegie studies of the professions[1-5] demonstrated the profound changes that can be achieved in professional education when leaders in the field find compelling evidence of both the need for positive change and the means to achieve that change, as well as documentation of aspects of professional education that are not accomplishing desired aims or adequately addressing societal needs.[6-11] Our study was designed to explore the positive aspects of excellence and innovation in physical therapist education and then consider how our findings might inform and lead to recommendations for enhancement and reform. Having the benefit of the results of the Carnegie studies when we designed this study meant that we could build on those findings to not only explore them more deeply in our investigation, but also to tailor our study to the needs of physical therapy. The approach we used focused on curricular and organizational factors linked to exemplary practices of clinical and academic programs.

We also worked from the assumption that one of the ongoing and acute challenges in physical therapy education is how to better integrate the teaching and learning that occurs within the classroom with the teaching and learning occurring in communities of practice in clinical settings. While the use of evidence-based knowledge is critical in practice, as the Carnegie studies[1-5,8] found, it is the students' ability to employ habits of mind or a sense of salience during practice that is also essential to professional formation. If we accept the assumption that the goal of physical therapy education is to improve the quality of care and health care outcomes for patients, then these kinds of questions follow: (1) What are the components of professional and post-professional education that lead to this outcome? and (2) What are the innovative teaching and learning strategies that facilitate the formation of a professional capable of delivering quality care? The clinical setting and community of practice is an essential element in fully understanding this process, as novices tend to adopt and internalize the values of the clinical environment in which they are immersed.[8,18,19]

In the Carnegie studies, teams of researchers from within each profession, scholars from the Carnegie Foundation, and investigators with expertise in higher education studied the 5 professions. The cross-professions design of the studies in the PPP initiative allowed for a common framework for understanding education in the professions based on the central purpose and thus there were some common research design features among the 5 studies. The design features that all of the studies had in common were: (1) use of a qualitative, multiple case study research design; (2) purposeful sampling to select exemplars of excellence in education in the profession; (3) review of existing literature from studies of the specific profession (4) onsite interviews and observations at each of the participating organizations and review of written artifacts; and (5) an *a priori* assumption that their investigations would consider 2 key features of preparation for the professions: the profession's signature pedagogy, and the role that the 3 apprenticeships of developing habits of head (the knowledge of the profession), hand (the complex skills of practice), and heart (professional formation), played in the preparation for each profession.[8,20,21] (see Chapter 2 for a detailed description of these features of the PPP studies.) Additionally, the research team for each study formulated questions that were more specific to the profession and thus there were some differences in methods across the studies that were based on those specific questions and the nature of each professions educational preparation. Some of the key differences were:

- Given the 5 professions were quite variable in whether they had components of workplace learning, such as preceptorships and residencies, they differed in whether and how they studied this aspect of professional education.
- How the research teams selected their sample differed given that there is a great deal of variability among the professions in the academic path to practice, from the relative uniformity of medicine

and law, the breadth of practice in engineering, the variability in the path to licensure in nursing, and the nature of faith-based education in the clergy.

- Some of the studies used large-scale surveys (eg, nursing) or accreditation reports (eg, engineering) to supplement their field observations, interviews, and review of print artifacts.

The number of institutions included in the field observation phase of the studies varied from 8 in the clergy, 11 programs at 6 schools in engineering, 16 schools of law, 14 schools of medicine, and 9 schools of nursing.

PHYSICAL THERAPIST EDUCATION FOR THE 21ST CENTURY

Our Journey

In the summer of 2008, 3 members of our research team (Jensen, Hack, Nordstrom,) along with the American Physical Therapy Association (APTA) staff members (Goldstein, Harwood), met with Drs. Lee Shulman, David Irby, and Bridget O'Brien at the Carnegie Foundation headquarters in Stanford, California. Dr. Irby was a co-director of the study of medical education and Dr. O'Brien was a member of the medical education research team. The Carnegie Foundation team thought that there was merit in a study of professional education in physical therapy and that the model used in the Foundation's PPP initiative, with its focus on shining a light on excellence and innovation to propel transformation, was proving to have the desired effect in the other professions. During that visit, we also concluded that our study needed to include academic and clinical education (CE) sites given the model of physical therapist education, the difference from the other professions in the Carnegie studies, and the importance of the integration between learning in the academic and clinical environment to prepare clinicians for practice. With the interest and support of these Carnegie Foundation leaders and scholars, our research team embarked on a 2-year process of designing the study and searching for financial support. Based on the funding levels for the Carnegie Foundation studies, the team estimated that $300,000 in funding would be necessary to fully support the study to include several academic and clinical sites comparable with those in the previous Carnegie studies. As often happens in education research, with the recent exception of the funding the Carnegie Foundation received for the PPP studies, external funding to the extent necessary to support a robust study was not materializing.

In November 2010, the APTA issued a request for proposals (RFP), entitled *Innovation and Excellence in Physical Therapist Academic and Clinical Education*, the purpose of which was:

> To solicit proposals for a program of research that will identify an innovative curricular structure, including didactic and clinical education models that may be replicated in the United States to meet the demands of a changing society. The research will be used to produce a publishable final report that provides a clearer vision of ways to evaluate and improve the quality of physical therapist preparation so that future graduates can best meet the needs of the populations they will serve and the societies in which they will practice.

The amount of funding available through the RFP was $50,000. Our research team saw the alignment between the study we were pursuing and the objectives in the RFP but realized that the scope of our study would have to be dramatically altered given the limited funding. We also realized that we would have to tailor the study to address the purpose of the RFP if we were to be successful in obtaining the APTA funding. Therefore, we scaled back the scope of the study to constitute a pilot study of one academic program and one CE site that would set the foundation for a future, larger investigation of physical therapist education. We received funding through the RFP and proceeded with the proposed study. Following completion of the first 2 site visits in 2012, the APTA funded an additional $12,250 to add 1 additional clinical site and 1 additional academic site. Subsequent funding from the

American Council of Academic Physical Therapy, and the Education and Orthopedic Sections of the APTA allowed the team to expand the study to eventually include 6 academic sites and 5 clinical sites, constituting a purposive sample comparable to the other Carnegie studies. With expansion of the study to more closely parallel those of the Carnegies studies, the richness of the qualitative data that emerged allowed us to address the purpose of the RFP from the APTA, while also investigating the 3 apprenticeships and signature pedagogy in the profession and add to the literature on excellence and innovation in physical therapist education. In response to the APTA request for proposals, the purpose of our study was to identify and describe the attributes of excellence and innovation in physical therapist education in the United States across academic and clinical settings. The specific questions were:[22]

- Which educational patterns and practices, curricular characteristics, are present in exemplar cases that result in the development of physical therapists who are prepared to meet the demands of a changing society and health care system?

- Which educational patterns and practices of professional education support the successful education of physical therapists in the presence of patients?

- Which of these patterns and practices are worthy of replication because they have the likelihood of leading to more effective and efficient delivery of physical therapist education?

As illustrated in our initial conceptual framework (Figure 3-1), we believed that examining the curricular and organizational characteristics of professional education across the continuum from entry to professional preparation programs through post-professional residency education would provide a broader, contextual view of the cases we planned to study. We strongly believed that finding a way to represent and understand the context of the case was critical as aptly argued by Shulman[23] you cannot look at education in isolation, as it is the power that comes from the other parts of the larger system where education both draws and contributes.

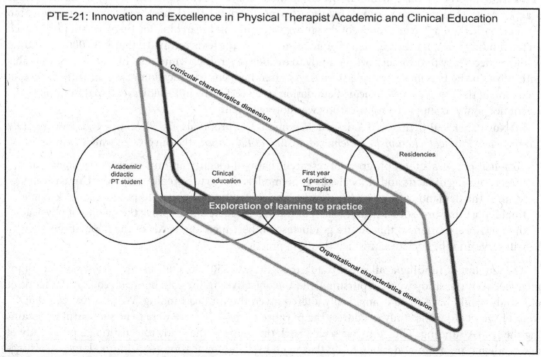

Figure 3-1. Original working model from the research proposal.

A detailed description of the study methods including (1) a summary of the national call for participants and selection process, (2) an overview of the general structure of the on-site visits conducted by the team, (3) an index of data collection instruments used during site visits, and (4) selected examples of interview questions for participants at the sites, is provided in Appendix B. The composition of our research team and selection of the purposive sample merit aree mentioned here because of the relationship to the prior Carnegie Foundation work and the findings that follow. Unlike the Carnegie research teams that included investigators from outside and from within each discipline, our research team only included physical therapists, all of whom have extensive experience in physical therapy education, clinical practice, and qualitative research. To address that potential source of bias and to assist in establishing the trustworthiness of our findings, we retained 2 consultants with expertise in education research and health professions education. We also employed an advisory panel comprised of representatives from the funding agencies and other stakeholder groups.[24] Given the results, recommendations for action and impact that the 5 Carnegie Foundation studies had in those professions and the potential to have a similar impact in physical therapist education, we knew that the criteria we used to select the purposive sample was a critical component of the research design. We developed the final selection criteria for academic and clinical participants in the study by (1) soliciting potential criteria from the education community, (2) considering the criteria in the APTA RFP and those used in the Carnegie PPP studies, (3) input from our advisory panel, and (4) review of evidence in the literature with attention to the purpose of the study and contextual factors in physical therapist education. A Delphi process was then used by the team to achieve consensus on the final selection criteria. The criteria for both the academic and clinical programs were as follows:[24]

Academic Site Selection Criteria
1. Acknowledged by a group of peers for excellence in physical therapist education
2. Physical therapist program with a breadth of CE from entry-level to active residency
3. Curricular structure that has integrated CE
4. Examples of interprofessional collaboration within the professional curriculum
5. Evidence of at least 1 example of innovative educational practice
6. A commitment to inclusion of groups that are underrepresented in physical therapy across faculty and students
7. Curricular requirements for student engagement in evidence-based practice and inquiry related to clinical practice
8. Research productive faculty

Clinical Site Selection Criteria
1. Acknowledged by academic affiliates and clinical agencies (peers) as providing excellent CE
2. CE site/program with breadth of CE experiences from entry-level preparation to active clinical residency(ies)
3. Opportunities for interprofessional collaboration and education within the CE program/site
4. Evidence of at least 1 example of innovative educational practice
5. A commitment to inclusion of groups that are underrepresented in physical therapy across faculty and students
6. Active clinical faculty development and mentoring program
7. Institutional commitment to health care professional preparation and education
8. Administrative support for CE activities

As the study expanded with more funding, the team added geographic distribution as a criterion for academic and clinical sites. Additionally, the type of academic institution (eg, private vs public, research intensive vs master's) were added to those criteria and, for the clinical sites, the type of clinical site was added (eg, academic medical center, community-based hospital, private practice). We had 2 national calls (2011 and 2013) for nominations and site selection that led to our final sample of 11 sites.

The 6 selected academic institutions represented diversity in terms of the type of institution, geography, size of institution and program, and role in residency education. The 5 clinical organizations chosen represented a diversity of clinical settings as well as geographic diversity. The profiles of the academic and clinical sites included in our final sample are found in Tables 3-1 and 3-2.

The research team, working from a sociocultural perspective on learning, used a multiple, qualitative case study design[25,26] and a grounded theory approach employing a constant-comparative method for within case and cross-case analysis.[25,27-29] The use of this design and analytic approach was similar to those used in the Carnegie PPP studies.[1-5] The research team of 5 experienced qualitative researchers, located in 5 geographic regions of the country, collectively had more than 150 years of experience in professional academic or CE. In addition, experienced educational researchers in medical education served as consultants to the team.

Like the Carnegie studies, our research study design was a qualitative case study design using a grounded theory approach that explored excellence and innovation in physical therapist education.[4,5] Case study design allowed us to explore, describe, document, and interpret what was happening in the teaching and learning environments across academic and clinical settings. An important element in case study design is the unit of analysis that represents the boundaries of the case.[25] Our unit of analysis was the organizational unit in academic settings (programs) and clinical settings (clinical entities). This structure allowed us to do both within-case and cross-case analysis (academic and clinical). The qualitative case study design uses data collection strategies well suited to exploring teaching and learning environments. This included observations of teaching and learning in classrooms, clinical teaching/learning activities, resident mentoring sessions; semi-structured interviews with administrators, faculty, students, and clinicians; and review of written artifacts and documents. We used a structured process typical of case study research starting with the creation of initial case records for each academic or clinical site that used a consistent structure (development of the case profile—organizational and institutional context), summary of data sources and sampling, and preliminary coding categories (learning for practice, organizational characteristics, people). These case records were then analyzed using an open coding process and then a detailed and comprehensive case report was written for each academic and clinical site based on a case report outline representing conceptualization of key constructs (culture, enacted curriculum, and professional formation).[24,30] An important step in qualitative case study research is the process of theory development done through pattern matching and the iterative process of explanation building. This comparing of findings and explanatory propositions from one case to another is a critical component of developing a conceptual model or framework.[25] We used the analytical strategy of pattern matching and explanation building[22] to examine how the elements of the framework fit our academic and clinical cases. We tested our assertions and eventually consistently found that the elements of excellence we had identified applied to all cases. The working conceptual model was stable after data collection from 8 of the 11 cases (5 academic cases and 3 clinical cases). The movement and evolution from our initial conceptual framework to our final model is described later in this chapter. Those transitions and transformations occurred as our data accumulated and our understandings deepened through ongoing within-case and cross-case analysis.

We employed several methods of verification to ensure dependability, credibility, and trustworthiness of the data.[25-29]

- The use of low inference data as all initial coding was done from verbatim transcripts of audio-recorded interviews.
- All individual interview transcripts were shared with the informant for review and comment to ensure an accurate account of the interview.
- Data triangulation occurred via multiple data collection methods including interviews, focus groups, document/artifact review, and field observations.
- Data were collected from multiple sites and numerous informants in all sites including students at multiple levels in their professional preparation, residents, academic, and clinical faculty, program directors, and faculty and administrators external to the profession.

TABLE 3-1

DEMOGRAPHIC DATA FOR ACADEMIC SITES AS OF VISIT DATE

ACADEMIC PROGRAM/ REGION	VISIT DATE	START DATE	CLASS SIZE	CORE FACULTY SIZE	RESIDENCIES	PHD PROGRAMS	INSTITUTION TYPE	LOCATION	CURRICULAR TYPE	CE TIMING/ PLACEMENT
1 Eastern	Mar 2013	1976	60	18 full-time 12 part-time	Orthopedics Sports Geriatrics	Biomechanics and Movement Science	Public, large, research intensive	Department of Physical Therapy College of Health Sciences	Traditional Systems-based	3 ICE experiences 7.5 months post-didactic work
2 Eastern	Feb 2013	1997	65 to 70	17 full-time 5 part-time	Orthopedics	Rehabilitation Sciences	Private, special-ized health sciences	Department of Physical Therapy School of Health and Rehabilitation Sciences	Case-based Systems-based	2 ICE experiences 5 months in 2 blocks within didactic work Year-long internship, 6 months after graduation
3 Eastern	Dec 2013	1984	60	14 full-time	Orthopedics	None	Private, masters	Department of Physical Therapy School of Medicine	Case-based using integrat-ed modules	8 weeks within didactic work 6 months post-didactic work

(continued)

TABLE 3-1 (CONTINUED)

DEMOGRAPHIC DATA FOR ACADEMIC SITES AS OF VISIT DATE

ACADEMIC PROGRAM/ REGION	VISIT DATE	START DATE	CLASS SIZE	CORE FACULTY SIZE	RESIDENCIES	PHD PROGRAMS	INSTITUTION TYPE	LOCATION	CURRICULAR TYPE	CE TIMING/ PLACEMENT
4 Midwestern	Jan 2014	1942	83	22 full-time 3 part-time	Women's Health Fellowship in Movement Science	Movement Science	Private, large, research intensive	Program of Physical Therapy School of Medicine	Traditional, systems-based	38 weeks in 4 blocks within didactic work
5 Western	Mar 2014	1946	94	25 full-time	Sports Orthopedics Neurology Pediatrics	Biokinesiology	Private, large, research intensive	Division of Biokinesiology and Physical Therapy School of Dentistry	Traditional, systems-based	Three 2-week blocks and one 6-week block within didactic work 32 weeks post-didactic work
6 Southern	April 2014	1960	55 (grow- ing to 75)	20 full-time	Orthopedics Sports Geriatrics	Rehabilitation Science	Public, large, research intensive	Deptartment of Physical Therapy College of Public Health and Health Professions	Traditional, systems-based	96 hours ICE 32 weeks within didactic work

ICE = Institute of Clinical Experience

Based on the categories used by the Commission on Accreditation of Physical Therapy Education.[31]

TABLE 3-2

DEMOGRAPHIC DATA FOR CLINICAL SITES AS OF VISIT DATE

CLINICAL PROGRAM/ REGION	VISIT DATE	TYPE OF SETTING	# OF SCHOOLS	STUDENTS PER YEAR	RESIDENTS	FELLOWS	# OF THERAPISTS AND CLINICAL SPECIALISTS
1 Eastern	Oct 2012	Inpatient Outpatient academic medical center (~2500 beds)	27	30	2	N/A	300 physical therapists 104 specialists
2 Midwestern	Nov 2012	Inpatient rehabilitation (96 beds) Outpatient rehabilitation	36	36	2	N/A	69 physical therapists 16 specialists
3 Southern	April 2014	Inpatient rehabilitation Outpatient rehabilitation Institute of higher learning (157 beds)	25	110	16	4	136 physical therpists 31 specialists
4 Western	Mar 2014	Outpatient Part of a 515-bed community hospital system	7	30	2	N/A	18 physical therapists 14 specialists
5 Northwestern	Aug 2014	Outpatient (80 clinics) Private practice (visited 2)	83	150	3 to 6	0 to 4	8 physical therapists 5 specialists (at sites visited)

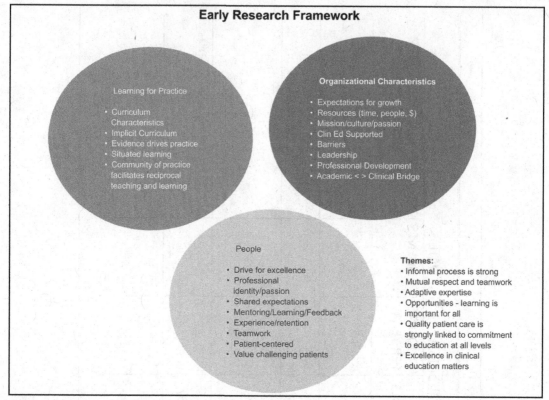

Figure 3-2. Early conceptual framework based on emerging findings.

- Multiple experienced qualitative researchers completed independent coding and achieved consensus on categories and themes through the testing of assertions and fit with the data.

The team used negative case analysis to look for disconfirming data that did not fit with our ongoing analysis and to confirm that our results reflected the preponderance of data. This strategy includes following up on surprises or unpatterns and examining not only what we were observing but also what we were not observing.[28]

The team also used peer review through our external research consultants, who provided a knowledgeable but outsiders' viewpoint, presenting emerging findings to peers, and inviting feedback from our advisory board as the study proceeded.[30,32]

EVOLUTION OF CONCEPTUAL FRAMEWORKS

One of the features of the qualitative inquiry approach employed in this study is the emergent nature of the findings that inevitably leads to an evolution of the conceptual framework that results from ongoing interpretation, synthesis, theorizing, and recontextualizing among the researchers.[33] As data were gathered and analyzed using open and axial coding from the growing number of cases, the team wrote case reports that allowed for data reduction and synthesis. Our research team, including the advice from the advisory panel and consultants, continuously tested assertions, found patterns, and built explanations to develop working conceptual frameworks in a progressive, iterative manner. As the number of cases grew, the team engaged in cross-case analyses to recontextualize the data to further refine the conceptual framework and develop the emerging theory. Once the study commenced, we developed the earliest conceptual framework (Figure 3-2) following the first 2 site visits. It had 3 large categories comprised of the teaching and learning environment where learning for practice was occurring, the organizational characteristics of the institutions including their missions and leadership, and the characteristics and commitments the people in the organizations brought to the educational endeavor.

As we gathered more data and observed the patterns among the cases, we continued to explore the inter-relationships among the categories found in the earlier model and generated a revised conceptual model (Figure 3-3). In this model, perceptions about what it meant to be a physical therapist embodying excellence and innovation became a foundational, central concept with connections to the organization context, the enacted curriculum, and the shared values and beliefs about learning for practice among the people in the clinical environment.

As it appeared that we were approaching saturation of our data toward the end of our planned data collection, we developed a third conceptual model that synthesized what we were observing at that point in the study, but this model was transitional and just an additional iteration on our way to the final model. Further cross-case analysis, and testing of assertions through discussion, consultation, and sharing our findings in multiple settings with different audiences, led us to our final conceptual model (Figure 3-4).

There are key features of the final conceptual model that merit explanation before the study findings are discussed in more detail in Chapters 5 to 8. The model represents physical therapist education as a totality rather than academic and CE separately, because we observed these key components of excellence in all our sites and with a high degree of interdependence between academic and CE (see Figure 3-4). We present the model here to serve as a unifying framework for the presentation of our findings. The model has 3 major dimensions: Culture of Excellence, Praxis of Learning, and Organizational Structures and Resources.[24]

The elements of the Culture of Excellence dimension were:

- Shared beliefs and values about the aims and importance of physical therapist education and practice; these shared beliefs engendered respect, trust and collaboration among participants in these communities of practice
- Leadership and vision that was shared throughout the settings; the leaders were attentive to the internal and external forces that influenced physical therapist education, practice, and research
- A drive for excellence with high expectations among all of the members of the community, including learners, residents, mentors, clinicians, and faculty members; they had a willingness to innovate and take risks in the service of continuous improvement
- True partnerships that were intentionally created bridges between the academic and clinical realms of physical therapist education and that recognized the critical interdependence of these realms for realizing excellence

The central component of the model—the Nexus—is the lens of the paired and highly valued aims of learner centeredness and patient centeredness that were pervasive in both academic and clinical settings and integral to how faculty, clinicians and mentors framed their work. This lens served as the conduit through which the culture of excellence was translated into the domain of praxis, where knowledge is transformed into meaningful practice through action. The shared commitment to the values of patient-centeredness and learner-centeredness were the foundation for the creation of a true partnership between academic and clinical sites that provided a coming together, or Nexus, for the important task of facilitating learning for practice through practice.

The right side of the model is the dimension, Praxis of Learning, where learning is the primary focus and where curriculum is enacted and embodied through action and interaction among learner and teacher grounded in practice. There are 4 elements in the Praxis of Learning dimension:

1. Signature pedagogy for physical therapist education with a focus on movement and the human body as teacher
2. Practice-based learning that provides authentic, situated, and powerful experiences for the learner in a variety of settings and across a diverse group of teachers and learners
3. Creating adaptive learners who are equipped to function in complex and uncertain environments and learn through unfolding experience

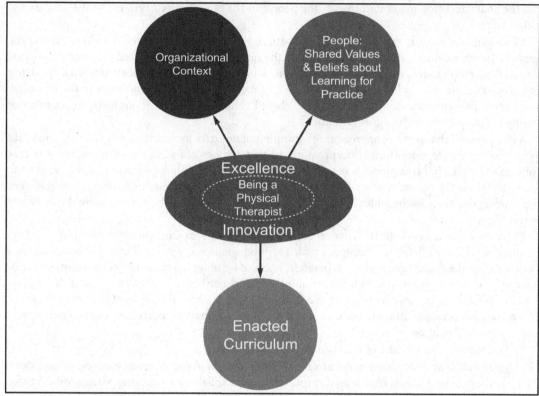

Figure 3-3. Revised conceptual framework demonstrating the relationships of key concepts.

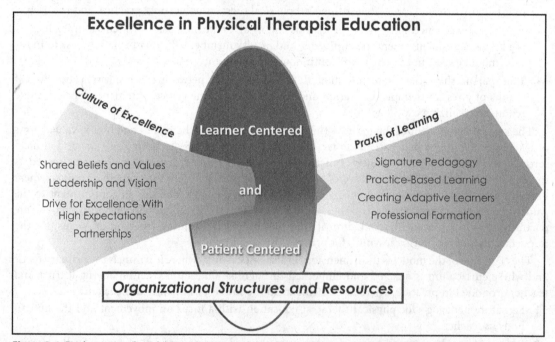

Figure 3-4. Final conceptual model representing excellence and innovation in physical therapist education.

4. Professional formation through which physical therapists learn and develop as moral agents in the context of the profession and society

At the bottom of the model is the supporting foundation of organizational structures and resources, which recognizes that these Cultures of Excellence, the Nexus, and Praxis of Learning do not occur in a vacuum. While we found that there was no one model for academic or CE that seemed directly linked with excellence, the development and wise use of resources within our exemplar organizations/sites was essential. The subsequent chapters in Part II will describe in further detail the evidence for each of these dimensions and elements in the model and discuss the implications for physical therapist education and practice.

REFERENCES

1. Sullivan W, Colby A, Wegner JW, Bond L, Shulman L. *Educating Lawyers: Preparation for the Profession of Law*. San Francisco, CA: Jossey-Bass; 2007.
2. Foster C, Dahill L, Goleman L, Tolentino BW. *Educating Clergy: Teaching Practices and Pastoral Imagination*. San Francisco, CA: Jossey-Bass; 2006.
3. Sheppard S, Macatangay K, Colby A, Sullivan W. *Educating Engineers: Designing the Future of the Field*. San Francisco, CA: Jossey-Bass; 2009.
4. Benner P, Sutphen M, Leonard C, Day L. *Educating Nurses: A Call for Radical Transformation*. San Francisco, CA: Jossey-Bass; 2010.
5. Cooke M, Irby D, O'Brien B. *Educating Physicians: A Call for Reform of Medical School and Residency*. San Francisco, CA: Jossey-Bass; 2010.
6. Benner P. Formation in professional education: an examination of the relationship between theories of meaning and theories of self. *J Med Philos*. 2011;36:342-353.
7. O'Brien B, Irby D. Enacting the Carnegie Foundation call for reform of medical school and residency. *Teach Learn Med*. 2013;25:S1-S8.
8. Colby A, Sullivan W. Formation of professionalism and purpose: perspectives from the preparation for the professions program. *University of St. Thomas Law Journal*. 2008;5:404-426.
9. Wegner J. The Carnegie Foundation's *Educating Lawyers*: 4 questions for bar examiners. *The Bar Examiner*. 2011;11-24
10. Noone J. Teaching to the three apprenticeships: designing learning activities for professional practice in an undergraduate curriculum. *J Nurs Ed*. 2008;48(8):468-472.
11. Cronenwett L., ed. The future of nursing education. In: *Institute of Medicine. The Future of Nursing Education: Leading Change, Advancing Health*. 2011;477-483.
12. Worthingham CA. The environment for basic physical therapy education—1965-1966: the academic or theoretical phase. *Phys Ther*. 1968;48:935-962.
13. Worthingham CA. The clinical environment for basic physical therapy education—1965-1966, Part I: Facilities. *Phys Ther*. 1968;48:1195-1215.
14. Worthingham CA. Study of basic physical therapy education: III, the clinical environment for basic physical therapy education 1965-1966, Part II: Staff. *Phys Ther*. 1968;48:1353-1382.
15. Worthingham CA. The 1961 and 1965 graduate of the physical therapy schools, part I: 1961 graduate, part II: 1965 graduates. *Phys Ther*. 1969;49:476-499.
16. Worthingham CA. Study of basic physical therapy education: V request (prescription or referral) for physical therapy. *Phys Ther*. 1970;50:989-962.
17. Worthingham CA. Study of basic physical therapy education: VI findings of the study in relation to trends in patient care and education. *Phys Ther*. 1970;50:1315-1331.
18. Black L, Jensen G, Mostrom E. The first year of practice: an investigation of the learning and professional development of promising novice physical therapists. *Phys Ther*. 2010;90:1758-1773.
19. Hayward LM, Black LL, Mostrom E, Jensen GM, Ritzline PD, Perkins J. The first 2 years of practice: a longitudinal perspective on learning and professional development of promising novice physical therapists. *Phys Ther*. 2013;93:369-383.
20. Shulman LS. Signature pedagogies in the professions. *Daedelus*. 2005;134:52-59.
21. Shulman L. Pedagogies of uncertainty. *Liberal Education*. 2005;91(2):18-25.
22. Jensen GM, Hack L, Gwyer J, et. al. National study of physical therapist education. Session Presentation. Presented at: American Physical Therapy Association Combined Sections Meeting; February 7, 2015; Indianapolis, IN.
23. Shulman LS. *The Wisdom of Practice: Essays on Teaching, Learning and Learning to Teach*. San Francisco, CA. Jossey-Bass; 2004.
24. Jensen GM, Nordstrom T, Mostrom EM, Hack LM, Gwyer J. A national study of excellence and innovation in physical therapist education: Part 1—design, methods, and results. *Phys Ther*. 2017;97:857-874.

25. Yin R. *Case Study Research: Design and Methods*. 5th ed. Thousand Oaks, CA: Sage Publications; 2014.

26. Patton M. *Qualitative Research and Evaluation Methods: Integrating Theory and Practice*. 4th ed. Thousand Oaks, CA: Sage Publications; 2015.

27. Corbin J, Strauss A. *Basics of Qualitative Research: Techniques and Procedures for Developing Grounded Theory*. Thousand Oaks, CA: Sage Publications; 2008.

28. Miles M, Huberman AM, Saldana J. *Qualitative Data Analysis: An Expanded Sourcebook*. 3rd ed. Thousand Oaks, CA: Sage Publications; 2014.

29. Merriam S. *Qualitative Research and Case Study Applications in Education*. San Francisco, CA: Jossey-Bass Publishing; 1998.

30. Jensen GM, Hack L, Nordstrom T, Gwyer J, Mostrom E. National study of excellence and innovation in physical therapist education: Part 2: call for reform. *Phys Ther*. 2017;97:875-888.

31. Commission on Accreditation of Physical Therapy Education. Aggregate Program Data, 2016–2017 Physical Therapist Education Programs Fact Sheets, CAPTE. http://www.capteonline.org/uploadedFiles/CAPTEorg/About_CAPTE/Resources/Aggregate_Program_Data/AggregateProgramData_PTPrograms.pdf. Published 2017. Accessed September 4, 2018.

32. Jensen GM, Gwyer J, Hack L, Mostrom E, Nordstrom T, Shulman L. Excellence in the health professions: what we have learned (Part I) and physical therapist education for the 21st century: research findings and recommendations (Part 2). Session Presentation. Presented at: American Physical Therapy Association Combined Sections Meeting; February 17, 2016; Anaheim, CA.

33. Morse J. Emerging from the data: the cognitive processes of analysis in qualitative inquiry. *Critical Issues in Qualitative Research Methods*. Newbury Park, CA: Sage Publications; 1994:23-43.

The Culture of Excellence in Physical Therapist Education
Where Values and Vision Begin

The pursuit of excellence in teaching physical therapists is one that must be consistently evaluated, in order to determine whether our processes create excellent or average practitioners. Teachers, collaboratively, including faculty, researchers, and clinicians, must discover how to create an environment that will model the goals set for our students. Teachers must comprehend their own meaning of excellence through traveling what Hansen[1] calls a teacher's *moral odyssey*. In doing so, faculty identify values and visions that can be articulated, translated, and developed into a culture desired by the community of learners. An identifiable Culture of Excellence is what we found in this research.

The first dimension of the Conceptual Model of Excellence in Physical Therapist Education focuses on creating, fostering, and authentically living a Culture of Excellence. Whether in the academic or clinical setting, each of our cases exhibited a deep commitment to cultures that foster excellence. What were some of the common characteristics of these cultures of excellence that we observed in physical therapist education?

We saw 4 elements that were essential to creating and fostering cultures of excellence that we will explicate in this chapter:

1. Shared beliefs and values
2. Leadership and vision
3. A drive for excellence with high expectations
4. Partnerships

Jensen GM, Mostrom E, Hack LM, Nordstrom T, Gwyer J.
Educating Physical Therapists (pp 39-57).
© 2019 Taylor & Francis Group.

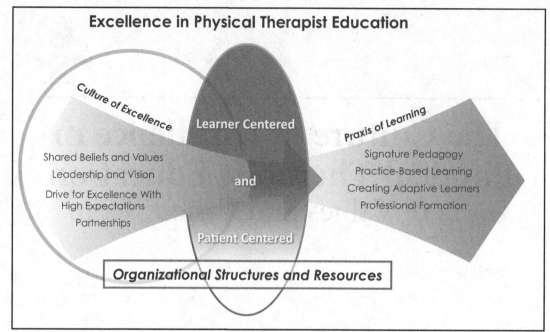

Figure 4-1. Model of Excellence in Physical Therapist Education: Dimension—Culture of Excellence.

As a clinical administrator shared with us:

I believe culture is everything. It all starts with culture; and culture comes from the top. Culture is about attitudes, and beliefs, and behavior, and if the organization doesn't believe in education—continuing education and research in training the next generation—it just doesn't happen. If that's a salient attribute of the organization's culture, then it does happen. I believe that everything that happens here—the way we treat each other, the way we act toward patients, what we value—it's all about the culture of the organization. We have a very strong culture here, and it does come from the top. Because we advocate training, and education, and research, we make time for it, we provide resources for it, we pay attention to it.

This dimension of the Culture of Excellence, located on the left side of Figure 4-1, is considered to be the catalyst that ignites the model. Excellence cannot be achieved without a commitment to building a culture that communicates the expectations for the entire learning community. In this chapter, each of the 4 elements listed will be described with supporting evidence and case examples.

SHARED BELIEFS AND VALUES

Health care practitioners and administrators are likely to be familiar with mission statements that communicate the values of the organization, be it universities, hospitals, outpatient facilities, or other settings. The first element in this dimension is the unique way these professionals choose to collaborate in identifying the most important shared beliefs and values in their community. These commonly held beliefs and values not only served as the foundation of their organization's mission, but they bound colleagues together with a passion for their work and created a common sense of purpose.

Some of our research sites had a broadly articulated value for innovation and excellence, while other sites identified more specific values related to, for example, research into human movement systems. We soon realized that each research site could articulate their shared beliefs and values, but these were not at all fully congruent across all sites. What was important is the presence of processes to develop these shared beliefs and values at each site. At each site, the participants described a variety of methods used to bring clinicians, administrators, and faculty together to create these shared beliefs. We found academic and clinical faculty typically made these values explicit through meetings, documentation, teaching, and modeling. Colleagues and students could describe the organization's values in interviews, for example, describing a strong belief in the importance of professionalism.

Evidence From Academic and Clinical Sites

In both clinical and academic settings, we found explicit expressions of the organization's missions, values, and beliefs in many formats. Mission, philosophies, and vision for the future were documented and personnel were familiar with these organizational touchstones. In some instances, the mission or values were written on a wall or on personnel badges. Because these external emblems of a mission and values are ubiquitous in organizations, we pursued these overt expressions of beliefs and values in interviews and focus groups, to determine the strength of commitment to these stated values and the mission. It was noteworthy that the people we interviewed, regardless of their position, not only related a common interpretation of the mission and values but described ways in which they were expressed through action in the organization. No matter what specific value was important in the organization, the path to creating and enacting the chosen values had common characteristics, including a high regard for mutual trust and respect for one another, no matter the level of the participant. The previous quote in this chapter by the clinical administrator describes a set of values that are pervasive in the organization, including how mutual respect among colleagues reinforces the importance of their culture.

In another clinic, the center coordinator of clinical education (CE) related how the shared values of teaching related to student learning:

> I think along with that I think that there's a lot of support for clinical education among the clinicians, that it's not something, "Oh, gosh, I've got another student. I have to take on another student." People, I think, are really invested in educating and teaching with the facility having really a strong teaching model that comes through loud and clear. Again, I go back to the high expectations that the clinicians have for students, and I think that that just is energizing for students. It's great.

In a different clinical setting, an administrator described the culture and the importance of collegial teamwork in terms not often used in an educational or clinical setting:

> It's the culture that we have created going back to the very, very beginning, the very first residencies, people understood that this was a group effort and this was a team we were building...It's about developing something, creating something that's bigger than any of us individually and the teamwork and the camaraderie. To work here, there is a citizenship or a stewardship or a contribution that you owe the organization that you're working in. It's not just 9 to 5, it's that you're part of the system. You are going to contribute. They don't have to all be leaders, but they have to have passion.

The academic faculties articulated the importance of building a culture that all members of the educational community participate in developing and modeling:

> Really everybody is open in the whole department and faculty...Really support one another, want to see everyone succeed, and has the same mission and purpose in place all across the board, regardless of your rank... That's transparent.

> I think we have a culture here in the program and across the University of growth and change...Another thing about the culture in the program is I think the soul of physical therapy remains central to us all...That makes for a much more cohesive organization. It makes for a commitment to the education of students. It makes for a commitment to patients if they walk in the door...One part of the soul is that we care about people and we care about each other...regardless of duties [in the program] people care about physical therapy and they're expected to know something about the world of physical therapy.

> It's a club. We're a really small club and we take care of each other because the better we are as a group, the better we are as individuals. This is a wonderful cadre of people to practice with, it really is.

The importance of shared beliefs and values was repeatedly shared in large focus groups containing academic and clinical participants. We observed the pride with which these professionals shared their cultural values, and the openness to conversation amongst learner, teacher, and administrator alike.

Envisioned Future for the Profession of Physical Therapy

The profession has a history of a code of ethics since 1935[2] and, as of 2003, a set of professional core values:[3] accountability, altruism, compassion and caring, excellence, integrity, professional duty, and social responsibility. These documents provide strong guidance for the development of ethical practice and professional values in learners as well as teachers. In our study, we observed faculty who promoted additional shared values for trust, respect, and collaboration among the entire community of learners. However, an explicit effort to explore and create the shared beliefs and values that underlie colleagues' work in clinical or academic settings are necessary. A lack of shared values and norms in an organization may limit the outcomes for innovation in the profession. At the extreme, faculty members may tolerate a culture of distrust and lack of respect within academic environments or between the academic and clinical environments. The professional community has yet to fully engage in the process of identifying and inculcating the shared beliefs and values that represent excellence in education, research, and practice in physical therapy. The lack of persistent inclusion of learners in the development of the Culture of Excellence in the organization is also of concern.

In a successful learning community, all members are fully engaged in the process of identifying and inculcating the shared beliefs and values that represent excellence in education. In excellent programs, everyone upholds and values the culture of the organization. That commitment sets the stage for many additional values and practices that are essential in today's health care environment. For example, the value for interprofessional education and for collaborative patient care may be developed through shared values that are considered to be innovative.

The profession may not completely comprehend the importance of the values of learner-centered teaching and patient-centered care. The unique variety of educational settings may stretch the faculty members' ability to adjust to these values. Or it is possible that these values of patient-centered care and learner-centered education are espoused but not lived if there is not accountability and shared understanding and investment in those values. These specific shared values will be discussed in more detail in Chapter 5.

These strongly shared beliefs and values of mutual trust, respect and collaboration, coupled with patient-centered care and learner-centered education, are crucial if academic and clinical faculty members are to work together to pursue excellence, and if learners are to adopt the beliefs and values of excellence modeled for them.

LEADERSHIP AND VISION

As it has for nearly a century, organizational leadership continues to receive attention in the popular press and in the literature, including leadership in higher education.[4] As emerging evidence is showing, leadership styles and personalities are less important to successful leadership than how leaders work with and through the members of their team, use systems-thinking to navigate the complex world around them, and lead with a clear vision for their organization. We had no a priori assumption that we would investigate the leadership styles and personalities of the leaders we encountered. Commonalities in leadership styles were not evident in our study. There were probably as many differences in style and personality as there were individuals in leadership positions. What we did observe across all of our settings was a commitment to fulfill their institutional mission and, in doing so, leverage that mission in order to support their institution and to become valued members of their institutions that were integrated into the institution's mission and direction. They also saw their mission in relation to advancing the profession's goals and responsibilities to society. They also expressed a clear, shared vision for their future and worked to facilitate team-based collaborations towards that greater goal. These leaders paid close attention to the internal and external forces and to the emerging trends that are influencing physical therapist practice, education, and research.

Evidence From Academic and Clinical Sites

We heard many of our participants discuss the creative energy of the faculty or staff who make it possible to fulfill their mission and strive toward achieving their shared vision. They often recognized the uncertainty inherent in the present and in the future environments of education and practice, what the constraints are, and the importance of accountability. One academic program faculty member described it this way:

> Everybody is trying to accomplish the same thing and trying to bring that commitment to the mission of trying to prepare physical therapists. What we're all trying to do, which is really an impossible thing, is to prepare people not for practice today but for practice 5 years from now, 10 years from now. That's the challenge. I think many, many programs have that commitment. The key is execution, of course. The key is figuring out ways to, on the one hand, allow people's energy and enthusiasm and innovative ideas to flourish, and on the other hand to harness that and keep people from getting too far off so to have this kind of controlled chaos of a situation. And I think we're constantly tipping from one side to the other in that process of trying to keep that in balance...I would say the most important aspect of that is that everybody on the faculty feel that they have both a stake and a voice.

We observed several examples of how the department linked its mission tightly to that of the larger institution in explicit ways that garnered them more support from executive leadership. One academic institution's mission focused on international and experiential learning and had a vision for strengthening research on campus. The physical therapy program revised its curriculum to strengthen experiential learning in diverse communities and added international learning experiences to its program to ensure that alignment was visible. A student comments:

> I think the experiential learning with the community service aspect helps as well. It's not just getting out there and helping the community and building rapport with people. It's also another way to show your professionalism as you're interacting with these people in different settings. I think they're kind of helping us to bridge that gap in all areas of our profession.

Students and faculty commented on how international learning experiences positively influenced the students' development as clinicians, particularly their clinical reasoning. A faculty member noted:

> ...last night [I was] with...3 students that have been in Jamaica a month and...their first patient with HTLD [Human t-Lymphotropic Virus]. It's a pretty common virus in Jamaica...I had students that came to Jamaica 10 years ago and they would have looked at me and said, "I don't know what that is." Then they would have implicitly blamed the curriculum, "You didn't teach us that," but that's not what happens now. It's almost like the unknown...is exciting, not scary or something...but they knew what to do. That's different than it was in the old curriculum where they would have abdicated responsibility and said, "The curriculum didn't teach us this."

In a series of interviews, the ability of the program to be an instrumental player in meeting the institution's research agenda was discussed from different perspectives, 2 from faculty and 1 from the program director:

> ...the ability of the leadership in the department and the faculty as a whole to read the institution and understand that environment and that culture and then make decisions about what they're going to do to lead and advance their interests while advancing the university's interests.

> But you're leading the university in a direction that it probably wants to go so they're holding this program up for other departments and schools to emulate.

> What we've had to push the institution to develop the kind of infrastructure that's necessary to support federal grants. It's been a struggle. It's nice to be a pioneer and able to do it.

This faculty also realized the importance of active participation in university governance and took leadership roles, a level of engagement that was appreciated by the dean and the program's director:

> I think the fact that we've got physical therapy faculty members on all the elective committees, often that the leadership roles, the chair [of] faculty council, things like that, is a good indication of the respect they've got across the entire campus, not just the sciences.

We're elected to committees, we're elected to university committees. That to me, you can't just do that with your own department. You have to have support from other departments to do that. I think that's an indication that they may be jealous, but they're respectful of what we've accomplished. They know we're hard workers.

When connecting the institution's mission to the program's mission and, ultimately, the core of the profession, there was often wide latitude in how that was transmitted from executive leadership. One current program director, speaking about the coherence between institutional mission and program mission, talked about the primary charge she had been given by upper administration:

...I've only ever been given one charge...and that is "do the right thing." I've heard it from 2 chancellors...That is the only thing I've been told to do, which could be on some days daunting...but most days I think it's...fun. I think it's fun because you have this enormous range of possibilities in one single obligation...I think mostly (doing) the right thing means a moral obligation.

Further light was shed on this in an interview with a senior administrator at the school level who connected it to the credo of health professions: "Isn't that what we're all supposed to do in health care? I mean that's the tradition of health care professionals." She elaborated that one of the things she has really noticed at the institution "...is that the desire to really strive for excellence is really just a part of our being here...Striving for excellence without being too egotistical...I think it goes along with the 'do the right thing'."

One of the clinics in our sample has the values of "Collaboration, Hospitality, Respect, Innovation, Stewardship, Teaching." While their written materials about the value "Teaching" emphasized teaching patients and clients, the clinicians and administrators also included teaching students and linked that to their mission and, more broadly, the profession. A clininical instructor (CI) stated:

I'm very proud of the practice that we provide and the care we provide our patients. I know that it's not like that everywhere. I hear stories of what it's like at other institutions, so I think to be able to share our practice, our beliefs, our professionalism with students, whether...It's beneficial if they stay on, and agree to stay in our department, but even if they go elsewhere. We have interns that have gone elsewhere, and they have brought those values with them to other institutions and have had an impact larger than our walls. I think it's great to be able to influence the future generation that way.

Perspectives on the importance of participation and development in leadership were evident in the clinical and academic settings, creating clear messages that leadership is a responsibility held by everyone. One clinician commented about leadership development:

...from a staff perspective and having been here for quite a while that there are a lot of different opportunities, either for staff to grow into leadership roles or to kind of pursue areas of specialty that they're really interested in...I think if you're patient and you communicate with your supervisors and you have an area that you really want to grow in clinically and develop a specialty that you have an opportunity to do that. I think that keeps us engaged and excited about our careers and that helps promote longevity and that excitement translates to students as well.

As noted previously, shared leadership requires shared accountability and responsibility to the mission and vision of the institution. Structures and functions also contribute to shared leadership, as one faculty member described it:

...we have a leadership structure. We have a system which empowers people to be leaders in the domains in which they're acting. And so we do have a structure. It's not real tight but we have a structure of semester committees, of curriculum committee, of an operations committee and a whole range of different structures that allow us a somewhat loose way to keep the whole thing cohesive. But all of the people who are operating in that structure are providing leadership. The key to leadership is not to have one person telling everybody what to do—that doesn't work. It's to have many leaders. And that's what we have in this faculty is a faculty of leaders, really. That's what we try to create. The idea here is to try to allow us to flourish but try to direct those energies in a cohesive way without stifling the creativity that's there. But in saying that, you have to realize that you can't do that without a faculty who is that committed to the process.

Envisioned Future for the Profession of Physical Therapy

The complex environments of health care and education require that leaders of the future have a shared, compelling vision in which practice, education, and research mutually reinforce and advance each other based on the leaders' deep understanding of the context of all 3. The profession should be served by visionary leaders in academic and clinical settings who value shared leadership to create a Culture of Excellence focused on achieving the program's and institution's mission and advancing the profession's societal responsibilities. Leaders co-create a shared vision for the future of physical therapy practice and education, grounded in the profession's responsibilities to society. True leaders are adept at realizing that the complex nature of practice, education, and research requires systems-based thinking and a reliance on creating a network of colleagues within and without their institution. Given the demands of the practice and education environments, there should be intentional development opportunities for promising leaders using diverse means.

The Education Leadership Institute (ELI) Fellowship[5] program of the American Physical Therapy Association (APTA) is making strides in preparing leaders that meet the profession's needs. We need more visionary, qualified leaders for our academic and CE programs toward excellence. Leaders must create environments in which shared leadership is the norm and the team focuses on leveraging the institutional mission to advance the profession's goals and responsibilities to society. Excellent leaders pursue knowledge of and engage in professional, national, and institutional policy development that leads to improvement and innovation.

A Drive for Excellence With High Expectations

When leaders believe it is good enough to conform to minimum standards from accrediting agencies or to achieve minimal standards, such as licensure pass rates, it places the future of the profession at risk, particularly if those beliefs are coupled with a predominant focus on parochial interests. Further along a spectrum towards achieving excellence are clinics and programs with systems for quality management or quality improvement. In those organizations, if the standards for assessment emphasize incremental improvement or are not attuned to the increasing expectations from the external stakeholders, it is unlikely they will achieve excellence. The academic and clinical programs we visited were characterized by cultures that continuously pursued improvement, but more importantly they questioned current practices, valued innovation, and embraced risk taking to achieve excellence. These excellent clinicians, educators, and leaders seemed to have adopted the mantra, "It is never good enough." That mantra compelled them to adopt innovative and creative means to improve their work.

Evidence From Academic and Clinical Sites

The drive for excellence was a pervasive and palpable characteristic in the environment of the sites we visited. The context of that drive was the importance for practice. As this program director described:

> When I came here, one of the big mantras that I heard all of the time from faculty and students, repeatedly, was this notion of not ever digressing to the mean. That just came up repeatedly and I had never heard that used as an expression used as often as it was used here. That sums it up a lot. We are going to train you to higher standards and educate you and encourage you, and hope that all of that, when you're on your own, sticks with you and that you continue to carry that forward—and that you never become complacent and not just be satisfied...that you keep reaching and stretching.

When the drive for excellence is pervasive in an organization, there is a mutually reinforcing phenomenon that can occur to promulgate constant improvement throughout the organization. One clinician had this observation of her experience at the organization:

There's a lot of creativity across the entire organization. I've been struck that when I have a challenge that I run into and I approach managers or people in other departments for their support, just how they really rally and exceed any of my expectations...In this organization I feel like people are really committed to excellence so when you bring them a challenge, they want to help you be successful so there's a sense of a real team approach—2 things that I really appreciate in this organization.

It was also recognized that the quest for high levels of achievement is not without risk. Previously in this chapter, one program's efforts to improve its curriculum were described like "controlled chaos" and that they were "tipping from one side to the other." Those feelings of disequilibrium were not uncommon, as one faculty member at another program eloquently captured his experience:

I can remember the first 3 to 4 years going, "These people never stop. They're like a shark swimmer. They just never stop thinking about the future." I thought I was going fast in my research. I thought I was a visionary thinker but you get in this culture and, we never talk about it, but it's a risky way to do business to continuously push the envelope, continuously ask, "Why? What are we doing right, wrong? What could we do better?"

One of the academic programs was in the midst of a complete curriculum revision. As one said, they were "blowing it up." As with all of our participating institutions, they were recognized for excellence, thus their radical change was not based on the need to address a serious problem. Also, it was not change for change's sake, but rather the recognition that recent literature on how to achieve deep learning for practice had outstripped their original curricular design. One of the leaders in the program described it this way:

Never being complacent with what you have, and always looking for the next thing to do, the next envelope to push, the next thing that's happening in the profession in education. It does take someone, at least one person, that keeps poking you a little bit about what else can you do?

During the discussion leading up to the change, there was disagreement and discontent that they worked through to reach consensus on the need to move forward. Ultimately though, they recognized that not every faculty member might be able to adjust to the new curriculum and they might lose valued faculty members, another risk of change:

I think that the faculty as a whole, as an aggregate, do embrace that and have enough cohesion to do it, but at the same time I think it's also going to help mold the faculty of the next 10 years here too as people come and see how we do teaching and learning here, they'll decide if this is the place for them or it's not. My experience has been some people don't prefer to teach that way.

Their drive for excellence was grounded in a passion for learning among the faculty members. Learners and clinicians had a thirst for learning that harkens back to the mantra, "never good enough," as one of the clinicians in an administrative role described:

You're striving for the hundred percent...We have 5 people going back for the DPT [Doctor of Physical Therapy] right now. So, even people who have been out 20, 25 years and you think of clinical excellence and customer service and the well-rounded person, it's them. Yet, they're going back for their DPT...we've never really achieved the pinnacle of excellence, we're always raising the bar. We're always growing, we're always changing. What's new, what's different. I mean, we're in the medical field, right? We're never going to reach that top pinnacle of excellence, because there's always something a little bit more.

Much like it not being change for change sake, it was not learning for learning sake, but connected to their mission, their responsibilities to the profession, and, most importantly, the connection to patients and how to improve the system. A center director of CE remarked:

We look for opportunities to learn and we look for that concept of continuous lifelong learning. Everybody's on that quest to continue learning, to continue to try and make themselves better as individuals but make the system better. It's not trying to make any one person better. It's really how can we make everything better. We spend a lot of time, a lot of my time is spent on professional mentoring and helping people move along their path and a lot of that is working on trying to get people to come back in and do more things. A lot of programs that we have are being performed by past residents and fellows.

At academic programs, the perspective of constant improvement of the curriculum was driven by the profession and the external environment:

I think [the curriculum committee] asked the question...and then the entire faculty—about 5 years ago, what is entry-level physical therapy? To which there is no final answer. Which is, I think, part of what you have to embrace. That is a constant question that's never settled. So, the group is constantly asking, what are we going to add? What are we going to delete? What is it that entry-level physical therapists need to know? And that's a tough question. But our practitioners really help us to answer that in terms of what's happening now. But I think the committee is also mindful of where should we be? Where do we want to see us in the future? And that balance of what do we need to do now to make sure our students are current has to be balanced with what do we want to see happening in the profession of physical therapy and in health care.

This faculty connected their curriculum and program to their clinical community as partners who helped drive their goal of meeting the future needs of the profession and health care.

There was also a deeply held sense of responsibility among these clinicians, educators, and clinician-educators to each other, their patients and learners, the profession, and society. One clinician commented:

Clinical education doesn't stop or start with students. It continues with the employees. If you can continue to educate someone who comes on board, they become a much better clinical instructor, so it's really constant what we do here, we are always going after more. We are always trying to prove the point…is what we do worthwhile, is it valid, and then I think that gets passed down upon students when they come through.

These practitioners and educators recognize that the status quo cannot be relied upon to continue because rapid, significant change is the norm. These leaders were creating environments that mutually supported practitioners and educators who took risks and held everyone on the team, including learners, accountable for advancing the shared vision for practice and education. In these institutions, individuals agreed to disagree and worked together to move their program forward.

With rapid changes in the health care and educational environments, physical therapy academic and clinical leaders need to be more engaged in policy development that will strengthen the roles of physical therapists in serving the population.

Envisioned Future for the Profession of Physical Therapy

Academic and clinical programs were characterized by a culture that continuously pursues improvement where current practices are questioned, innovation is valued, and risk taking is embraced to achieve excellence. Conformity to minimum standards, sometimes based on parochial interests, is often considered good enough. In these excellent programs, everyone looks beyond minimal standards and local opinions to guide their quest for excellence. They are never satisfied with the status quo and are willing to take risks.

PARTNERSHIPS

The profession of physical therapy realizes the importance of developing excellent learning opportunities for students and residents in both the classroom and practice settings, as do the health care professions of medicine, nursing, and many others.[6] Accomplishing this goal in physical therapy often requires the pairing of independent organizations or institutions, such as universities and hospitals, to build a level of partnership among these groups.[7,8] While these partnerships are vital, the resources needed for educating learners can be limited. One of our most powerful findings in this study was the strong, intentional bridges and critical interdependence among the academic and clinical worlds. The partnerships we observed had a positive impact on both the academic and clinical enterprise. The previous 3 elements we described, shared values, leadership, and a drive for excellence, are elements that clearly enhanced the culture of these successful partnerships, demonstrating a culture of mutual trust, respect, and collaboration. The institutions seeking excellence in teaching were benefitting from the shared resources of partnerships, including academic and clinical faculty and leaders.

Evidence From Academic and Clinical Sites

The primary type of partnerships observed in our study was between academic faculty and CE faculty. In some instances, the physical therapists with primary roles as clinicians in health care organizations external to the universities were given academic titles, benefits, and, in some cases, were compensated for their teaching. In other settings, the partnerships depended upon volunteer time provided by the clinical site. Many of the academic faculty also had clinical practice opportunities in addition to their primary roles in teaching, research, and administration. Faculty practices developed by the university or academic medical center were found in 4 of our 6 academic sites. These faculty practices served to provide patient care in an outpatient setting, and in all faculty practice settings, students were assigned to practice with faculty members or full-time clinicians. These onsite or closely located faculty practices provided resources for integrated CE and were required as part of the students' curriculum.

The faculty practices are just one example of a partnership with mutual benefits. Other partners sought clinicians with expertise to teach in the classroom or clinical laboratory, and in exchange, academic faculty members would engage clinicians to participate in research studies or in discussing the literature or practicing clinical skills. Academic faculty who direct the CE curriculum were often teaching the CIs at various clinical settings, a clear mutual benefit to the students and the CIs. Regardless of the format of the partnerships, the administrators and leaders in both settings commented on the importance they placed on the partnership, and the pride they expressed in the mutual trust of their colleagues.

> I think the continuation of making sure that our clinical partners are heard, and that we work closely with them. I think…that leadership has had that understanding from the very beginning.

> …a better word might be a better partner in terms of who we are and how we can cooperate with each other. Our philosophy here is that we don't want to be a dumping ground for universities to take on their clinical education. We want to be a partner with the universities, to carry out clinical education, which means that when curriculum development comes around, we want to be, at some point, at the table. Being an equal partner with them for the education of those students.

> That's why I really think that it's got to be a partnership. There's got to be a strong collaborative relationship between the clinical entities where the students are doing their rotations, and the academic institutions. Where the 2 of them have a mutual agreement. This is what we're trying to create, this is how we're going to go about doing it, and this is the effort that we're equally going to put into this.

The partnership collaborators were quite clear about the importance of a fair and equitable format for their work. These examples were quite striking, given the potential barriers that could stand in the way of innovation and learning in both clinical and academic sites. Administrators, faculty, and clinicians found ways to clearly identify the benefits for each setting, and as the partnerships grew, so did the benefits to each party. In interviews with faculty and clinicians, we heard of the great value in "transit across the bridge" of these educators between the classroom and the clinic as these examples from 2 academic sites and 2 clinical sites illustrate:

> Here, it's very collaborative. I think the researchers have a great respect for the clinicians…they're using the clinicians to do that, the interventions or they're using clinicians to drive their questions, to help formulate their questions…I think there's a healthy mutual respect for the different sides of the profession and part of that is mutual respect for the work each side does, but I think there's also a mutual respect for the people.

> …people who serve as clinical instructors or some other clinicians within these facilities are invited preferentially, to come to campus to be lab instructors. Because we want them to see what our students…are taught, and we're wanting them to help keep us in check…Having that bridge is really, really important, because we use many programs; I'm sure we use a lot of alumni for CI's. When they're not alumni, they don't really understand our philosophy and it's really nice to have them get a handle on our philosophy…

> We are challenged to have the right outcomes and to prove administratively or in other creative ways our worth, but we know what we do is important, how we do it, and so to be at the academic site in front of students and be serious and committed and explain to them what it is that they should expect when they come [to the clinic] is invaluable. I don't know how much more integrated you could be than academic, clinical, and faculty going both ways so that students understand what it is that we do both there and…here.

Several of the staff, as you probably already heard, not only teach Clinical Ed here at [institution name], but they also teach at universities.

The typical leader of the partnerships between academic and clinical settings in physical therapist education has been found in the academic setting. However, we observed strong leaders in the clinical settings who described a vision and charted a course that benefited the clinical sites. In one setting, the Vice President of Rehabilitation described his desire to increase the number of top student physical therapists completing internships at his clinic, and he facilitated this by providing local low-cost housing for them. In this example, the clinical administrator was leading the new partnerships:

We made a very intentional decision that we wanted to really increase the diversity in our student pool that was here. We have a wonderful collaborative relationship with 2 of our PT schools here...We also want to see very diverse students from all over the country. We went out there and started actively trying to recruit some of the best of the best from schools around the country and one of the barriers is a lot of kids simply cannot do that if they don't have an affordable place to live.

In group interviews, students consistently offered appreciative comments on the partnerships they observed first in their academic program. The academic and clinical faculty demonstrated collegial teaching during lectures or clinical laboratories. If an academic faculty member had roles in research or administration, the clinical faculty members provided additional learning experiences. Once the students had met the clinical faculty in a CE setting, seeing them in the classroom created an enhanced opportunity for learning:

...one of the things that I really love is that we get outside clinicians that we get to know really well, that come in as adjuncts, in our labs. You see the way that they practice, especially when patients come into our labs, and you see the tensions that they discuss, and you see that sometimes it is okay to hang in the tensions.

The partnerships we observed included a significant role for clinical educators who facilitated the presence of current or former patients to participate in the academic classroom. These encounters provided an example of practice-based learning in an academic setting, and the mutual benefits to students, faculty, and patients were clearly identified.

Envisioned Future for the Profession of Physical Therapy

From every perspective, we observed the major impact of effective partnering, but this is likely not the case throughout all institutions and organizations involved in physical therapist education. While leaders in academic and clinical settings must pursue the substantive resources needed to support excellent partnerships, they must also foster the culture of collaboration that helps all educators identify the mutual benefits within the partnership. Some educators may identify CE programs as the sole partnership aspect of the academic institution. A much broader approach to the development of partnerships is needed to enhance the Culture of Excellence in learning and patient care. Too often, a separation exists among faculty. Prominent examples of this include unequal relationships between academic and clinical faculty and between researchers and teachers.

Two Paradigm Cases That Illustrate the Embodied Pursuit for Excellence

Clinical Paradigm Case: A Mission That Grounds the Culture of Excellence

A CE site was identified by the research team as a center of excellence for learning and patient care. It is selected as a case study for elucidating the elements of the dimension of Culture of Excellence. The 4 elements of the Culture of Excellence contain a significant amount of overlap, and therefore, we provide 2 paradigm cases—1 in a clinical practice setting and 1 in an academic setting—that highlight all of the elements composing the Culture of Excellence: shared values and beliefs, leadership and vision, drive for excellence with high expectations, and partnership.

The clinical case setting is a major community, not-for-profit hospital in a suburban area of the West Coast, with a 500-bed hospital and several outpatient settings, focused on musculoskeletal, pediatric, and rehabilitation care. Over 50 physical therapists work in the inpatient care setting and over 18 physical therapists work in the outpatient settings. The health setting supports learners in physical and occupational therapy, speech-language pathology, and nursing, and physical therapist residents in orthopedics and sports physical therapy.

Mission is intensely valued in this setting, which is identified as a faith-based health care system. The mission is:

To improve the health of communities and to share God's love by promoting healing and wellness for the whole person.

Despite the culture of the faith-based health care system, no clinicians are required to follow any aspects of the history or current activities of the church. Instead, the mission becomes an intense commitment to the values expressed in the mission statement. The practitioners, students, and physical therapists alike, refer to the community as a family with a clear, explicit expression of support and.collaboration:

This is cheesy but Will and I both have this experience. This is an extremely tight group. A lot of people say, "Oh, our staff is a family." This staff is a family and...not only do I know that I could go to somebody and they will help me but I feel comfortable with them. —Student Intern

Managers and leaders in staff interviews ensure that candidates understand a mission that impacts duty to patients as well as colleagues:

We carefully interview...the whole department, much of the medical center, we want the right fit. We want a person that fits and is going to uphold our standards, our culture, and our mission. It is a rigorous interview process here because we're looking for the right fit. We're not hiring warm bodies to go get a job done. We're hiring somebody who fits and believes in and is going to really promote our mission here.

It has not been worth it to me to just hire in a therapist to get patients in. There have been times through the years as I've helped grow this department where we've had to hold out for the right person to add to the team.

The mission may be considered unassuming, but the shared values of the community are translated into excellence in teaching and patient care, which will result in high patient satisfaction. Managers and administrators commented:

Well, it starts with our mission. Everything about why we're here. This is our mission. We're a non-profit base and it certainly drives the culture here in the hospital. I think it starts at the core.

When a kind of a consistency across the group, you know you're kind of working together for this common mission, and you have kind of these common values and goals that you can kind of share with one another, then I think that does have something...we go together to weddings and birthday parties, and our kids' birthday parties, and I mean, there's very much a sense of community and family amongst my staff.

We are very mission driven and that spans out to clinical education, as well as general patient care. I think we have to do that; it's for the generations coming up. It's for future health care. We would be remiss, I think, in our profession if we didn't.

In addition to a shared commitment to the health care system, students, clinical educators, and residency mentors identify other shared values for professional development. Learners and teachers alike model behaviors that each group finds to be important to their professional careers:

We're working on professional behavior and how to carry yourself as a professional, not as a student and making sure that they get that they need to be that professional presence in front of their patient all the time. —Clinical Instructor

I think there's a lot of ownership on the staff and that these are the people that are going to join our profession and so we need to have that trust in their skills and their abilities and we're going to do everything we can do if they're not already at our standards to bring them up to those standards. —Manager

Today when you ask, "Well, what if someone doesn't want to be a CI?," it's really not the case here because it's made very abundantly clear that that's part of your job and most people who come here are here because they want to do the clinical education part of it. —Resident

I think the office culture is the really important part and you can just tell people you're passionate about education, both about learning new things and about teaching. That acceptance makes you feel more comfortable sharing but also just when you come into an environment where everybody else is excited about education, about going to con-ed, about having students and teaching students, you become more excited and it becomes this snowball effect. —Resident

What do your students take away from this setting? "I would say that I would hope that they would have an unquenchable thirst for knowledge to get so that they keep learning, so that they don't think that just because they left here and graduated school that they know everything." Do you think your whole group models this? "I'm pretty sure that we do." —Clinical Instructor

The community of administrators, clinicians, and students describe the intentional drive for excellence in this setting. The practitioners seek excellence in their own specialty areas, and in their teaching. The clinical site has a long history of contributing CE opportunities for student interns from a variety of universities. The center coordinators of CE participate with a regional CE consortium, and all physical therapists complete the APTA CI course, and are required to teach students, which they do willingly. The clinicians and managers commented:

Well, the thing is, that's important to our profession. I have a responsibility, the medical center or really us in the medical center or rehab team have a responsibility to our profession, whether it's physical therapy, occupational therapy or speech therapy. We want to be known for our excellence. We want to be known for clinical instruction to be excellent here so that we therapists have graduated and are out there, "Oh, I was trained in the best center possible."

That was my first thought is just, we need to make sure our clinical staff are excellent so we can provide excellent instruction.

We've never really achieved the pinnacle of excellence, we're always raising the bar. We're always growing, we're always changing. What's new, what's different. I mean, we're in the medical field, right? We're never going to reach that top pinnacle of excellence, because there's always something a little bit more. To grow, to change. Somebody came in with a new idea. I think we are excellent, because we're continuing to strive for that excellence.

I think that's something that's ingrained to us at this medical center that even though, let's say, our target is 90%, but we always shoot for 100%. That's not OK to be where everybody else is. Even though the benchmark is there, our benchmark is 0 falls.

Individual clinicians pursuing excellence often design new programs or initiatives, and the leadership supports this type of generative thinking. This support from the medical center and the individual leaders is key in envisioning improved outcomes for patients and for learners.

When we have something, new programs, come up, whether its pediatric program or driving programs, specialties, we have a lot of people that jump to try and get part of that because they know we're going to let them. Even outside of that, if we have a program that we're starting, we will take extra money out if it's not part of the clinical to make sure that they are set up for success. And it's rare when we don't have somebody just jump-we probably sometimes have too many people interested where we have to actually pick from a list. We have clinicians that are just wanting that—to start a program or be part of an innovative something that the hospital's doing.

I think the other thing, too, is that we—I know it's what we hear—is that there's always something coming around the next turn. Something that we're doing or developing or a new program. I think that we really have that culture here that we're not stagnant in any way and that we're always—like the Director said—achieving or going back to school or we don't have that program and really support the staff in that.

The health system has several managers and directors serving in leadership roles for clinical and teaching services. The student internship program at the site has grown to give more learning opportunities across the inpatient and outpatient settings. The leaders had a vision to enhance the educational opportunities for student interns in physical therapy as well as occupational therapy, speech language pathology, and nursing, and this created interprofessional teamwork activities.

To me, this is a great clinical experience and we've had students that have come to do an acute or a rehab rotation and then moved on to do an outpatient or vice versa. We have this great multi-disciplinary structure here so, to me, obviously I'm the Director, that's very important. Each individual discipline has their strengths and their purpose and I think this is a great opportunity for students to learn that and to mix and be a part of that team and working together as a team.

The importance of leaders who can envision the future aspects of excellence for physical therapy is a vital component for developing a Culture of Excellence. The managers envisioned the resources required for developing 2 clinical residencies for physical therapists, in orthopedics and sports physical therapy, with the support of the directors and health system administrators. All members of the community agreed that the benefits of the residencies are significant:

> We have the support of the administration here at the hospital. When [he] brought to me this-we want to have a residency program here-and I brought it to the COO, there wasn't a question of "wait a minute that's going to decrease productivity and cost us money." It was really embraced as "yes, this is what our hospital is about." It is evidence-based practice. It is providing excellent clinical care and having a residency program just fit in with really our philosophy at the hospital.

> And they all mentor each other, also. It's like therapist to therapist, they mentor each other. It's like, oh, they've got a skill and then they work one-on-one with each other to help develop that skill in the other therapist.

> I think we all take teaching very seriously here. We do. I think we are very dedicated and we...I think we're proud.

> Again, for me, being a mentor to me is a thing I take seriously and I don't want to...I don't make light of it.

> I think you've probably caught on to the fact that everyone here is very proud of what's been built here and have put in a lot of time and effort into it being excellent and I think if you're not up to the challenge, it would not be beyond someone to be like, "Listen, you do need to do something better for your student. This is not okay." I think what I've noticed, and I don't know if this is the same for everyone, but because clinic hours had become such a big part of PT school, clinicians who were newer or out are more welcoming and more prepared to take students.

The residency mentors in the clinic provide didactic classroom work for the residents, and they also partner with residents training at other clinical sites. The residency mentors and CIs also participate in the academic setting by presenting lectures and clinical laboratories. A strong partnership between the CIs, the center coordinators of clinical education (CCCE), and the directors of clinical education (DCE) at the universities provides important communication for enhancing the CE program:

> I know the consortium has a sense like a clinical education forum, like quarterly that we can go to. That influence and that's where you meet all the other DCEs of that programs. You develop that kind of a relationship. Also, really, the type of students that we're getting, we can say...I could honestly say, I could talk to the DCE and say, "Gosh, what is going on with your program?" Kind of thing. We're seeing a decline in the students' quality.

> Our CIs can make recommendations back to [the CCCE] and he can pass on to the next site of things that the student still needs to work on.

Coda/Epilogue

This clinical paradigm case provides a glimpse of a clinical setting that is strongly mission-driven, where expectation for excellence in patient care and teaching is intensely explicit. This culture provides an excellent example of the necessary elements to facilitate teaching in clinical settings, including shared values and a drive for excellence. Creating a strong mission statement depends on the vision and leadership of the entire staff. In this setting, the importance of partnering for excellence allows the clinical and academic sites to create innovative programs that include interprofessional projects for clinicians and students. The health care system finds mutual benefits in these partnerships, for example, sharing clinicians' expertise in both the classroom and the clinic. The pursuit of fair and sound partnerships, and the clear sense of pride in excellence for all members of the community; these are vital elements to enhance the Praxis of Learning in this clinical setting.

Academic Paradigm Case: Creating a Culture of Excellence Where Partnerships Are Central

The purpose of this case is to highlight the dimension of a Culture of Excellence with a focus on how this academic program created a culture in which partnerships and shared responsibilities for those partnerships was the norm. In this case, the partnerships occurred at many levels within the department, across the university and with its clinical partners in the community.

The physical therapy department in this case is part of a multi-disciplinary college at a large, research-intensive university. In addition to the DPT program, the department offers an interdisciplinary PhD in rehabilitation. They have a department chair and a Director of the DPT program.

This university had a mission matrix (Table 4-1) illustrating the relationship between the key components of the mission at the university, college, department, and DPT program. As one moves from the broader mission of the university to the mission of the department and program, what is notable is the relationships among teaching, scholarship, and practice and their importance in making a difference in people's lives. Despite this being a research university, the emphasis is on the fundamental importance of teaching and the importance of collaboration, service and partnerships. The DPT's mission is:

> *To prepare students to become physical therapists that embrace evidence-based physical therapy practice, meet the multifaceted health needs of patients, consumers, and society, and participate in professional and community service. To fulfill this mission, we create a stimulating and collaborative environment that promotes education, research, service, and leadership.*

They identify excellence, diversity, integrity, respect for human dignity, teamwork, and social responsibility as the pillars of their philosophy and program outcomes. Their beliefs about optimal learning are person-centered, (eg, fosters growth of the individual personally and professionally, is safe, inclusive, respectful, caring, collegial, and ethical). It describes their beliefs about collaborative learning among patients, students, clinicians, and faculty thus clearly establishing the values that support shared responsibility, partnerships, and learner and patient centeredness.

Their dedication to creating the culture of a shared commitment to being good partners to support excellence begins with people who are connected to the mission and who focus on their purpose. As the director of the DPT program put it:

> *I think we have good people, which sounds simple, but a lot of it is that we have really good people that tend to be focused on finding the solution and less concerned with battling each other. I know some people like to battle each other. I think the leadership that was spoken of the tone that [the Department Chair] set 10 to 12 years ago really has been followed. One of her mantras is that you're involved in all 3 missions of the university if you work here...but that's an expectation. You're going to meet...with [2 faculty members] who are basic scientists who have NIH level funding but, because they are in our department, they have more teaching responsibility than they would if they were in the physiology department.*

The commitment to the entire mission and collaboration begins with who the department hires, as this faculty member explained:

> *So, we're really trying to bring in the person who is going to contribute to the community, instead of picking someone you know is going to be great at one part but is going to let down on the other part. Then that also sets up that person for failure in an environment like this. You have to be willing to engage. But we have someone who's open to the administration like [Department Chair], who's saying anything is possible. We can do just about anything; let me hear what your ideas are. Some people are really excited about that, some people are really intimidated by that. The people that don't fit well in that system usually don't stay here very long, but our turnover hasn't been that great.*

The faculty do not let perceived barriers stand in their way of the need to work together, because, as this faculty member explained, they are passionate about what is best for their students and the need to prepare the best physical therapists:

> *I always find this, the collegiality, that just the willingness of everyone that jumped in whether they're on a research track, whether they're located over [at the nearby affiliated clinic] most of the week to find the time that we're going to get together and do this because of the importance of the education of the students and that being the primary focus is that this is their opportunity to grow and become best and real physical therapist. I feel that passion driving everyone, that that's why everybody puts aside that time to make it happen. I think as a people we have very much of a "can do" attitude. We look for solutions and we are willing to work together. There's a culture just of working together independent of where you are or who you are to come up with a better solution. I think pretty much everybody who sits here very much has a "can do" attitude.*

TABLE 4-1			
MISSION MATRIX			
UNIVERSITY	**COLLEGE**	**DEPARTMENT**	**PROGRAM**
The university welcomes the exploration of its intellectual boundaries and supports its faculty and students in the creation of new knowledge and pursuit of new ideas.	The mission of the college is to preserve, promote, and improve the health and well-being of populations, communities, and individuals.	The mission of the department is to advance rehabilitation practice and science.	The mission of the DPT program is to: Prepare students to become physical therapists that embrace evidence-based physical therapy practice; meet the multifaceted health needs of patients consumers, and society; and participate in professional and community service.
Teaching is a fundamental purpose of this university at both the undergraduate and graduate levels.	To fulfill this mission, we foster collaborations among public health and the health professions in education.	We do this through education and mentorship.	To fulfill this mission, we create a stimulating and collaborative environment that promotes education.
Research and scholarship are integral to the educational process and to the expansion of our understanding of the natural world, the intellect, and the senses.	To fulfill this mission, we foster collaborations among public health and the health professions in research.	We do this through basic and clinical research.	To fulfill this mission, we create a stimulating and collaborative environment that promotes research and embraces evidence-based physical therapy practice.
The university serves the nation's and the state's critical needs by contributing to a well-qualified and broadly diverse citizenry, leadership, and workforce.	To fulfill this mission, we foster collaborations among public health and the health professions in service.	We do this through service to the profession and communities.	To fulfill this mission, we: Create a stimulating and collaborative environment that promotes service and leadership; meet the multifaceted health needs of patients, consumers, and society; and participate in professional and community service.

Ultimately, this department has intentionally and successfully created a culture in which outstanding faculty value each other and no single faculty role is perceived to have more importance than another, whether it be research or teaching. The department chair was explicit about the need for everyone to have the sense of being equally valued and carried that through in how she managed by not allowing people to buy out their teaching and avoiding a 2-tier system.

That culture among the faculty is then transmitted to the students through a shared sense of belonging and purpose. One of the faculty members described it this way during the focus group:

One of the things I think is culture is very important, so you have not only diverse faculty who have their separate strengths...and you've been hearing [about] excellence, so one of the things you have a collection then of people who all are really great at what they do. They work well together and [this is] the culture then that leads...for the students. There's an expectation that the students participate in that and so the sharing isn't just among faculty or among faculty and clinicians; it's also between faculty and the students and that's the culture of excellence.

One of the department's administrators, when talking about their culture, related it to their high expectations of each other and of students, saying that "you never get to where you want to be, because you're always trying to go further. And the students get that too."

Thus, this department had a shared commitment to the mission clearly linked to their students and the DPT program as the central reason for their existence, even though they are a research-intensive university. Much like excellent leaders in other institutions, this department chair was able to read the institutional environment and leverage her and her faculty's expertise to become more important to that mission. The university had an initiative to invest in 8 key areas, including neuroscience, global health, and metabolics. The department's expertise in neuroscience and muscle biology aligned closely with these initiatives and the department chair became a leader of one of the task forces. The department chair described her role as a partner this way:

I felt that my number one job was to network, linking with other disciplines and other opportunities, and be at the table...I think that as people saw doors opening, I think that they realized, "Wow, they do want to sit at the table with me and look now what we can do together." If I would say, "What is the part that I contributed?" that probably was the part, not being afraid of other disciplines. Going and knocking on the door and saying, "Hey, you want [to] do this together?", and "Here's what I have to offer," and "I would like to work with you on this."

She was clear what it meant to be a good partner in the interdisciplinary work that was occurring at the university:

Good partners do not mean that it's in one direction. It means it goes in both directions. I think I'm always conscious of being a good partner, because it only works long-term if there's a 2-way street. There's a benefit both directions...Being a good partner is having something to offer, being reliable in your commitment, being consistent in your performance, and being somebody, they can count on...These things don't develop overnight. It's not because you did one good thing; therefore, you have a relationship. Your relationship builds over years of being there. I think, also, having confidence that you have something to offer. I think there is people that have things to offer, but may not be so confident in that...I think it is being willing to pick up the phone, or go meet and find common ground, right? I mean, it's all finding common language. I think each field has kind of its own language, and that's where your comfort zone is...and you create a bridge...I remember having similar discussions saying, "Look, we partner with them in research and as a consequence they'll be able to help us in our educational mission." I think that's true.

A faculty member recognized that these partnerships that reached across departmental boundaries and across different disciplines were not without risk, but, as he says here, they saw the potential to learn as over-riding those risks:

For my perspective too, I think across all the themes I think there is a culture of embracing partnerships and collaboration and...I think often faculty are concerned about reaching out and maybe not knowing certain things. I think as a faculty we collaborate with lots of different disciplines. We embrace diversity and so this willingness to go learn something else and work together for a better solution I think is something that's true, I think, across the different disciplines where we work together.

There was definitely a pragmatism behind this collaboration as it garnered attention, prestige and resources for the department. As the department chair said, "at the end of the day, I represent the department. If the department was promised money, then I'm going to fight for that with everything I got until that money is in."

The way in which this faculty valued partnerships extended into their clinical partnerships as well. The department chair said that the message to create more partnerships "came from the top." During the visit to this campus, we had focus groups with clinical faculty and interviews with the Director of CE and with the Director of Rehabilitation at a nearby health system with hospitals, rehabilitation, and outpatient centers. That health system is on an academic medical center campus with a teaching mission. As one of the clinical faculty members described it:

And for me, it is our mission. And we're a teaching hospital, and I find that people that are motivated to learn and to participate with students gravitate toward that teaching hospital setting. This is a prime place to do it, because we're so intertwined.

As this chapter has illustrated, mission is central to how people thought about and valued their work and it was evident through their actions. It was evident that the academic and clinical faculty recognized that it has taken time and a steadfast commitment to creating a meaningful partnership.

But the fact that we're sitting at the table and we're talking about these things frequently throughout the year, versus having to reach someone and never getting an answer. It's evolved over the past 6, 7 years to something I think is special...think it's become more of a collaborative effort between us and [the university], as far as it's a win-win. We help support the academic avenue, and they support the clinical avenue. From a business standpoint, these students are already trained. They know the system, they know us.

A member of the academic faculty described the importance of the partnership with their nearby clinical partners this way:

I would say...from my perspective [they] are a very willing clinical partner in the education of our students, at least that I've seen since I've been here, and leadership of the health enterprise, you have health itself, academic and the clinic mission continue to try to integrate the clinical practice side of [system] and the education mission of the university I think has been phenomenal, even you starting to see that trickle down to the staff and leadership and willingness to embrace innovative ideas about educating students in the clinical environment...

The health system has physical therapy residency programs at many of its sites. These residencies are operated by the health system, not jointly with the physical therapy program. The director of the rehabilitation center and residency program put it this way:

That program is really, I think, been a model for how we can improve post-professional education. It's allowed us to have an even greater collaborative effort, with the school of physical therapy. Things with co-teaching, working together on various research projects, and it's actually resulted in us hiring several [of] those graduates, and they come...to work for us.

Besides doing the work of creating a relationship in CE and residency education that benefited both partners, the academic program holds CE summits during which the clinical and academic faculty could jointly explore innovative ways to improve the students' education:

The other key area is, just these summits we've been having, have allowed us to have discussions on how we can be innovative in the clinical education, particularly here at [Institution Name]. With the therapy students in the entry level program and evaluating different models on how we can optimize their educational processes they go through, they go through their clinical rotations.

The faculty in the program also recognized the value of the partnership and the synergy it brought to their department:

It's hard for me to imagine how we could do all that we're doing without that collaboration. It adds a lot of richness, that diversity, anywhere from some of the residents that I work with. They're carrying forward actually on the frontlines of some of the most innovative spinal cord injuries here that we're pursuing from a research perspective. They're doing things in the clinic and I'm meeting with them. At the same time, some of their patients are coming to our classroom and visiting. That exchange we don't...I'd say we need to grow that aspect here.

The Director of CE might have best summed up the nature of their collaboration, responsibility, and partnership when he said:

When I think of excellence, I think it's something great and it's a wonderful benefit because it's what makes us excellent in clinical education. I'm grateful for it, believe me, and I'm proud of it. We couldn't do it, clinical education, without their support with the number of students that we have. I know it's not an expectation everywhere, but I think it should be. I think it's good for our academic faculty to be out in the facilities. That's the other thing I think that's really phenomenal around here. You're not asked to do things that are impossible. When you are asked to do things, that you have the resources to accomplish them and do them very well.

Coda/Epilogue

This case illustrates the importance of leadership, the centrality of mission, clarity of purpose, and the importance of the enactment of the mission and the underlying values to create partnerships that garnered support and created opportunities for faculty, clinicians, researchers, and students. The lessons embedded in this case apply regardless of whether the institution is public or private, large or small, research intensive, or a master's focused. These themes are also relevant in any organizational structure for the department or DPT program. The fact that the university was on a campus with an academic medical center might be perceived as a built-in advantage, but the relationships between the university and health system were not consistently conducive to these partnerships. Sometimes university and medical center politics and the complex nature of their relationship presented barriers to creating their partnerships. However, none of the players let these barriers dissuade them from their purpose. While partnerships within the university were absolutely aided by the department chair's reputation in her discipline, she also skillfully led the department, built relationships, and provided the faculty the support they needed to allow them to flourish and learn in the demanding university environment. That skillful type of leadership is valuable in any setting to lead with vision.

CONCLUSION

In this chapter, we have focused on the first dimension of the Conceptual Model of Excellence in Physical Therapist Education: The Culture of Excellence, along with 4 elements. In the 11 research sites, we observed teachers in all roles to be highly focused on creating a Culture of Excellence for their institutions, and for their learners. The learners we observed were clearly growing into the Culture of Excellence provided for them. A sense of pride within the entire community illuminates their future goals. This dimension of the model suggests the importance of developing a Culture of Excellence that will facilitate growth in the profession of physical therapy. Without shared values, leadership, drive and partnerships, it may be quite difficult to advance the profession and physical therapist education.

The next aspect of the conceptual model will elucidate the importance of the Nexus. This component of the model will set the stage for growth and innovation in the Praxis of Learning dimension. In the Nexus, 2 shared values observed in our work, a concurrent commitment to learner-centered teaching and patient-centered care, are highlighted. These shared values will be discussed in Chapter 5.

REFERENCES

1. Hansen DT. The moral is in the practice. *Teaching and Teacher Education*. 1998;14(6):643-655.
2. Swisher L, Hiller P. The revised APTA code of ethics for the physical therapist and standards of conduct for the physical therapist assistant: theory, purpose, process and significance. *Phys Ther*. 2010;90:803-824.
3. American Physical Therapy Association. *Professionalism in Physical Therapy: Core Values*. http://www.apta.org/Ethics/Core/. Accessed February 2, 2018.
4. Kezar AJ, Carducci R, Contreras M. Rethinking the "L" word in higher education: the revolution in research on leadership. *ASHE Higher Education Report*. 2006;31(6).
5. American Physical Therapy Association. Education Leadership Institute Fellowship. http://www.apta.org/ELI/. Accessed February 2, 2018.
6. Jette DU, Nelson L, Palaima M, et. al. How do we improve quality in clinical education? examination of structures, processes, and outcomes. *J Phys Ther Educ*. 2014;28(1):6-12.
7. Applebaum D, Portney LG, Kolosky L, et. al. Building physical therapist education networks. *J Phys Ther Educ*. 2014;28(1):30-38.
8. McCallum CA, Mosher PD, Howman J, et.al. Development of regional core networks for the administration of physical therapist clinical education. *J Phys Ther Educ*. 2014;28(1):39-47.

5

The Nexus
Bridging Our Academic and Clinical Worlds

Critical to our Model of Excellence in Physical Therapist Education is the central component, or Nexus, a metaphoric lens, where the paired and highly valued aims of learner- and patient-centering in the educational enterprise come together in both academic and clinical realms. The Nexus serves as an important bridge or conduit between the academic and clinical realms and facilitates the translation and transportation of the Culture of Excellence into the domain of Praxis of Learning—where knowledge is embodied and transformed through action and interaction. The Nexus is also a resource for the development of true partnerships between academic and clinical sites that enable a coming together for the important task of facilitating learning for practice through practice.

We use the metaphor of a lens in the model because lenses have the capacity to gather and change light and bring clarity to what we see. As light passes through a convex lens it refracts and converges to a focal point. In our model, the Nexus is represented as a convex lens composed of 2 concurrent commitments to learner-centered teaching and patient-centered practice (Figure 5-1). In our conceptualization, the 4 parallel and critical elements in the model dimension, Culture of Excellence, pass through the lens of paired commitments to learner- and patient-centering, to converge on the focal point of facilitating learning for practice—our dimension of Praxis of Learning. The importance of the Nexus, or coming together, of a combined focus on learner-centered teaching and patient-centered practice cannot be overstated. These 2 shared viewpoints are integral to the Nexus and are necessary for excellence in physical therapist education to be realized in both the academic and clinical environments. In this chapter, we define what we mean by the terms *learner-centered* and *patient-centered* and then provide evidence from our study that illustrates these paired commitments in action.

Jensen GM, Mostrom E, Hack LM, Nordstrom T, Gwyer J.
Educating Physical Therapists (pp 59-74).
© 2019 Taylor & Francis Group.

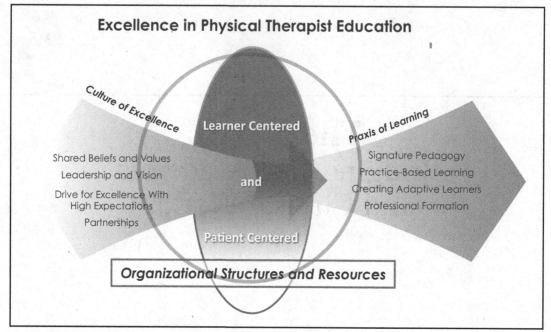

Excellence in Physical Therapist Education

Culture of Excellence

Learner Centered

and

Patient Centered

Praxis of Learning

Shared Beliefs and Values
Leadership and Vision
Drive for Excellence With
High Expectations
Partnerships

Signature Pedagogy
Practice-Based Learning
Creating Adaptive Learners
Professional Formation

Organizational Structures and Resources

Figure 5-1. Model of Excellence in Physical Therapist Education. The Nexus of the paired commitments to learner-centering and patient-centering is a central component and critical for the realization of excellence.

What Does Being Learner-Centered Mean?

Building on the educational philosophy of John Dewey and the progressive education movement with its focus on learning through meaningful experience,[1] being learner-centered means that attention is focused on the learner and the actual and possible learning that might occur in the teaching-learning environment, rather than primarily on the teacher and what is being taught.[2-4] As Weimer[4] has described it:

> Being learner-centered focuses attention squarely on the learning; what the student is learning, how the student is learning, the conditions under which the student is learning, whether the student is retaining and applying the learning, and how current learning positions the student for future learning…We make the distinction between learner-centered instruction and teacher-centered instruction as a way of indicating that the spotlight has moved from teacher to student. When instruction is learner-centered, the action focuses on what students (not teachers) are doing.[(pxvi)]

It is important to note that learner-centering or learner-centered teaching does not infer that the teacher-learner interaction is merely transactional; that is, it is not about student as a consumer or customer.[5] In such conceptualizations, education can become viewed as a product and educators would focus on satisfying their customer, providing them with what they want or need.[4-6] The task of teaching for learning, however, is far more difficult than merely providing a product or transmission of knowledge. In learner-centered environments, the task of learning is a mutual endeavor between teacher and learner and conjoint engagement and shared responsibility seeks to cultivate a thirst for learning and develop skills for lifelong learning that the student can then carry forward in the absence of direct instruction or guidance.[4,6]

One caution that should be raised regarding interpretations of what it means to be learner-centered dates back to the early 20th century as articulated in John Dewey's treatise on progressive education and critique of traditional education, *Experience and Education*.[1] In describing his new philosophy of experience as education, Dewey warned that a focus on the learner and the learning that might ensue through experience did not mean that the teacher abdicated responsibility for shaping experiences and the environment so that they indeed promoted learning and development; freedom of the learner and experience itself, while elements of his philosophy, were not, in and of themselves educative.[1]

> The belief that all genuine education comes about through experience does not mean that all experiences are genuinely or equally educative. Experience and education cannot be directly equated to each other. For some experiences are mis-educative. Any experience is mis-educative that has the effect of arresting or distorting the growth of further experience.[(p25)]

Dewey's philosophy and theories of education have had a profound effect on pedagogical practice in the 20th century and continue to do so today. Unfortunately, some (mis)conceptualizations of learner-centering have focused primarily on learner direction and active learning without serious attention to the role of the teacher in shaping the nature and aims of activity in the classroom. An understanding of learning as a process, not a product, emphasizes the unfolding nature of learning over time; a process that leads to change not only in knowledge but also change in beliefs and behaviors. Learning is not something done to students but is the direct result of students interpreting and responding to their experiences, past and present, conscious and unconscious, as all learners (students and teachers) engage in the learning environment.[7] As Dewey suggested, it is not merely the experience itself that promotes learning, it is what one makes of the experience.

So, you might ask, exactly what does learner-centered teaching look like? How does it differ from traditional models of teaching and the presumed learning that ensued? In brief, Weimer[4,6] suggests that there are 5 key features of learner-centered teaching that distinguishes it from other forms of teaching.

1. The role of the teacher changes from that of wise teller or transmitter of knowledge to that of wise guide or facilitator of learning. Thus, the focus shifts from what the teacher is doing to what the learners are doing—what meaningful tasks or activities they are engaged in.

2. The balance of power and control of the learning environment moves from solely residing with the teacher, to one that is more shared and distributed between teacher and learner depending on the subject matter, situation or learning activity. It is easy to understand how relinquishing power and control can be unsettling to teachers; it requires a great deal of adaptability because unanticipated and unpredictable situations are sure to arise—ones that can make teachers feel vulnerable.

3. The notion that content coverage must drive what a teacher does and that more is better, shifts to the aim of uncovering content with goals of not only expanding a knowledge base, but also developing skills that set the stage for learning across life-span.

4. Both teacher and learner have the responsibility for learning. The expectation for this shared responsibility is made explicit and cultivated by a teaching/learning climate that moves students away from passivity and dependence on the teacher to one that promotes learner intrinsic motivation and self-directed learning.

5. Finally, the purpose of and processes used to evaluate learners and learning change. The purpose of evaluation moves from determining mere mastery of content or attainment of skills as a measure of what has been learned (often through grades on an examination), to a deliberate focus on how that content or those skills have been integrated and can now be used and adapted in situations that require them. As for the processes of assessment and evaluation of learners, these move from being solely the purview of the teacher and primarily used for summative purposes, to more activities designed to provide formative feedback to learners with the sources of such feedback coming not only from teachers but also from peers and the learners themselves. The latter emphasizes the importance of reflection in the development of meta-cognitive processes and ongoing self-assessment of learning.

In our study, we saw frequent examples of such learner-centered teaching in both academic and clinical settings. We will turn to detailed descriptions of those examples in the pages to come in this chapter.

What Does Being Patient-Centered Mean?

A term far more familiar to physical therapists, patient-centering means that the needs and goals of the patient are always in the foreground when clinical decisions are being made about care. It means that therapists must listen carefully to the patient and seek an understanding of their life and illness experiences to inform therapist decisions about patient care. The World Health Organization (WHO) has developed a framework and guidelines for measuring health at both an individual and population level.[8] The *International Classification of Functioning, Disability and Health* (ICF)[8] framework, focuses clinicians' attention to an individual's health status, activities, and level of participation in social roles, in the context of environmental, external, and personal, internal, factors that influence those things. The ICF clearly underlines the importance of patient-centering in addition to drawing attention to the social and societal factors that affect health.[8] The primacy of the patient in determinations about the actions of physical therapists and the nature of care they provide is codified in the American Physical Therapy Association (APTA) *Code of Ethics for the Physical Therapist*[9] and the APTA *Professionalism in Physical Therapy: Core Values* document.[10] In particular, Principle 2 in the Code of Ethics emphasizes the moral obligation and fiduciary responsibility of physical therapists to act in the best interests of their patients. The importance of patient-centeredness is further emphasized by the Triple Aim[11] and both patient- and learner-centeredness are critical elements of the Interprofessional Education Collaborative core competencies.[12]

The focus of the ICF framework and the other documents referred to previously is on the provision of patient-centered care. A question pertinent to our discussion in this chapter and throughout this book, however, is: What does patient-centered teaching and learning look like in academic and clinical environments where physical therapist education occurs? The simple answer is that a patient's needs, wants, and goals are always brought into view when teaching and learning about patient care. Furthermore, the patient's needs and goals are considered in the broad biopsychosocial context in which they exist. Patient-centered teaching and learning requires that such considerations are made visible and explicit as future physical therapists develop their clinical reasoning and decision-making skills and as practicing therapists refine and advance their reasoning processes. In this chapter, we provide the reader with some illustrative examples of what patient-centered teaching and learning looked like at the academic and clinical sites we visited during our study. We share evidence from participant interviews and field observations; you will hear the voices, and hopefully be able to visualize, the actions and interactions of both teachers and learners at the level of professional and post-professional preparation as they develop and strengthen their capacity to provide truly patient-centered care.

The Nexus: Teaching and Learning That Is Both Learner-Centered and Patient-Centered

We found evidence of a concurrent commitment to learner- and patient-centering in all of our sites and suggest that it is a non-negotiable requirement for achieving excellence in physical therapist education. While one would suspect that academic environments are more learner-centered overall, in those sites we found an intentional focus on patient-centered care that was ubiquitous and central to curricula and the design and implementation of learning experiences and the development of learning environments. Likewise, in our clinical sites, where patient care is the primary mission, there was also a robust commitment to learners and learning within the organizations and to the learning and preparation of the next generation of professionals. The evidence we present here is drawn from both academic and clinical sites and includes data from organizational documents and artifacts as well as field observations and interviews with participants.

Evidence From Clinical Sites

Perhaps the Nexus of learner- and patient-centering is best captured in the following quote from a participant at one of our clinical sites. This health care system provides clinical education (CE) experiences for students from many schools during their professional (entry-level) preparation. It also has an acute care internship program and 2 residency education programs. The system provides clinical services in a variety of venues from inpatient acute care and teaching hospitals to sub acute rehabilitation facilities and outpatient settings. When asked why they host physical therapist students during a focus group interview, one participant responded this way:

Professional responsibility primarily. I think when you are a dedicated clinician...you have a responsibility to the next generation of clinicians and to the patients that we treat. And the best way to ensure excellent patient care is to excellently train students in the clinic. And our organization and the different sites that we work with, I think helps toward our individual and group mission of providing the best possible patient care and outcomes that we can. It's not just an individual treatment session but it is looking forward into the future—and the best way to ensure that is to train students in an excellent fashion in the clinic. So, we take that mission, I think, very seriously. It is a responsibility that we all have. It informs our own practice. I think it makes our own professional life more of a rich experience. It pushes us in lots of different ways

In addition to what we heard and directly observed at many of our clinical sites, the mission statements for those sites also explicitly blended commitments to the delivery of high quality patient care and fostering learners and learning within the organization. The following statement is from a private practice that provides primarily outpatient services in numerous clinics:

[Our organization is]...dedicated to providing high quality, patient-centered rehabilitation. We are committed to the professional growth and development of employees to best meet the needs of our patients, referral sources, and payers. We strive to provide creative and innovative delivery systems to maintain the most efficient outcomes-based rehabilitation services.

As a learning organization, [this company] strives every day to improve our clinical expertise through education, mentoring and shared experience. We believe in the lifelong goal of always finding ways to improve and passing that insight along. [Our organization] has earned a reputation as a leader in rehabilitation by our positive outcomes with patient treatments and a nurturing environment that empowers professionals to develop into exceptional healthcare providers. It is my goal to honor the vision of our founders by continuing to develop [our organization] as the rehabilitation provider of choice; the company that best improves the functional lives of its patients. Companies that remain in business for over 50 years do so for a reason. They have shown that meeting the needs of both the consumer and their employees ensures they will be around to continue the legacy for future generations.

At another institution, a large rehabilitation center that provides both inpatient and outpatient services, the core values for that organization link patient-centered care with involvement in teaching future generations of physical therapists and physical therapist assistants.

[Our] Hospital's core values are collaboration, hospitality, respect, innovation, stewardship, and teaching. We believe physical therapists and physical therapist assistants are able to develop and embody these core values by serving as clinical instructors for PT and PTA students completing clinical rotations at [our] Hospital.

The definition of the core value of teaching, at the center is "We recognize every moment as an opportunity for mutual learning, and strive to share our knowledge and skills with our co-workers, those we serve, and the broader community." At this same center, one of the participants in a focus group interview with a variety of clinicians and administrators described how the WHO-ICF model has influenced the nature of patient care and framed the commitment to patient-centering at this rehabilitation center:

[We've] always been patient care focused. We've done a lot of education on the WHO Model. We believe in it very strongly and so we promote it. I think it really does promote a transdisciplinary approach because for us, I think, real rehab is about returning people to life, and that's that participation piece in the WHO model. How do they participate in those life roles? We start there—say, who is this person, how do we get

them participating in their life? Then rather than focus so much on discipline specific goals we're focused on patient goals. We look at the patient and say, "What do they need to do to return to being a mom, or teacher, or whatever their life role, or an athlete, whatever it might be."

Another of our clinical sites has created an Institute of Higher Learning to foster staff professional learning and development and to support clinical, residency, and fellowship education. The institute is viewed as an important complement to the clinical services provided by the agency. In a description of the CE philosophy for the agency, the commitment to excellence, patient-centering, and learning is clearly articulated.

All health professions are founded in response to the health care needs of individuals and society. Attitudes and beliefs about the quality of life, the nature of health and illness, and man's [sic] right to reach life's full potential are implicit in its philosophical tenets. As a practitioner in a healthcare profession, we seek to maintain, improve, or restore dignity and health through the delivery of quality clinical services. A pursuit of excellence, as well as a commitment to service and the helping process enables the clinician to function as an integral part of the health care team. In addition, it is the expectation of [Institution Name] for all of its clinical staff to embrace and commit to lifelong learning and professional/career development.

At this clinical site, a great deal of effort has gone into the creation of academic-clinical partnerships like those described in Chapter 4, that help to meet the paired aims of patient- and learner-centering.

Evidence From Academic Sites

As mentioned earlier, while one might expect that a primary focus in academic sites would be on the learners and learning, a concurrent commitment to patient-centering is never out of view. At one of our academic programs, a faculty member described how that commitment is integrated across the curriculum and into one of the courses she teaches:

Patient-centered is a core value [in our teaching]...What we've done in our course and it's consistent with others [faculty members] here is that we're trying to be patient-centered so we're looking at it from a whole point of view..."Here's the patient–what do they say? What's the patient identified problem? What might be some non-patient identified problems?" We're starting from that point of view.

At another of our academic institutions, the co-occurrence of patient-and learner-centering came into sharp focus when an academic faculty member and resident mentor described her approach to mentoring: "You have to have both brains going at the same time." Here, the mentor was explaining the nature of her work with residents in the presence of patients. This triad of individuals—the patient, resident, and mentor, were in her view co-learners engaged together in the co-production of clinical knowledge. To make such an endeavor work and to serve both the patient's and the learner's needs, she needed to be closely attuned to the patient's presentation and the learner's performance concurrently; that is, she needed to use both brains, her patient-centered brain and her learner-centered brain.

This description, which accurately matches a field observation of the same mentor in action, resonates with descriptions by Shulman[13] and Irby[14] of the many forms of knowledge and understanding it takes to be a good clinical teacher (Figure 5-2). Not the least of these are knowledge of the discipline and patients (in this case, physical therapy clinical knowledge) and knowledge of pedagogy and learners.[13,14] Furthermore, these forms of knowledge are framed by, and must be employed in, variable contexts that may change from moment to moment and situation to situation. Thus, understanding of context is also critical.[13,14]

Of interest was the fact that this resident mentor, and other advanced clinicians like her in several of our sites, also teach in the professional preparation (entry-level) program at this university. Thus, they must shift frames when teaching in the context of the clinic or in the classroom. This particular mentor felt that her work with residents had shaped, in significant ways, the way she taught and worked with learners in earlier phases of their professional preparation. In fact, she thought that one turning point in her development as a mentor was when she translated the strategies and process she was using for resident mentoring in the clinic into classroom teaching:

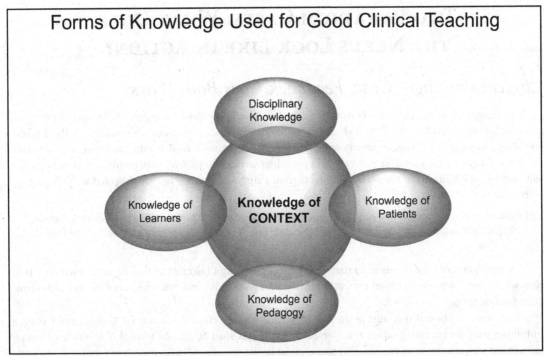

Forms of Knowledge Used for Good Clinical Teaching

Figure 5-2. Forms of knowledge used for good clinical teaching. In physical therapy, disciplinary knowledge is the academic and clinical knowledge foundational to physical therapy. (Adapted from Irby DM. Excellence in clinical teaching: knowledge transformation and development required. *Med Educ.* 2014;48:776-784.)

I think, how I really learned it [mentoring] was when we took this process, we pulled it back into the entry-level program. I was able to recognize how little they [the students] were synthesizing the material. It made me realize, I need to ask more questions at more key times. I want to know—our students learn that you put a towel in their waistline and it makes them [the patient] feel better, but why?...That was an aha moment for me—where we need to be better at getting them to talk to us about their thought processes [while in the classroom].

The latter is a key point because it shows the reflexivity in this program between the various levels of education going on; teaching and learning in the residency and fellowship post-professional programs folds back onto the nature of teaching and learning in the professional program in the classroom and the clinic. At many of our sites, we observed individuals who concurrently assumed several roles related to the educational endeavor; that of advanced clinician and role model, gifted instructor or mentor in the clinic, and classroom and/or laboratory teacher. A faculty member at another of our academic institutions highlighted the value of having residents in the classroom:

...our residents are also teaching in the program, so they serve as exemplars for the students—"Hey, this is what I want to be." A significant number of our full-time and part-time faculty are former residents [at this institution].

The importance of the presence of such individuals who fulfilled dual or multiple roles at our sites will be discussed further in Chapter 6 on the Praxis of Learning.

To illustrate the power of the combined commitment to teaching and learning that is both patient- and learner-centered we provide 2 paradigm cases—1 from a clinical site and another from an academic site.

Two Paradigm Cases: What Does the Nexus Look Like in Action?

Clinical Paradigm Case: Feedback Goes Both Ways

The following case is drawn from one of our clinical sites that provides CE experiences for students, interns, and residents in a broad array of clinical sites. This health care system included an academic medical center providing inpatient acute care, inpatient acute rehabilitation centers, skilled nursing facilities with subacute rehabilitation units, and several outpatient clinics providing services for patients with a wide variety of diagnoses and conditions. Recall part of the participant quote from a clinician at this agency highlighted at the beginning of this chapter:

> *I think when you are a dedicated clinician…you have a responsibility to the next generation of clinicians and to the patients that we treat. And the best way to ensure excellent patient care is to excellently train students in the clinic.*

This quote forecasts the Nexus of learner- and patient-centering illustrated in this vignette based on a field observation and interviews with an exemplary teacher, John (pseudonym), and the intern he was mentoring, Brian (pseudonym).

John is a senior clinical specialist at the agency. He has been in clinical practice for 19 years and has been with this agency for his entire career as a therapist. During this span of time he worked in a variety of venues early on but within a few years he found his niche—what he described as his primary interest and love—in acute care. Recognizing his enthusiasm for and expertise in the management of patients after trauma, acute illness or surgery, the agency created the position of Acute Care Team Leader for John. Subsequently he became even more interested and involved in the management of patients with cardiovascular and pulmonary conditions and became an American Board of Physical Therapy Specialties board certified clinical specialist in that area.·In his role as Acute Care Team Leader, John serves as a resource person for and mentor to students and other staff members working in intensive care units and other aspects of acute care. He is also responsible for running a special interest group for acute care that involves regular educational and professional development offerings available to staff across all the agency sites and is involved in the clinical effectiveness quality improvement initiatives in the acute care areas in the system. Working with other colleagues, John was instrumental in the envisioning and development of an acute care internship program for which he currently serves as the clinical lead. The internship idea and program was developed in partnership with some local universities and the program had been active for 7 years at the time of our site visit. The 6-month program involves 3 months when a student is completing a terminal clinical experience in their professional curriculum and then the student moves into an intern position for an additional 3 months following graduation and licensure. During the internship, learners work as a new graduate staff therapist for 20-hour weeks and the remaining 20 hours are spent with a mentor, like John, who supervises and works with the learner to advance their clinical knowledge, skills, and reasoning.

Brian is currently completing this acute care internship program. Now, as a licensed therapist and intern, he has rotated across several services and worked with advanced clinicians and mentors in the areas of neurology, oncology, and cardiothoracic surgery. John is his mentor in the latter area and the field observation described here was a 45-minute session during which Brian and John were working with a female patient who had undergone cardiothoracic surgery a few days earlier. She also had other medical conditions and complications, including acute renal failure and atrial fibrillation. This patient was not known to John, so he had asked Brian to do a review of her chart and be prepared to report those findings to him at the beginning of the session.

As the session began, Brian and John are outside of the patient's room. They exchange information about the patient based on Brian's chart review and John asks some focused questions around data that would shape the plan for the session. Brian appears to know what is expected of him regarding his reporting; he discusses the patient's history and comorbidities, information in the chart from the last physical therapy visit, and pertinent laboratory values, including a low platelet value. Based on this pre-briefing, John asks Brian, "What's the plan?" Brian lays out a plan for close monitoring and ambulation and John agrees. John defines their respective roles during the patient encounter: Brian will be the lead therapist and John will act as his aide, assisting with equipment, transfers, and ambulation as requested and necessary. Before proceeding into the patient's room, John and Brian assess information available on monitors outside the room and discuss those findings, including an irregular QRS wave on the electrocardiogram, and the implications for the session. They also talk with the patient's nurse inquiring about how the morning went for the patient.

Upon entering the room, the patient is seated in a chair. As planned, Brian takes the lead asking questions of the patient, especially around her current functional status, and explains the plan for the session. John functions as an aide, helping with preparation and set-up and occasionally interjecting a question of his own to the patient. Brian checks the patient's vital signs, including blood pressure, and indicates some concern over those; he discusses this with John who reassures him that it would be safe to proceed. With Brian leading and John following with her IV pole, the patient walks approximately 20 feet and returns to her chair without incident. Once seated, Brian talks with the patient about her postoperative precautions and asks her to repeat them. John asks Brian to also discuss a likely discharge to a skilled nursing facility for continued recuperation and therapy. After a period of time, John steps in to ask the patient more about her current status, physically and cognitively. He asks, "Do you feel like yourself?" and the patient responds, "No, not really." He observes some lower extremity edema and asks the patient if she has heart failure to which she replies, "No." John also tries to help the patient understand that her discharge to a skilled nursing facility is meant to be a temporary, not permanent, transfer.

After John and Brian leave the patient's room, they complete a debriefing session, reflecting on what they have just experienced and thinking forward for this patient and others that Brian might encounter. Noting that the patient seemed lethargic, John asked Brian some questions about why she might have been slow to clear some of the narcotic analgesics she was on following surgery. They discuss the impact of acute renal failure on drug clearance and John encouraged Brian to learn more about how comorbidities could influence the rate of recuperation for patients like this. Brian asked John about causes for heart failure and the 2 of them discuss this further. Finally, John suggests some ways to talk with patients about the need for other services after discharge and stresses the importance of this patient's understanding that such services are intended to be temporary and are meant to help her return to previous levels of function.

In a follow-up interview after the observation, Brian was asked whether the nature of interactions between John and Brian that we saw were fairly typical of his work with John and other mentors. Brian confirmed that they were.

> *But with this, as far as this interaction goes, between me and John, I mean, very typical. As far as pre… he'll kind of set me up with some things to think about, some questions. We'll kind of go over some of the things past medical-wise. We'll get into the room and it varies patient to patient…But then outside the room we'll end up talking similar to today, sometimes a little more, sometime a little bit less, just kind of more thought provoking questions. And maybe, if you saw this…what would you expect to happen? So kind of just taking the step further of not just what did we see in the room, but why did this happen. How would you respond? What would you do? And he's really good at those really thought-provoking questions that you need to think critically about, not just what you saw, but maybe…why would that be going on? But to compare that to other mentors, It's fairly similar.*

As a result of this mentoring and thoughtful questioning during his internship, Brian noted that he felt his clinical decision making had dramatically improved.

> *But I do feel like my clinical decision making, at this point, without question is above and beyond anything I would even expect for it to be at this point in my career, only a couple of months out of school really.*

Brian commented on the central role of feedback that goes both ways in his development as a clinician at this agency. He noted that feedback among members in this community of practitioners who highly value teaching and learning and are committed to delivering high quality patient care is ubiquitous in this agency. As a student and now intern, Brian felt that expectations were clear and that he was respected and listened to as his learning experiences unfolded.

I feel like one of the great things that I wasn't anticipating coming into this rotation is that the feedback, especially here…is that the feedback here holds a lot of weight both ways. They want to know just as much how I feel things are going as they feel things are going…I can have a very open relationship with all of the mentors I've had. That I can say, "Hey this really worked for me. This didn't work for me." I feel like they just—they're really—they value that information…and it makes for a great learning experience. Because when you feel like you're being listened to, you value the change as much as they do. I'll be willing to change what I'm doing if they are as well.

Finally, Brian noted how much he valued the willingness of the staff at the agency to welcome him, help him, and respond to his questions.

I could stop anybody in the entire department and they're more than willing to not just answer a question but to explain their answer…Everybody's willing to help all the time…it's been pretty remarkable in that sense…I feel like education, I think, plays a pretty big role here. And I think they value…the teaching experience of it. Like I feel like the people here are good about recognizing that if somebody has a question, it's not just a question for no reason—that most of the times it's related to clinical care and they see the importance of it. So, they'll take the couple minutes to explain why you're doing something or willing to answer pretty much anything as far as clinical-related.

In a post-observation interview with John, he reaffirmed Brian's observations and comments. He was committed to an approach to clinical teaching that set out clear expectations for learners, used assignments, pre-briefings and debriefings, and probing but non-threatening questioning as tools for advancing learning. He had learned through his own previous personal experiences and mentoring that it was important not to butt-in in some, though not all, cases when the student was trying to interact directly with the patient. At that time in the encounter, he felt it was important to provide guidance and support to the learner when indicated but not take over a session unless it was absolutely necessary for the well-being and safety of the patient. He passes these insights along to the clinical instructors and other mentors who work on the acute care team.

It's the hardest thing really for clinical instructors that are in acute care and very fast paced to do-is step back when you don't have to butt in…and I talk to them, the clinical instructors, very openly about this…this is how it's going to be very hard for you because you can see so quickly and so clearly where you want to go and you have to let the students and interns [make] their way in a non-unsafe way because that's the only way they're going to learn and if you keep going in, first of all then the authority in the clinical scenario gets confused. I mean you do want to try and encourage your students to take responsibility and ownership and if you keep jumping in…you set the groundwork but then you have to step back, and you really have to let the process go…

John also talked about the importance of the mutual exchange of feedback between instructor/mentor and learner that Brian had discussed as a facilitator to his learning. John felt the same way about the importance of feedback for his own self-monitoring and development as a teacher. He talked about this when he observed students who weren't carrying over lessons learned into other situations and the importance of feedback in determining the learning diagnosis and solution in such cases.

…but if he [a learner] is not carrying over what we have asked him to do, then you have to figure out, like in any clinical instructional scenario, why you are not carrying over? (A) is it my fault? Have I not explained it clearly and why it's so important? So, kind of figure out a different way to say that, or (B) did you understand what I said but didn't prioritize it as much as I thought you should, so let's figure that gap out…

Finally, John emphasized the importance not only of advancing his students clinical knowledge and skills, but the critical importance of attention to the patient and their wants and needs of patient-centering.

You [the student] have to see who is this lady, who she was, what you're recommending, why you're recommending it, what the problems are to her, limits to her mobility so you better incorporate that…I mean if you come back at the end of the day and tell me, you know what, I walked this patient down the hallway, she had a Foley [catheter], oxygen, IV, heart monitor, she was in A-Fib and I got her back safe. That's great, that's good, but I'm not going to be as excited when you are doing that at 6 weeks. I want to know who that lady was, what were the physiological problems and how you interacted with her so that I know it was successful interaction. You [not only] got her back safely, you talked about discharge, you talked to the right people [about needed services].

Coda/Epilogue

In this paradigm case, we illustrate an encounter between an exemplary clinical teacher/mentor, an intern, and a patient they were working with in an acute care setting following cardiothoracic surgery. As expected, the most important focus in this clinical setting is on the delivery of high quality patient care. In this center, however, the drive for excellence in patient care is closely linked with a passion for teaching and fostering learning and professional development for students, interns, residents and all staff members. The members of this community view ongoing learning as fundamental to their professional responsibilities and their obligation to meet the needs of society. Clearly, the intern described in this case, appreciated and was benefitting from the combination of a learner- and patient-centered approach to his development as a new clinician. In addition, this case is an example of many of the features integral to conceptual models of learning through participation in the workplace put forth by Billet[15,16] and elaborated by O'Brien.[17] Here we have a picture of a workplace where (1) relationships within the community promote participation and foster learning; (2) the sequencing and selection of work tasks and activities is paramount in teaching and learning; and (3) the sociocultural norms and nature of the workplace and organization shape what and how learning is occurring. The workplace learning model and its implications for our study findings will be discussed further in future chapters.

Academic Paradigm Case: Practice-Based Evidence Is the Heart of the Matter

This case is drawn from one of the academic sites we visited. The mission for the professional Doctor of Physical Therapy (DPT) Program at this institution is:

To prepare physical therapists to be responsible health care providers who demonstrate core professional values, address the needs of the individual across the lifespan, and embrace evidence-based and patient-centered practice.

In the view of the faculty and department leaders, a key factor contributing to the realization of this mission is a shared vision and accountability toward achieving it; the DPT curriculum, and its outcomes, are seen as the responsibility of the whole faculty. The entire leadership team talked about how one of their roles is to harness the creativity of the faculty to move them toward a common goal. The Department knows what it wants to accomplish but has room for discussion and alternative paths about how it is going to get there. One participant in a faculty focus group described it this way:

Everybody is trying to accomplish the same thing and trying to bring that commitment to the mission of trying to prepare physical therapists. What we're all trying to do...is to prepare people not for practice today but for practice 5 years from now, 10 years from now. That's the challenge. I think many, many programs have that commitment. The key is execution, of course...I would say the most important aspect of that is that everybody on the faculty feel that they have both a stake and a voice. And I think that that's something that we've tried to do here is to make sure that when we move forward with changes in our curriculum and all that that we are really getting everybody's involvement and input into it.

Collectively the faculty have designed and organized a curriculum with the end in mind around several key concepts: (1) an agreed upon definition of entry-level physical therapist practice; (2) an inclusive understanding of movement and movement analysis as a foundation for practice; (3) interprofessional education; (4) explicit attention to professional formation; and (5) patient-centeredness and the importance of practice-based evidence as a cornerstone for clinical decision making. They pay close attention to formative assessment of students and have specific processes to support student learning. They explicitly acknowledge and implement student-centered, active-learning, pedagogical approaches that promote student learning. CE experiences are integrated throughout the curriculum in all 3 years, and the clinical faculty see themselves as integral to the program. The faculty describe the curriculum as highly integrated and owned by the entire faculty; no one course is owned by the core faculty member for that course. There are semester- and thematic-based curricular groups that meet and discuss what they are doing and how the students are responding. This regular involvement with other faculty members is a clear expectation.

For the purposes of this chapter on the Nexus component of our model, the remainder of this paradigm case will focus primarily on how the key concept of patient-centering is threaded through and emphasized across the curriculum in combination with learner-centered approaches to teaching in the classroom and clinic. In this case, we hear the voices of faculty members and of students completing the DPT program.

Patient-centeredness is addressed in explicit ways in classes, laboratories, and clinical experiences throughout the program. The program has an active faculty practice and 4 residency programs that are highly valued by the students and faculty because they bring current, active clinical expertise and practice into the classroom experience, thus deepening the clinical context for student learning. The formal CE curriculum begins in the second semester of Year 1. In the description of the curriculum that follows, we use the language/terms of the program to describe the sequence and names of CE courses across the curriculum. During the first 2 years there are three 2-week clinical practicums and two 6-week clinical affiliations. During the third year, there is a 16-week full-time clinical clerkship and a 16-week part-time (3 days/week) advanced clinical clerkship paired with an integrated patient management seminar. The last of these clerkships is when students, guided by clinical and academic faculty, complete an integrated patient project.

The faculty pay close attention to how they frame and define evidence-based practice so that it is conceptualized as practice-based evidence, when implemented by students and new graduates, with attention to patient needs and concerns at the heart of this approach to evidence. The faculty discussed how students need to be able to interpret and apply the evidence available to them in the literature based on what a particular patient brings to the clinical visit; it is not the scientific evidence alone that drives clinical decisions. The faculty acknowledge this is not an easy shift for students to make, but it is the way physical therapists practice. This patient-centered approach is also at the heart of movement analysis as the foundation for physical therapy. One has to begin with the problems the patient brings to therapy and start with an examination of the related movement disturbances that are affecting their lives, function and meaningful participation.

Several of the faculty members described how this approach is emphasized in the integrated patient management seminars and project:

> But the evidence that I'm bringing in is the patient evidence so...they're looking at qualitative life issues. But they also have [to] tie in what intervention are they doing and they have to let the patient drive where they're getting the evidence from. That's been a change. We tweak that project a lot...they were finding evidence and then wanting to apply it to their patient as opposed...to practice-based evidence...This semester in our latest tweaking we're meeting with all the students after they have met with their patient the first time. Even though they have a faculty mentor who is out there with them, we're driving the discussion of how the evidence fits in...They paint a picture for me of what their patient looks like and we really talk about what are you going to do for this patient because you only get to see [them] 2 or 3 times.

The director of the DPT program talked more about how the faculty work to help the students develop a more inclusive view of evidence-based practice. That view goes well beyond searching the literature, though important, to combining that knowledge with the needs of the patient and the deep clinical expertise that advanced clinicians bring to the equation to make the best decisions about patient care. Here he discusses how many students come to clinical experiences with good skills in accessing and identifying scientific evidence, but few clinical practice and judgment skills early on:

> Our students and I think students anywhere, in their defense, all they have when they go on to [clinical experiences]...I mean, if evidence-based practice is the best available evidence they [have]...If they have no clinical strengths, then of course, they're going to lean very heavily on the evidence or what they've been told. So, we're trying to get them to listen to the patients and we're trying to get them to listen to the clinicians who have those strengths and to learn from them. That's like where the practice-based evidence comes in. Because our faculty, particularly in the clinical courses, they're all practicing clinicians, they're able to inform them [the students], again, from their daily practice.

There are explicit efforts to support and encourage student-centered learning that the faculty members have adopted. They have a commitment to use formative assessment of the curriculum and of their teaching to improve their processes and outcomes. They also use formative assessment of student learning to improve their teaching as well as to identify means to support students from matriculation through completion of the program.

[We] came up with the rule that every lesson would have a student-centered active thing. Now it's gone from that being a piece of every lecture to that being the majority of the lesson and then a little bit of lecture if I feel like I need to give them some basic information...I asked them how the course is going, what's helping them learn, what's not...Every year, I change my course based on that feedback...I really try to take it [to] heart what they have to say because they're pretty invested...Mostly, they're right, I find, when you really think about it...I try to change anything that they give feedback on it...The first time I do things is a big risk. I get butterflies in my stomach...I do debates, scavenger hunt, and I get, "How do I do this?" It's so uncontrolled. I don't know what's going to happen. I find halfway through every lesson, I'm like, "This is what I do. This is so much fun," because their eyes are bright and they're engaged. One thing I have to give up is you don't have to finish every lesson. Sometimes I don't finish all the content and then I just figure out a way to deal with that.

These paired commitments to learner- and patient-centering were not lost on the students in this program; they were recognized, applauded, and integrated. In focus group interviews with students from all 3 years in the entry-level program, participants consistently reported that they benefitted greatly from the experience and expertise of their faculty and felt that they were readily available and willing to assist their learning and development. They felt supported but also challenged by faculty to become lifelong learners and owners of their own future growth as therapists. And they clearly got the take home message about being patient-centered and embracing practice-based evidence in their clinical practice. The following are some responses from students regarding the biggest lessons learned through their participation in this program and components of the program that they felt contributed most to their learning and development as future therapists.

The whole thing behind evidence-based practice...Not exactly like, yeah, I'm learning how to do research, do articles. But more of enabling you with the tools to continue your own learning, and facilitate your own learning...We want you to continue to be in charge of your learning even after you graduate. So, I think that's one huge thing that's going to make the biggest impact [for me].

Several students commented on how the intermittent clinical practicum experiences and the integrated patient project advanced their learning and kept the patient front and center in decision making about care:

Three 2-week rotations. Even though that's a small little slot though, it's nice to kind of have that break from sitting in the classroom, and being able to apply it immediately to the clinic, and get that real-world experience. And then bring that back to the classroom...

For me, this semester we're doing an integrated project, so each group has a patient that we're actually working with. And it's been really awesome, because we've learned certain techniques for our patients, and like 3 days before I got to see the patient and actually use it. And in class I was like, "Oh, this would never work. I don't think I would ever use this in the clinic." And then we used it on our patient, and it was really awesome. So, kind of just having that opportunity to practice everything you sit in the classroom all day and learn about is really awesome.

...the integrative project that [another student] was talking about. With the treatments that we're doing with our patient, we have to have evidence related to it or behind it. Also, to integrate it with the clinical practice perspective, patient perspective and put all of that together. So just kind of all that coming together into one project, that pulls a lot of coursework in the semester together.

...the 2-week clinicals, I bring it back to that...and the integrated project we're working with a patient. I find myself looking at our notes from class with a different perspective. It's not like in undergrad where I'm just studying for a test. I'm like, "How can I help this patient?"

One of the biggest things for me is I really appreciate that most of our professors are practicing PTs. So, when they teach us something in the class, they'll give us patient cases that are real, actual patients that they've seen, and we can even see videos of them sometimes...You can hear what our professors did with them in the clinic, and why they did it. It just helps bring it all together so much more easily...

As a final question in one of the student focus groups at this site, an interviewer asked participants to summarize in a few words the type of therapist that they felt the faculty and their experience in this program had helped them to become. This question encouraged a chorus of responses, but the most frequent are captured in the brief quotes that follow:

Lifelong learners. I mean if I had to sum it up in a few words, that would probably be it.

And we've been taught really strongly to be patient centered, and the ICF model, and that's sort of embedded in this program. It's always thinking about goals, and always checking in with your patient that what you're doing is important to them, and that they're buying in and that they feel competent. You know, all the things that are so important for learning and all that process. And making sure that you're just designing a program that is for that patient. You're not just coming up with something ahead of time and trying to force it upon someone or something like that.

I think too, they also want us to advocate. Advocate for our patient, advocate for ourselves, and for the profession.

I'd say there's also a lot of emphasis from our professors on empowering our patients...Because we can only do so much, and they can't come to us forever. So, we have to really get our patients to understand that. They're not coming to us for a quick fix, we're just giving them the tools to go on with their lives healthier.

I think another...big idea is to treat the whole patient...Taking into consideration their likes, dislikes, hobbies, everything.

Coda/Epilogue

In this paradigm case, we hear the voices of DPT program leaders, clinical and academic faculty, and students that articulate and illustrate the Nexus of paired commitments to learner- and patient-centering in the context of an academic program and setting. The program faculty explicitly identified, embraced, and enacted these aims. They took risks in their teaching to create classroom learning experiences that closely resembled the descriptions of what it means to be learner-centered provided at the beginning of this chapter. They kept the patient front and center in their conceptualization of what evidence-based practice really means and demonstrated a deep valuing of practice-based evidence. The students clearly heard and benefitted from these paired commitments; they got these messages loud and clear as they proceeded through their professional preparation at this institution. The delivery of such strong messages was facilitated by the availability of a faculty practice and many clinicians filling dual roles as academic faculty and practitioner, by the presence of residents and resident mentors, through the early and continuous integration of clinical exposure across the curriculum, and by the collective agreement and ownership of faculty to live and model these ideals.

Envisioned Future for Physical Therapist Education

As discussed in Chapter 4, in the physical therapist educational communities we studied that are characterized by a Culture of Excellence, there are shared beliefs about the value of learner-centered education and patient-centered care that are integrated through new pedagogies and partnerships, by faculty who teach with a focus on both the learner and the patient in academic and clinical settings. In physical therapist education for the future, these beliefs and values are not only shared, but transformed into explicit and paired commitments that are articulated, visible, and enacted on a daily basis by all faculty, regardless of primary role, in all educational endeavors and environments. The Nexus of learner- and patient-centering provides a critical conduit for the translation of a Culture of Excellence into the domain of the Praxis of Learning. In our vision of the future, faculty will seek out and strengthen opportunities to model and promote interprofessional collaborative patient care and interprofessional education of learners at multiple levels, which will further serve the shared values of patient-centered care and learner-centered teaching.

CONCLUSION

In this chapter, we have focused on the central component of our Model of Excellence in Physical Therapist Education. The Nexus of the paired and highly-valued aims of learner- and patient-centering in the educational enterprise that constitutes physical therapist education in academic and clinical realms. This Nexus, or coming together, of these 2 aims is critical for excellence to be realized. It is important to note, however, that these aims in and of themselves, while laudable, must be transformed into commitments that inform and create intentional action by members of the community in educational settings. Such action is what allows a Culture of Excellence (the first dimension in our model) to grow and flourish and what facilitates learning for practice through practice in our second dimension of the model, Praxis of Learning. Readers will note the presence and importance of learner- and patient-centering in both of these dimensions as discussed in the preceding chapter and the chapter to follow. This is precisely because of the criticality of the Nexus—these paired perspectives and commitments are diffused across both dimensions as represented by the lens in our model.

Perhaps a few examples of such diffusion, drawing on Chapter 4, will clarify. The first element in the Culture of Excellence dimension was shared beliefs and values. Among those shared beliefs and values were learner-centeredness and patient-centeredness. Yet, these were 2 among other shared values such as mutual respect, trust, collaboration, and teamwork, that sowed the seeds for the cultivation of a Culture of Excellence. Thus, while learner- and patient-centering were 2 of the espoused values in the communities we studied, they were some, but not all, of those shared beliefs and values. Similarly, the last element described in the Culture of Excellence dimension was partnerships. While the true partnerships we observed at many of our sites would not have happened without the joint valuing of and commitments to learner- and patient-centering, there is more to the creation of such partnerships than just commitment to those aims. Thus, these shared commitments enabled, but did not ensure, that creative partnerships would be envisioned and strong bridges would be built between academic and clinical settings for advancing physical therapist education and achieving excellence.

Finally, it is worth noting that both learner- and patient-centering are necessary for the Nexus and excellence to occur. While each of these are important, they are not sufficient on their own to create excellence. In reality, there are many clinical sites that provide quality patient-centered care that are not learner-centered nor do they take learning in the organization as essential to its mission. Likewise, there are no doubt many physical therapist educational programs that take learner-centering and teaching and learning very seriously, but the commitment to patient-centering may be less visible or implicit vs prominent, persistent, and explicit, in curricula or in the classroom.

REFLECTIVE QUESTIONS

- In your educational environment, where, when, and how do you see learner-centered teaching occurring? Give some specific examples.
  - Is it implicit or explicit? Is it part of the visible or hidden curriculum in your setting? How could learner-centering be enhanced?
- In your educational environment, where, when, and how do you see patient-centering occurring? Give some specific examples.
  - Is it implicit or explicit? Is it part of the visible or hidden curriculum in your setting? How could patient-centering be enhanced?
- In your educational environment, where, when, and how do you see learner-centering and patient-centering co-occurring? Give some specific examples.
- What factors (ie, individual, institutional, professional, or societal) facilitated the concurrent enactment of learner- and patient-centering?
- Are there factors that are constraints or impediments to concurrent learner- and patient-centering in your setting? What are they? How could they be modified or changed?

REFERENCES

1.   Dewey J. *Experience and Education.* New York, NY: Macmillan Publishers; 1938.
2.   Hafler J, ed. *Extraordinary Learning in the Workplace.* New York, NY: Springer Publisher; 2011.
3.   Schumacher D, Englander R, Carracio C. Developing the master learner: applying learning theory to the learner, the teacher, and the learning environment. *Acad Med.* 2013;88:1635-1645.
4.   Weimer M. *Learner-Centered Teaching: 5 Key Changes to Practice.* San Francisco, CA: Jossey-Bass; 2002.
5.   Albanese M. Students are not customers: a better model for medical education. *Acad Med.* 1999;74(11):1172-1186.
6.   Weimer M. *Learner-Centered Teaching: 5 Key Changes to Practice.* 2nd ed. San Francisco, CA: Jossey-Bass; 2013.
7.   Ambrose S, Bridges M, DiPietro M, Lovett M, Norman M. *How Learning Works: 7 Research Based Principles for Smart Teaching.* San Francisco, CA: Jossey-Bass; 2010.
8.   World Health Organization. International classification of functioning, disability and health. https://www.cdc.gov/nchs/data/icd/icfoverview_finalforwho10sept.pdf. Published 2018. Accessed September 4, 2018.
9.   APTA. Code of Ethics for the Physical Therapist. https://www.apta.org/uploadedFiles/APTAorg/About_Us/Policies/Ethics/CodeofEthics.pdf. Published 2013. Accessed September 4, 2018.
10. APTA. Professionalism in Physical Therapy: Core Values. http://www.apta.org/uploadedFiles/APTAorg/About_Us/Policies/Judicial_Legal/ProfessionalismCoreValues.pdf Updated December 14, 2009. Accessed September 4, 2018.
11. Triple Aim Institute for Health Care Improvement. http://www.ihi.org/engage/initiatives/tripleaim/pages/default.aspxTriple AiM. Accessed September 4, 2018.
12. Interprofessional Education Collaborative Expert Panel. *Core Competencies for Interprofessional Practice: Report of an Expert Panel.* Washington, DC: Interprofessional Education Collaborative; 2011.
13. Shulman L. Those who understand: knowledge growth in teaching. *Educ Res.* 1986;15:4-14.
14. Irby DM. Excellence in clinical teaching: knowledge transformation and development required. *Med Educ.* 2014;48:776-784.
15. Billet S. *Learning in the Workplace: Strategies for Effective Practice.* Crows Nest, New South Wales, Australia: Allen & Unwin; 2001.
16. Billet S. Constituting the workplace curriculum. *J Curriculum Studies.* 2006;38(1):31-48.
17. O'Brien B. Envisioning the future. In: Hafler J, ed. *Extraordinary Learning in the Workplace.* New York, NY: Springer; 2011:165-194.

The Praxis of Learning
Opportunities Abound

The central focus of our research and this book is on excellence in education and how to improve our ability to educate the next generation of physical therapists. A foundational premise in education is understanding the critical importance and interdependence of teaching with student learning. The challenge in professional education is that it involves both *learning what* and *learning how*, which requires students to learn with supervision and guidance through experiential learning in the workplace. We found that learning for practice through practice was a primary focus of curricula across all academic and clinical settings. Whether the teaching and learning occurred in the academic setting or clinical setting, the curricula were both enacted and embodied through interactions grounded in communities of practice. While we found many examples of excellent teaching across academic and clinical settings that can be explained through the application of key learning concepts and educational theory, we found that often these teachers did not have the language nor understanding that would connect their good work with educational theory and research.

In this chapter, we focus on our model dimension Praxis (practice) of Learning and expand on each of the 4 elements in this dimension (Figure 6-1):

1. Signature pedagogy
2. Practice-based learning
3. Creating adaptive learners
4. Professional formation

Jensen GM, Mostrom E, Hack LM, Nordstrom T, Gwyer J.
Educating Physical Therapists (pp 75-93).
© 2019 Taylor & Francis Group.

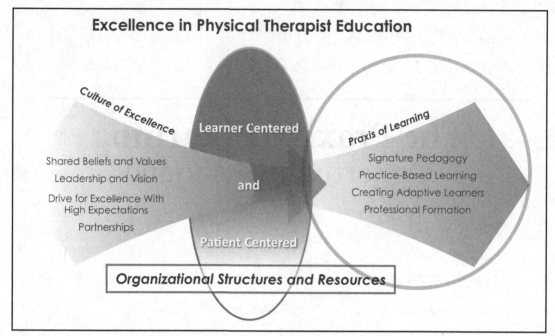

Figure 6-1. The Praxis of Learning from the Model of Excellence in Physical Therapist Education.

SIGNATURE PEDAGOGY

Signature pedagogies in the professions are characteristic forms of teaching and learning. They are fundamental ways that students, novices, are instructed about the major domains of professional work (to think, to perform, and to act with integrity).[1] In the Carnegie Preparation for the Professions Program (PPP), a signature pedagogy was identified for each profession studied as described in Chapter 2. There are 3 structural dimensions of signature pedagogy: (1) a surface structure that includes the concrete, operational acts of teaching and learning; (2) a deep structure that reveals assumptions about how best to impart knowledge and know-how in that profession, which also includes the application of underlying rationale or theory; and (3) an implicit structure that is a moral dimension, often tacit, reflecting a set of beliefs about professional attitudes, values and dispositions.[1] Shulman and colleagues later identifies a fourth structural dimension, that he refers to as the *hidden* or *shadow structure*, which represents the absent features of the pedagogy, those that are missing or are only weakly engaged.[2] While our research revealed many examples of the operational acts of teaching and learning and provided some insights on how academic and clinical faculty focus on connecting analysis of movement with patient function, there is much more to be understood about the moral dimension of our signature pedagogy as well as what may be the shadow side or absent dimension in our signature pedagogy.

These structural dimensions for signature pedagogy cross the 3 fundamental components or apprenticeships of professional education, to think (habits of mind), to perform or do the work of the profession (habits of hand), and to act with integrity (habits of heart), the ability to conduct ourselves in ways that meet our moral obligations and exercise wise judgment in the face of uncertainty. This multidimensionality of professional education is critical because it is not just about knowing and doing—it is about ways of being—it is preparation for doing good work in the service of others. These pedagogical signatures tell us a lot about the personalities, dispositions, and cultures of the field. They are often unique to the field but also applicable across professions[1-3] (Figure 6-2).

In physical therapy, movement is readily embraced as central to the profession and we would be quick to identify movement as central to teaching and learning in physical therapy. The evidence in this next section is drawn from both academic and clinical sites and demonstrates how we see the dimensions of signature pedagogy for physical therapy.

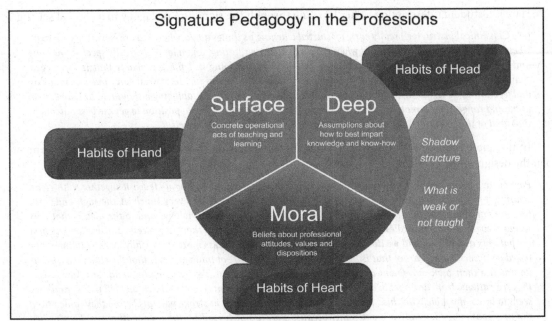

Figure 6-2. Signature pedagogies in the professions.

Evidence From Academic and Clinical Sites

We observed a dominant and pervasive focus on the human body as teacher. We repeatedly observed teachers helping learners to focus on what they could learn through close attunement to the human body: what they could *see* about movement and function by close observation of the body; what they could *feel* about morphology and movement through their hands and skilled touch; how students learn to move their bodies skillfully, safely, and efficiently while facilitating patient movement; and what they could *hear* about movement and function through close listening to their patients and what they said about their bodies. The last of these is important because it calls attention to our definition of the body in this signature pedagogy. The human body as teacher is more than what is taught and learned through the physical body and the patient's movement and function, it is also the embodied life and illness experiences of the patient captured through careful listening to patient stories. This signature pedagogy was evident whether the student was in the anatomy laboratory, learning in clinical laboratory sessions from his or her own body, working with a peer or instructor, or working with patients. In the following quote, a resident mentor describes her approach to helping a resident develop this keen sensitivity to movement through observation and touch:

> When she [the resident] said, "I'm not seeing the breathing." It's learning [sic] your eye to look for timing, speed, change in movement, and then learning to be able to put your hands on them and feel it. That takes some time. A lot of times, we won't see it in the clinic, and then we'll take in a video of something. You can see it when you have no other information in your head and you can just focus on what you're looking at on the video.

The excerpt that follows from a field note is taken from an observation of a laboratory session focused on teaching and learning about musculoskeletal examination procedures. Here, we see how central analysis of movement was in the teaching of these skills:

> In this laboratory session on the shoulder, the session is grounded in a patient case shown through media. Analysis and discussion of the patient's shoulder movement by the class then becomes the structure for student review and practice of critical and appropriate examination tests.

Here is a student's description of her learning through the signature pedagogy in a clinical setting:

(My CI [Clinical Instructor]) really early on started teaching us things about when you are elevating your arm, when the scapula begins to move and when the clavicle starts rotating, and a lot of the really specific anatomy and biomechanics behind what we are doing and why we are doing it. I think probably that is the biggest change I've seen in myself as I have stopped thinking about things...as just like, what can I put my hands on and feel how to do it, but also am I doing this most effectively for if I'm mobilizing a shoulder, do I have them at the end range of their motion...am I mobilizing them in the most optimal position to get the best outcomes, that kind of thing. I think that would be the biggest change I've seen in myself.

In the quote that follows, academic faculty shared a view on the critical importance of movement on the design of the curriculum:

Part of the idea of pushing movement analysis to first semester and having us teach it together with clear, clearly-established differences in terms of our patient appearances...he's very much at the high-end, athletic patient management, and I'm working with patients with neuropathology...and so the idea is that they would recognize that, regardless of the diagnosis, we utilize the same thought process, and we look at how the patients are moving and we do decisions about what then to assess more specifically, or how to intervene based on observation...Part of that is the experiences in your part of that course, is that the students actually do practice their own movement and analyze their own movement...We're using the iPad, but they have... they see patients from day one. Every one of our labs, we have patients come in. I actually tell them...and they seem to be comfortable with this...that the idea that they're looking at stroke patients before they understand the neuropathology is really a great thing, because they're not biased by the neuropathology. They're just thinking about the movement, and so they are seeing patients that they haven't studied, well in advance of understanding that.

Paradigm Case: Reflections on Movement for Health and Life

This case is drawn from one of our academic sites. The educational program has a long history of developing curricula and teaching/learning experiences around the central concept of a human movement system and the mission statement for the program is "Movement for health and life." There is an onsite clinical practice providing physical therapy services and supporting clinical education, residency, and fellowship programs at the institution.

Here we share an example of mentoring for learning and a description of some pedagogical strategies, including the signature pedagogy, the *human body as teacher*, oriented around the subject matter of human movement and function. The paradigm case is drawn from (1) a field observation of a resident mentor, Tara (pseudonym), and a women's health resident, Carrie (pseudonym), as they worked with a returning client; and (2) a follow-up interview with the mentor. The resident had completed almost 6 months of her year-long residency. Tara first invoked the metaphor of mentoring as a dance. As illustrated in the following case, this description was consistent with our observations and the metaphor then carried through into the follow-up interview.

The observation consisted of a 10-minute pre-briefing session with Tara and Carrie, followed by a 45-minute re-examination and treatment session with a long-standing returning patient. During the pre-brief, Tara and Carrie exchanged ideas about what they hoped to accomplish during the session, and Tara used questioning liberally to determine what Carrie would be asking about, looking at, and palpating or testing for as she worked with the patient. Most of the responses to the questions were followed by another familiar refrain: "Why?"

As the treatment session unfolded, Tara, Carrie, and the patient seemed comfortable with each other and there were frequent exchanges between the 3 of them (verbal, visual, and positional) a triadic dialogue and dance. Tara did pose questions to Carrie throughout the session; the questions were directed at exploring what Carrie was hearing, seeing, feeling, and thinking about the patient's presentation and what she might offer in the way of intervention and education around those observations. There were also times when Tara was silent and stepped back from the encounter, other times when she stepped in to engage in joint problem-solving based on verbal or nonverbal signals from either Carrie or the patient.

In the interview following the observation, Tara talked about her use of questioning as a pedagogical strategy and how she decides when to employ that strategy or not. "I think I asked more questions than I always do, but I also know...she (Carrie) is ready to get pushed. She's right at that...she's not quite halfway, but she's really going to cross over where she's really going to be at a much higher independent thinker. We...talked about it after you left the room. She was, "That was great!" She loved it. Tara continued, "Commonly, I'm a little bit more aware of not wanting to get the patient concerned about why I'm questioning the resident so much in front of them. This patient was familiar with Carrie...and the rapport was already there. It's definitely a dance that you have to play."

The mentor also talked about her own positioning and movement relative to the mentee and patient as they went through the session: "You saw us sitting in front of a triangle format. That's a common thing. I'm a little off to the side and maybe a step behind the resident in order to be, they're the one in charge and I'm just here as a consult. It intuitively happened where I commonly position myself a little more passively as I can in order to just be able to take it all in and let them keep their rapport going."

When we asked, "How do you decide when to step forward and when not to?" Tara replied: "If I think that they're going to miss a really important detail, then I may try to bring it in. You have to watch how they're processing. I always try to read the resident as to—does it look like the're going to ask another question or not, or does it look like they're ready to move on in their process? Are they finished with this phase...? It's watching them, trying to read them..."

Referring back to the session we had just observed, Tara then discussed one of the moments when she needed to step in to help Carrie refine her observation and manual skills: "When she said, 'I'm not seeing the breathing.' It's learning [sic] your eye to look for timing, speed, change in movement, and then learning to be able to put your hands on them and feel it. That takes some time."

Recognizing that such fine attunement to the human body and movement through touch and vision takes time and is a complex skill, Tara also mentioned that she uses videos to help hone observation skills for her mentees: "A lot of times, we won't see it in the clinic, and then we'll take in a video of something. You can see it when you have no other information in your head and you can just focus on what you're looking at on the video."

Finally, when Tara was asked about her own learning to be a mentor, she responded: "I think I learned to dance...Sometimes you just learn it. You don't recognize your own learning."

Coda/Epilogue

The pre-briefing session here is part of the signature pedagogy and sets the scene for what is to come. Tara's questioning and guidance draws Carrie's attention to the search for the most salient features of the patient encounter unique to physical therapy: What will she inquire about and listen for regarding the patient's current function? What will she be observing in terms of the patient's body and movement? What will she be palpating and testing for as she examines the patient?

As the actual therapy session proceeds, we see the patient's life experience and body as both subject and object, and the therapist's body as instrument; it is a diagnostic tool and a treatment tool and often diagnosis and treatment can occur through our own movement in addition to that of the patient. The triadic exchanges occurring between mentor, mentee, and patient really do evoke the metaphor of a dance; the movement and engagement of all participants creates a choreography of practice, teaching, and learning in the clinical encounter.

Finally, when Tara is talking about how she is trying to help Carrie better detect changes in breathing patterns and trunk movement through her eyes and hands, she notes that one tool for teaching this can be the use of video analysis outside of the actual client encounter to help Carrie focus and refine her observations. Here, Tara is sensitive to the effect of situational complexity and cognitive load (without naming it as such) on the potential for learning at a particular time for that particular resident. The use of video analysis as a teaching tool raises an important point: the patient/the body in this signature pedagogy can also take symbolic forms. The patient/body can be textual as in a paper case, or it can be images, models, videos, or peers; but the richest, most interactive and emotionally engaging form of the signature pedagogy comes through actual client encounters.

Envisioned Future for the Profession of Physical Therapy

Given our strong consensus in the profession on the role of movement in the work of the physical therapist, the profession is benefiting from a focused look at movement, including use of shared language, what movement means, and how to apply it in education, practice, and research.[4] The signature pedagogy of human body as teacher provides the profession with a structure for further study into how movement is the unique subject matter of pedagogy in the teaching and learning of physical therapists. Academic and clinical educators engage in explicit analysis and application of our signature pedagogy in teaching and learning. The 3 structural dimensions of signature pedagogy—surface (concrete, operational acts of teaching and learning), deep (assumptions about how best to impart knowledge and know-how) and implicit (moral dimension and set of beliefs about professional attitudes, values, and dispositions)—can guide this work.

As signature pedagogies highlight distinctive features of teaching and learning in the profession, there may be a shadow side, a fourth structural dimension, in forcing certain kinds of learning into limited structures of teaching based on our current beliefs. Signature pedagogies are not a static pre-scription for how we must teach, as they can change over time as the conditions of work and the nature and norms of practice change. For example, the Carnegie PPP study of medical education identified the signature pedagogy in medicine as teaching at the bedside.[5] As hospital stays shorten and more and more care is delivered in alternative ways and settings, this pedagogy is likely to change. Signature pedagogies can also privilege one dimension of professional work and education over another. Here is an example from the PPP study of legal education: The signature pedagogy in legal education was socratic dialogue around a case and the texts of the law.[2] This was very effective for teaching students how to think like a lawyer but far less helpul in helping law students develop clinical skills and a strong moral foundation (habits of hand and heart)—in preparing them to do the work of a lawyer.

In our envisioned future, educators and researchers investigate all the dimensions of signature pedagogy in the profession, as emerging technologies provide opportunities and challenges related to how we teach about movement. We also suggest that this signature pedagogy, while prevalent in our observations, is generally more tacit and implicit than explicit. We lack a clear definition and shared language about key concepts—not only about the pedagogy itself but also about the content—the role of movement and the movement system as organizing elements for curricular design and decision making about teaching and learning approaches. This lack of shared language and understandings means that these important aspects of physical therapist education are underexplored and underdeveloped. We need to shine a brighter light here as we believe that there is great opportunity for further investiga-tion on physical therapy's signature pedagogy, including a closer look at the 4 structural dimensions (surface, deep, implicit [moral], and shadow).

We found that this signature pedagogy was a pervasive and powerful form of teaching and learning in both clinical and academic sites. It has much to say about what counts as knowledge in our field and how things become known, and it teaches the choreography of practice.

PRACTICE-BASED LEARNING

The concept of learning for practice through practice provides an important goal for all profes-sions. This concept is grounded in a rich body of theory and research across disciplines on the power of situated learning through which the student has frequent opportunities to engage in authentic, practice-based learning experiences in diverse communities of practice.[6-15] These sociocultural theo-ries of learning suggest that professional expertise develops through the interaction with and in the communities of practice. The experiential opportunities help students learn the practice by engaging in activities and ways of doing, thinking, and being in the profession through their participation in practice. This focus on learning for practice is done early as it creates a scaffold for contextual and continuous learning, learning that sticks.[8] There is no single recipe for designing and implementing an excellent curriculum. The facilitation of the learning process that is done through a true collaborative partnership between academic and clinical communities is non-negotiable. A community of practice and learners that includes a diverse group of professional and post-professional learners (ie, entry-level students, residents, fellows), provides an opportunity for continuous reflection on and in the teaching and learning environment. This integration of learners at various levels results in a unique layering of teachers and learners and fosters reciprocal teaching/learning and role modeling among members of the community.

In all the sites we visited, the importance of learning for practice through practice was a driver in the curriculum and for the development of learning experiences. We found that faculty and learners were frequently engaged in early, authentic, practice-based learning experiences. There were vibrant faculty clinical practices tht supported teaching and learning in the entry-level curriculum, residency education, and clinical research in 5 of the 6 academic programs we visited. The sixth program had a robust, long-established interprofessional community outreach program that students were engaged in early on; and the program was working on building a faculty clinical practice. The value of learners' access to patients transcends the application of knowledge and skills. Through access to patients, learners experience first-hand the value of highly contextualized learning that occurs in a community of practice where patient care is central. This dominant focus on practice-based learning was also grounded in the use of evidence in driving practice across all sites.

The power of participation in practice-based learning experiences in communities of practice was recognized as a valuable resource for teaching and learning. It can also create tension because, while practice-based experiences are high impact, they are also unpredictable, introducing a potential loss of control of the curriculum. What can that messiness or uncertainty contribute to teaching and learning? What are we teaching for? How can we take advantage of the unpredictability that is inherent in practice to better prepare professionals for their future work? Shulman argues that we must recognize that "practice-based is not practice-imprisoned" learning.[16] The process of learning to be or act like a professional goes way beyond content knowledge.

Given the power and promise of practice-based learning for physical therapists, we must ask ourselves about the preponderance of ways that we still teach, especially in the professional preparation phase of education. How much of what we do in the curriculum and the classroom is driven by content? *What gets measured most when assessing learning?* This is not to say that content isn't essential; it is. It just isn't sufficient; it benefits from being embedded in the practice and situations of use. While the people we observed in our study were doing really good things, they often lacked a shared language for talking about those things and a deep understanding of learning theory and research that could inform and strengthen what they were doing.

Evidence From Academic and Clinical Sites

Here a student describes the impact on learning from faculty and students having access to a practice-based environment:

> *I just talked to that professor. I stopped at that class and asked him if I could observe and he said "sure, no problem." It was wonderful because he knows what I'm learning [in the clinic]. He knows my knowledge base and he welcomed me in…The other opportunity was to have currently practicing clinicians who are immediately accessible (working in the faculty practice) coming into the classroom to teach and using recent clinical examples…*

The following quotations from a variety of participants represent the centrality of practice in the learning environments we observed:

> *I think being able to be in the clinical setting just makes things more relevant. If you learn something specifically about a patient with a patient, with them right there in front of you, you're never going to forget that thing. Whereas, half of what you listen to in a lecture you're not going to retain. I think being able to be there in the moment and make things so much more relevant, I think it's kind of cool. —Clinical Instructor*

> *We are very evidence based…because our therapists are involved in research and always asking the question. We expect our students to ask the question. Well, why are you doing that? Where is the evidence? Is the evidence not there? Where is your outcome measure? We are expecting that. —Administrator*

I really enjoyed being able to be immersed in the hands-on learning experience, starting the first semester, unlike some programs where you start later on in your first year or second year and so on...you can practice hand skills and start applying clinical decision-making models that you have learned; there is nothing like seeing true barriers, psychosocial and economic, to get a real appreciation. You have classroom learning on it, but that just extends so much. You are seeing patients that are at such a high risk for certain injuries because they are using their bodies like machines in certain jobs, or they can't get there any way but walking...It is a very good education in that sense. —Student

We go to independent living centers. It's a group of 12 students from each of the seven disciplines. The faculty from each of the disciplines rotates so we don't stick with the group, but the group stays together, and they meet an elder and they go back 3 times over 2 semesters. They meet each other, and they learn...what everybody's scope is. They meet as kind of social and then we go, and we meet the elder...these are people who are in definite need of intervention. We do a team assessment of polypharmacy, cognition, function...PT will do any kind of gait assessment, any kind of mobility assessment. We never know what we're going to get...Then they [the learners/team] put together a plan and we give the plans...we send the plans to physicians. We give it to the facility, but the big thing is to be in the home because they don't know how to get to do home visits and to work with the team. Then we're supposed to be facilitators. —Faculty

Paradigm Case: Layers of Teaching and Learning In Situ

We enter a relatively small outpatient clinic with 5 physical therapists, including the clinic director. The clinic itself is in a vibrant urban downtown location with an open, airy warehouse feel to the large gym space, bordered by private booth areas on one side. This particular clinic is one of many owned and operated as part of a larger company with a long history of delivering physical therapy services in a private practice setting and involvement in physical therapist professional and post-professional education.

The characters (pseudonyms) in the story we will encounter include:

- Robin is a recent graduate, now intern, at the clinic. She has been at this site for almost 1 year, first as a student working with her CI for half of that time, then graduating and becoming a licensed physical therapist, and now as an intern/new graduate at the site. Through this transition she has continued to work with the same supervising physical therapist who is now identified as her mentor in this early phase of her career.
- That mentor is Janet. Janet has been a therapist for 8 years and has worked for this organization since starting her career. In that time, she has completed an orthopedic/manual therapy residency and became a certified orthopedic manual therapist and is currently pursuing a manual therapy fellowship. Thus, she is both a mentor and mentee in this clinic.
- Bob is Janet's mentor for the fellowship she is completing. Bob is a therapist with decades of experience who serves as director of mentorship and fellowships within the organization and he will be mentoring Janet today.

We will also meet 2 patients, Katherine and Beth (pseudonyms) who will be introduced as they enter the story.

Act 1

As the observation begins, Robin welcomes her returning patient, Katherine, and escorts her back to a private booth. Katherine has been seen by Robin for approximately 2 months. She is a cash-paying patient. She is a dancer, yoga practitioner, and walker who values mobility but has been experiencing lower extremity malalignment and pain that has limited her desired function. As Janet sits in the booth and quietly observes, Robin asks Katherine about her current status and progress, does a brief manual check of her left foot and ankle, and both Katherine and Robin note improvements. She discusses her plan for advancing Katherine's program today and within 5 minutes they move to the gym area and begin standing functional activities with Robin providing tactile and verbal cues to facilitate dynamic arch support. During this time, Janet stands to the side and provides very brief and intermittent cues and once interjects to encourage Robin to shift her hand position slightly to facilitate muscle activity.

After about 10 minutes, the patient describes one exercise that she is having difficulty with and Robin, Janet, and Katherine move to the stairs to explore the step downs that are the culprit. Now the trio engage in 10 minutes of joint problem solving focused on movement as they tweak form and postural control strategies while verbalizing what they are doing and why, and explain how these strategies might be used during walking and in various yoga poses.

As the patient practices these new strategies and then rests, Janet calls a time out. She and Robin head to the computer to look at Katherine's current program and discuss possible deletions, additions, and progressions in her home program. Janet asks Robin several questions and pushes her to determine treatment priorities and specify those in addition to identifying desired frequencies, repetitions, and cues for performing exercises and activities.

Soon thereafter, Katherine joins Robin at the computer and they discuss new exercises, others that can be discontinued, and reminders or cues for when to do prescribed activities. During this exchange, Janet steps back and to the side to hand the lead back to Robin. As the session concludes, Robin asks Katherine if the current plan makes sense to her and if it is doable; the patient affirms this, and they agree on a return appointment in 2 weeks for a recheck.

Immediately following the session, Robin and Janet move to a booth for a 5-minute debriefing. The debrief starts with a familiar question for both, "How did that go?"

Robin self-identifies things that went well and sticking points especially around decisions regarding program progressions and adaptations. Janet reinforces some of the feedback she provided during the session and gives a few recommendations about specificity of questioning and cues for the patient. She reminds Robin to always consider "What does the patient absolutely need to be doing?" and what is non-essential, so that the patient can safely and effectively transition away from therapy to independent performance and pain-free function. The debrief session concludes with positive feedback to Robin, especially related to tying the program to desired activities for the patient, like walking and yoga.

Act 2

This observation and debrief was followed by an interview with Robin and then later Janet. Their comments provide insights about the nature of teaching, learning, and mentoring that was occurring in this session and throughout the time that Janet has been working with Robin.

Both Robin and Janet experienced a shift in the nature of instruction and degree of supervision over the course of the year: from closer supervision and guidance when Robin was a student, sometimes structured around activities such as completion of the clinical performance instrument, to participation as a new graduate/intern who is being mentored in her early professional career. In this organization, it is the expectation that all new graduates and employees are mentored; but for Robin these early months of the internship have consisted of several hours of formal 1:1 mentoring each week in addition to informal opportunities to engage around practice issues. The big shift occurred for both of them with the realization that once Robin was a licensed therapist, ultimately her patients were *her responsibility* and the patients were looking to her for guidance and quality care.

In addition, the last half-year has seen the introduction of a Clinical Reasoning and Mentor Case Report Form developed by education directors and staff in the organization to specifically develop and enhance clinical reasoning processes for all staff and for therapists in the residency program. The form provides a structure for therapist pre-thought or individual pre-briefs before bringing key clinical cases and questions to their mentor. The forms are completed and provided to the mentor prior to meeting to discuss the case. Both Robin and Janet have found that the use of the form often helps the mentee refine her reasoning process and answer her own questions. As Robin put it, "there have been several times when we never actually talked about [the case], but just writing everything down and organizing it in that way helped me to kind of reason through what I needed to do and then go in a different direction with the patient."

Another transition during this year for Robin and Janet has been the increased emphasis on engaging in evidence-based practice as an individual responsibility, in addition to being a shared and collective responsibility within the organization. Robin realized that one habit that she had in her life in general, and in clinical practice specifically, was that when seeking additional ideas regarding the management of patients, she would seek that information from others. Now, she says, "when I'm seeing a patient and I'm wondering about things…I don't just automatically think: 'I'm going to ask someone about this.' Instead, I immediately think, 'OK, I'm going to look this up. I'm going to see what the evidence suggests.'"

In discussing the observation session with Robin, she was easily able to reiterate the take home message from the session: "The biggest thing that I got today…is being really, really aware of making the therapy people are doing on their own, doable [and meaningful] for them or else it's not going to be therapeutic." Lesson learned.

Robin is truly grateful for the excellent teaching and mentoring she has received from Janet and felt that one of the things she has most benefitted from is her use of challenging and guiding questions as a teaching strategy. The constantly asking: Why? What are the goals? The hows? Not just do this, try this responses. She also felt it made a big difference that Janet is actively being mentored even as she is serving as a mentor. She is a mentee and a mentor. She exemplifies a love of learning and growing professionally and shares that desire through her excellence in and passion for teaching.

Janet confirmed this passion in our interview with her. She loves teaching patients, she truly enjoys teaching students, and mentoring staff and residents, and she loves learning and being mentored now as she is pursuing a fellowship. In fact, this commitment and passion is now being translated into a new developmental track within the organization, a mentorship track that will offer an alternative to, or supplement to, a leadership track for advancement of therapists within the organization. It will concurrently meet the demand and increasing need for mentors as the staff and number of residents grows within the organization.

Janet highlighted that she especially loves teaching and learning in the context of clinical practice: As she put it, "Being able to be in the clinic just makes things more relevant. If you learn something about a patient, with them right there in front of you, you're never going to forget that…I think being able to be there in the moment makes things so much more relevant. I think it's cool."

Act 3

A little later in the day, we observed Janet working with a complex patient while being mentored by Bob. The patient, Beth, was a returning patient for Janet with a long and complicated history of multiple types of headaches, cervical and thoracic pain, and vestibular dysfunction and symptoms. The latter of these concerns was still unfolding and being explored. In fact, when one of the interviewers asked Janet, "What are you seeing her for?" She said, "Well, how long of an answer do you want?"

The details of the entire session won't be described here, but it focused primarily on manual assessment and therapy of the upper quarter with close attention to the patient's verbal and non-verbal responses to treatment and the therapist's clinical observations as they proceeded through the session. Bob observed closely and only occasionally offered a brief observation, question, or suggestion to Janet.

The treatment session was followed by a 10-minute debriefing between Bob and Janet. It started with the question of the moment: "So much history with this, how do you differentiate some of that?" (ie, the multitude of symptoms and impairments) That question invited a cascade of thoughts and hypotheses that Janet had about the relationship between the physical findings, what she was feeling with her hands, the patient's history, and the nature and variability of Beth's symptoms. Bob listened carefully and affirmed her reasoning process with occasional observations of his own; observations that usually matched those of Janet. Interspersed with the observations and positive feedback came the questioning that pushed Janet to articulate her thoughts, reasoning process and actions for Bob: "Good to go over her exercises first when she's not too tired…What did you think about her form on most of those?" Janet and Bob then discuss this.

Later, Bob asks: "I was just wondering if it's maybe too much to have her neck in that position?" So collaboratively, Janet and Bob consider alternatives.

After one technique, the patient needed a period of quiet rest. Bob, who was less familiar with the patient, says: "You let her lie there for a while, which was great, and let her calm down a bit to see how things were going." Then he asks all-important questions: "What if she wasn't doing well? What would be your approach…Where would you take that?" Together they consider the possibilities.

The debrief session concludes with positive feedback on the management of this complex patient but ends with another thought-provoking question: "Next steps?"

Coda/Epilogue

Through this vignette we see many of the elements of the enacted, embodied curriculum in this rich clinical practice and learning environment and organization. We see patient- and learner-centering. We see multiple layers of teaching and learning, of mentoring and being mentored, in the context of clinical practice. We hear and see a focus on evidence in practice, with patients, as well as research literature, serving as sources of evidence. We see a focus on the development of sound clinical reasoning fostered some by curricular structure and tools, as well as pedagogical strategies of questioning, coaching, and guiding. We see dynamic and formative assessment of learners including patients, a recent graduate and intern, and a fellow. They are all learners embedded in a complex practice environment; they are learning *for* practice *through* practice, and collectively create a powerful teaching and learning community.

Envisioned Future for the Profession of Physical Therapy

There is no debate that physical therapist education embraces the centrality of integration of clinical practice, clinical cases and clinical experiences as critical to the preparation of physical therapists. A focus on learning for practice through practice, when done early in the curriculum, creates a scaffold for contextual and continuous learning—learning that sticks. While there is no single recipe for designing and implementing an excellent curriculum, the facilitation of the learning process through a true collaborative partnership between academic and clinical communities is non-negotiable.

The concept of learning for practice through practice is grounded in several robust learning theories on the power of situated learning and is supported by a rich body of educational research that spans many disciplines and professions. This concept provides an important goal for the profession and professional education. To realize this goal, we need to have a broader and deeper understanding of learning theories and the learning sciences to enhance, extend, and exploit the affordances and opportunities inherent in practice-based learning. Equally important, we need to better understand the constraints to learning in those environments so that we can address those as well. We need to consider whether prevailing models of content-driven, or model-driven, or structure-driven curricula, with an emphasis on formal knowledge, are the best way to prepare physical therapists of the future. Concurrently, we need to consider whether the predominance of physical therapist preparation programs that offer only entry-level education is in the best interest of our learners and profession. A community of practice and learners that includes professional and post-professional learners provides an opportunity for continuous reflection on and in the teaching and learning environment that is not available when only professional (entry-level) education is offered in academic or clinical environments.

CREATING ADAPTIVE LEARNERS

In professional education, we are not only preparing our learners to apply their knowledge and skills in practice, but more importantly, they are learning problem solving and clinical reasoning in uncertain conditions. Effective clinical reasoning and decision making in the face of uncertainty requires new learning, adaptability, innovation, and creativity. If we accept the premise that the goal of professional education is to prepare practitioners who become experts, then the premise of that education is fundamentally altered by our understanding of what it means to be an expert. Expertise is not a static concept, or something achieved at a given point in one's career; experts do not become so by years of experience or the gathering of credentials.[17,18] Rather, growth toward expertise is an ongoing, dynamic, and developmental phenomenon that continues across an individual's professional life. When expertise is viewed as a developmental phenomenon, theory and research suggest that expert clinicians move beyond what has been referred to as *routine expertise* to *adaptive expertise*.[9] Adaptive expertise is characterized by effortful and continual learning and innovative problem solving that is essential to practice in uncertainty.[7,9] Ongoing research on learning in professional education focuses on how educators can foster the development of adaptive learners. A focus on excellence and high expectations provides the essential, fertile ground for the creation of adaptive learners, especially when teaching and learning occurs in situations that mirror the complexity and uncertainly of practice. Adaptive learners engage in continuous learning, including situational and self-awareness and assessment, embrace feedback, adapt to and function in uncertain environments, reflect on and learn from unfolding experience, and incorporate new learning into practice.

A deeper understanding of the core concepts and underlying educational research on the development of adaptive learners is essential to the design of innovative and excellent didactic and clinical curricula. The evidence suggests that teaching/learning environments that embrace the discovery and use of evidence and explore and create experiences that facilitate learners' ability to manage decision making in uncertain conditions are more likely to prepare adaptive learners and thus promote the development of adaptive expertise. If one accepts that effective clinical reasoning must occur in the uncertainty of practice, then the development of students and therapists' clinical reasoning abilities demands well-crafted learning experiences that are grounded in established teaching and learning strategies based on what we know about how learning occurs in complex, often unpredictable environments. Learning about reasoning and thinking requires that the learner gains the metacognitive skills necessary for engaging in ongoing critical self-reflection. Teachers who are designing learning experiences through which learners gain these reasoning and metacognitive abilities must also exhibit these same attributes when reflecting on their own teaching, the learning environment, and their learners.[6,7,9]

We observed faculty promoting the developmental skills, attributes and dispositions that characterize an adaptive learner, particularly by placing students early on in situations where they can safely struggle with the complexity and uncertainty of practice. We also observed learning environments where the presence of teachers and learners at multiple levels of professional and post-professional preparation (as described previously in our discussion of practice-based learning) provided a learning context for fostering reflection and innovation in response to the inevitable challenges that arise in clinical practice. These individuals frequently exchanged feedback, engaged in mutual inquiry around challenging situations, and demonstrated reciprocal teaching and learning on a regular basis.

While the academic and clinical faculty members we observed demonstrated a basic understanding of the important aspects of the teaching and learning environment that facilitate the development of students' and residents' clinical reasoning skills, they did not all articulate or demonstrate a depth of understanding of the underlying pedagogical and critical learning concepts pertinent to most effectively creating adaptive learners.

Evidence From Academic and Clinical Sites

In the following quotations, some students and an intern describe some critical features of the learning environments in which they were embedded that contributed to their development as adaptive learners. The first quotation comes from a student completing an early integrated clinical experience in a faculty practice connected to the academic program in which she was enrolled:

> I'm in my first clinical rotation downstairs right now. It's the scariest, most stressful and rewarding thing I have ever done in my life. So, I have a new patient every half hour which is exhilarating. It's as stressful as it is…it's also almost stress relieving that I know once I go out and do externships and clinical rotations at other sites, I'm going to feel so much more prepared for having made mistakes while I was here but also for having professors and clinical instructors who knew exactly what we had in classes so far, what we should be expected to know, and how to go about expanding our knowledge base so that we could be evidence-based practitioners as we go out into the workforce.

One student with a background in education described how the structure and sequence of learning experiences in his program had helped him:

> …they employ spiral scaffolding…they use that idea throughout the 3 years in the units and they use their zone of proximal development, so they introduce terms. They put things at a space, a distance that you can reach and then return [to those terms and concepts]…at a greater intensity and details later on, and so I really liked that. I also liked that it's broken into 3-week segments, so they use chunking [of information].

Finally, an intern describes how her clinical teacher has pushed her to be a more reflective and adaptive learner:

I've always been much more confident in working and doing mobilization and teaching and hands-on things rather than sitting down and clinically reasoning through a patient case or reasoning through a plan of care and things like that. That's what's really helpful for me as having her there and asking me those questions of, "Okay. Why are you doing this? What is the goal of doing this?" Not just, "Can you teach this exercise?" kind of a thing. That is what [my instructor/mentor] has always done a fantastic job of when I was a student and now, later on, because she is being actively mentored, so she knows what works really well and what doesn't work well from an instructor kind of point of view. She has always done a really good job of challenging me and making me work a lot harder that way.

Academic and clinical faculty provided evidence of continual emphasis on deep learning and the ongoing assessment of learning so critical to facilitating the development of sound clinical reasoning and adaptive learners. In the following quotations we hear from both academic and clinical faculty how intentional they are in asking those second and third order questions to get insight into student's thought processes.

The depth of clinical reasoning. I think it takes a certain kind of person to form that bond and make the most of that kind of relationship, but it's the depth of clinical reasoning, it's the depth of knowledge, the design...It is a community of people that never take no for an answer...I need to learn more about this...
—Academic Faculty

We are direct with students...It is not a secret. We say "We are going to be looking at the skills you need for acute care so that psychomotor aspect. We are going to be looking at your knowledge base, cognitive skills that you have, what you know, related to acute care, how you are going to apply it. But probably most importantly we are going to look at your affective domain and how you are receiving feedback. —Clinical Faculty

I think the themes that are consistent, [in my teaching]...are trying to get a sense of what their thought process is and what their clinical reason is and why they're doing what they're doing. I think sometimes that is maybe more important than how they're doing what they're doing. Maybe their joint mobilization isn't the most effective or most skilled, but sometimes the why they're doing what they're doing is, I think, more important to kind of get at and help guide than the actual motor skills. Those will come with time, but if the reasoning skills aren't there, I think that's a bigger deficit. —Clinical Faculty

Paradigm Case: A Clinical Instructor With a Three-Track Mind

This case is drawn from our observation of a CI and a student who are providing care to a patient and his wife. The CI and student have been providing care for this inpatient for several weeks. The case illustrates the teaching strategies utilized by the CI, and the episodes of uncertainty experienced by the student. Following the observation of the treatment session, the researchers interviewed both the physical therapist and the student.

The gym is large and filled with numerous mat tables and exercise equipment, patients, family members, staff, CIs, students, residents, and mentors. The high ceilings help to dissipate the noise. The patient, Karl, is rolled into the gym in a wheelchair by his wife, Joanne (pseudonyms), and you are struck by their extreme differences: Joanne, petite and about 5'4"; Karl, well over 6' with a large frame, likely over 250 pounds. Karl is in his 40s and is recovering from a stroke, his right arm moving with the help of his left. He carries a knee splint in his lap. As Joanne speaks with Karl, you notice he has difficulty replying to her comments.

Cindy and Megan are sitting on a mat table waiting for Karl to arrive. Cindy, the CI, has 25 years of experience as a physical therapist and Megan, the student, is in her final 4 weeks of her first 4-month internship. Megan and Cindy have discussed a plan for Karl's treatment today that includes exercises to improve his walking and balance, and involves getting Karl onto a mat table on his hands and knees, with the goal of exercising his hip muscles and facilitating his right arm movements. Cindy agrees to let Megan direct the session, with Cindy acting as her aide, as it will clearly take 2 people to help Karl today.

Megan and Cindy greet Karl and Joanne, and Megan explains to Karl that they will start their session today with exercises on the mat table. Both student and CI guard Karl closely as he takes a few steps from his wheelchair to the edge of the mat table. Megan instructs Karl to place his hands on the mat and bring his knees up onto the mat. Karl has great difficulty performing this, while both Cindy and Megan support him. Megan tries several suggestions for Karl to place his knees on the mat table, but nothing is working. Gently, Cindy suggests that Megan lower the mat table to allow Karl to get his right leg onto the mat. This works and Megan proceeds to instruct Karl on his exercises. Karl struggles to maintain his balance while on his hands and knees, and Cindy invites Karl's wife onto the mat to help. Now Cindy is supporting Karl's left side, Joanne his shoulders, and Megan his right side. Megan instructs Karl to extend his right arm, and he repeatedly replies by raising his right arm off the mat, causing Megan to strain to support him. Cindy sees the frustration on Megan's face, the worry on Joanne's face, and again she intervenes to help Karl understand what to do. Cindy touches Karl's left arm, which is fully extended at the elbow, and asks Karl to make his right arm look like his left arm. Karl follows Cindy's directions, and Megan can proceed with her exercises. The tactful cueing that Cindy has given Karl has helped Megan correct her instructions for Karl, but Megan is losing her confidence in this treatment session.

After the treatment session with Karl ends, Cindy reflects on her teaching during this patient treatment session. She realizes that the plan Megan developed for this treatment session was challenging. Cindy says, "This morning, we put ourselves out on a limb. This is not something we've ever done before, and that's why I was very much a part of it because I felt like not only would Megan need some directions, but for safety reasons we would just have to be ready for anything. Karl is just a little bit impulsive. He thinks he knows what you want, and he doesn't always recognize what the consequences of a quick movement might be especially with regard to the right side. He has had some issues with falling out of bed when his wife attempted to transfer him. We're doing everything that we can to avoid any more incidents because they are such confidence destroyers."

Cindy reflects on Megan's performance in this session. "Megan kept telling Karl to extend his arm and he kept thinking that she meant reaching and she figured it out, but I gave some quiet cues to help him know that the elbow needs to be straight and underneath him. Sometimes knowing how to cue the patient is something that I find students need. With Karl, a lot of demonstration really works best and that's what Megan resorted to and it made a big difference. Megan's been here a while. With the simple patients, she anticipates well. With more difficult, impulsive patients when you are doing something new, you're not quite sure how [the patients] are going to respond...I think that's where experience just really helps because I'm able to anticipate a lot better, but I try not to just cue every step of the way."

As a CI, Cindy reflects, "...nobody likes criticism...students always feel like they're doing something wrong and it may not be wrong, but there might be a better way." Cindy noticed that Megan forgot to lock Karl's wheelchair while she was putting his splint on his knee. "It just makes sense to lock the wheel," Cindy muses. "There are times where I definitely would make a big deal out of something that was a major safety risk and I would do it but in private. Or, I would try to express this feedback through comments to the patient, for example, I would say to Karl, 'Karl, you have to make sure that you lock your wheels before you get up.' But even then, the student will hear this as a criticism. So, when I shift the feedback to the patient with a goal of providing it to the student, it gets complicated...It's like treating 2 patients when I have a student with me."

Megan also has some time to reflect after her treatment session with Karl. She is aware that it did not go as she had hoped and that Cindy had to provide more guidance than she expected. Megan says, "This happens to me a lot with Cindy because Cindy gives me the feedback before I get the chance to correct the patient or do it differently. I was just ready to put the mat table down when Cindy told me to do that." Every now and then Megan will ask Cindy if she could back off a little bit. "I appreciate just a little bit of space to flounder before Cindy jumps in" Megan comments. When she asks Cindy about this, Cindy seems familiar with that feedback from her former students, "every student has told me that!" Megan realizes that Cindy wants to get the best results for the patient, and she can many times provide less assistance than she does, which allows the patient to do things more independently. Megan reflects on a changed attitude toward Cindy's teaching methods. "I'd like a little more independence, but really, I've taken to looking at these situations as just an important mentoring opportunity."

Coda/Epilogue

In this case based on a field observation and follow-up interviews, we see a clear example of uncertainty in the patient, family member, and student; thus, the 3 tracks that the CI must safely manage. The CI was willing to take a risk with her student and patient, and she was confident that she could ensure the confidence and safety of the patient and the patient's wife. The clinician demonstrated her adaptive skills as various problems developed for the student, providing a model of unexpected but correctable outcomes. The clinician allowed the student to safely struggle with a complex activity, until support for the patient was clearly needed. Adaptive learners must learn to manage more than one safety concern at a time. For example, at one point, the clinician realized that the patient's wife appeared frightened, and so was asked to come onto the mat table to help her husband. The student may not have recognized the benefits of inviting the patient's wife to assist, while she tried to solve her current problem, but the clinician recognized the importance of this clinical decision.

Adaptive teachers and learners in a clinical setting like the one described in this case, have a golden opportunity to learn from one another and teach one another. In the interviews following the observation, both Megan and Cindy spoke of the importance of learning in the setting of uncertainty. The patient is impulsive and large in build, and these characteristics must be understood by both clinician and student. Cindy's values for patient primacy is quite evident, and she is willing to be clear on this with her student. This is teaching that allows the student to understand the value for professional commitment to patients. The student engaged in reflection after the session, identifying the errors she made. Megan, while at first concerned that Cindy corrected her during the treatment session, appears to have embraced the feedback she received and demonstrates her self-awareness. These characteristics set her on a path toward becoming an adaptive learner.

Envisioned Future for the Profession of Physical Therapy

Continued research on learning in professional education is an important knowledge base for all educators in the profession. A deeper understanding of the core concepts and underlying theory that helps us understand more clearly the development of adaptive learners is essential to the design of innovative, excellent didactic and clinical curricula. The learning environment embraces the discovery and use of evidence and finds ways to facilitate learners' ability to manage decision making in uncertain conditions. The development of students' and therapists' clinical reasoning abilities demands well-crafted learning experiences grounded in teaching and learning strategies that are supported by educational theory and research. The ability to facilitate the critical skills of metacognition demands an ongoing process of critical self-reflection by both learners and teachers.

Consistent with the profession's commitment to evidence-based practice, teaching and learning also needs to be evidence-based. The profession needs intentional development of physical therapist educational researchers who can provide such evidence for the profession and address urgent problems of learning in the profession.[19] Researchers need to understand and explore the teaching and learning strategies that best prepare adaptive learners who can assume responsibility for their learning through openness to feedback, self and situational awareness grounded in strong self-monitoring skills, and a lifelong commitment to learning. A central focus for faculty development activities should be on development of adaptive learners.

PROFESSIONAL FORMATION

Society recognizes that a profession and its members have access to a unique and complex body of knowledge that is not commonly held among members of the society and, when used appropriately, benefits individuals and society. Thus, society grants the members of the profession a great deal of autonomy in exercising that judgment. In return, society expects that the profession and its members place the best interests of the people they serve and society above those of the professional and the profession. The professions have a commitment to serve a public interest in what Colby and Sullivan call an *essential compact*.[20] Professional formation includes the important element of moral formation that prepares students for understanding their professional responsibility to serve and act as moral agents.[21-24] Moral agents have the responsibility to act on behalf of others and the discerning judgment to exercise that responsibility. Moral agency goes beyond the outward manifestations of professional behavior, such as dress, to the heart of a physical therapist's intention and responsibility to place his or her patient's interests first and to have a critical voice in protecting the most vulnerable in our society.[22,25] Acting on our societal responsibilities requires that health professionals go beyond moral agency at the level of the individual; it also requires that they work to remove social injustices that affect health.[22,23,26,27] Students need to be ready to take on the responsibility to meet the needs of society through advocacy, volunteerism, and participation in community- and population-based efforts that seek to improve health in communities and society as a whole.

Evidence From Academic and Clinical Sites

We found strong evidence from clinicians, faculty, and administrators about the centrality of professional responsibility and a commitment to the provision of high quality care for the patient in all that they do. Patient primacy and doing good on behalf of the patients we serve is viewed as a guiding principle for decision making and action. This principle is illustrated in the following excerpts from organizational artifacts or interviews conducted with a variety of participants:

All health professions are founded in response to the health care needs of individuals and society. Attitudes and beliefs about the quality of life, the nature of health and illness, and man's [sic] right to reach life's full potential are implicit in its philosophical tenets. As a practitioner in a healthcare profession, we seek to maintain, improve, or restore dignity and health through the delivery of quality clinical services. A pursuit of excellence, as well as a commitment to service and the helping process enables the clinician to function as an integral part of the health care team. In addition, it is the expectation of [Clinic Name] for all of its clinical staff to embrace and commit to lifelong learning and professional/career development. —Organizational Documents

Professional responsibility...I think when you are a dedicated clinician, regardless of the site, you have a responsibility to the next generation of clinicians and to the patients we treat and the best way to ensure excellent patient care is to excellently train students in the clinic. —Clinician

Patient-centered is a core value. If they are going out patient-centered and empathic and dedicated to...learning. —Faculty

One part of the soul is that we care about people and we care about each other...regardless of duties. —Program Director

All of our decisions really are based on patient care. It's always been patient care focused... —Clinicians

Because we want them [our students]...there are professional behaviors that we hold ourselves to, that we expect our students to have the same professional behaviors. It's not just professional but it's also spiritual and the nurturing portion of it. We just want them to be good people really that are caring, that are excellent not just clinically but also as part of customer service representative and as part of being a good soul, a good person. —Center Coordinator of Clinical Education

In addition to this strong evidence of a commitment to developing learners' professional identity and a sense of professional responsibility focused on the provision of high-quality, patient-centered care, we also observed many instances of community outreach and community-based activities at our academic sites. Even so, such activities often seemed focused on meeting curricular goals rather than meeting the profession's obligation to address larger societal needs.

Paradigm Case: The Power of Doing, Knowing, and Being

In this paradigm case, we see just how critical the clinical practice environment is for the learning and integration of students engaging in not only doing and knowing but also the critical dimension of professional formation-being.

Doing, knowing, and being, it all has to happen in the act of clinical practice. The voices of clinical administrators and clinicians in the clinical site described here expressed their strong, unified consensus on their commitment and responsibility for the development and formation of the next generation of professional colleagues. This means they held high expectations for members of the community in terms of their professional knowledge and performance as well as evidence of their commitment to acting as, being, a professional. When they bring new people into the community, they explicitly share these expectations. Involvement in clinical education is one of the expectations and is seen as professional development and formation for everyone, as seen in these comments from a focus group of clinicians:

> *Clinical education doesn't stop or start with students. It continues with the employees. If you can continue to educate someone who comes on board, they become a much better clinical instructor, so it's really constant what we do here, we are always going after more. We are always trying to prove the point...is what we do worthwhile, is it valid and then I think that gets passed down upon students when they come through.*

These professionals are involved in all aspects of education and learning from clinical practice, participation in research projects and ongoing special interest groups, and active engagement in state and national legislative work that affects the delivery of quality health care. One cannot be in this community of practice and not notice the passionate commitment of the physical therapists for preparation of the next generation. When asked why they participate in clinical and residency education, one individual in a focus group interview put it this way:

> *Professional responsibility, primarily. I think when you are a dedicated clinician, regardless of the site, you have a responsibility to the next generation of clinicians and to the patients that we treat, and the best way to ensure excellent patient care is to excellently train students in the clinic. And our organization and the different sites that we work in and the colleagues that we work with, I think helps towards our individual and group mission of providing the best possible patient care and outcomes that we can. It is not just an individual treatment sessionsession, but it is looking forward into the future and the best way to ensure that is to train students in an excellent fashion in the clinic. So, we take that mission, I think, very seriously. It is a responsibility that we all have. It informs our own practice. I think it makes our own professional life more of a rich experience. It pushes us in lots of different ways.*

When they hire new staff in this organization, or when they welcome students or residents, there are clearly articulated expectations for the provision of high quality patient care, along with the expectation that those new members of the community demonstrate commitment to their role and responsibilities as a professional. Among those responsibilities will be a teaching role in the future. Evidence of the success of this aspect of professional formation is seen in what residents say about their experience at this site:

> *They instill this in you when you're a student but I feel like physical therapy is a lifelong commitment as far as education and I think that you're doing your patients a disservice if you're not staying up on evidence-based practice, you're not up-to-date with the literature, and there's something to be said for years and years of clinical experience but there's also something to be said for understanding what's out there, what's the research showing. A combination of both, I think, is going to make you an awesome therapist and make you a more skilled clinician so that you can ultimately give better care, and I feel like that is not only wrapped up in this mentoring but also within this organization. It's instilled in you that you have to be up-to-date on what's going on—if you're not, you're really out of the loop because I feel like every therapist out there could tell you why they're using this special test, or why they're not using it, or what their rationale is or what their reasoning is and support it with some type, if you went out there and asked, some type of article...So, I feel like that's what I'm going to take from it [the residency program] and hopefully give back to the mentoring program in the future.*

Coda/Epilogue

The workplace and community of practice described in this paradigm case is a robust learning environment for learners as they interact with professional colleagues who demonstrate daily what it means to be a professional. We cannot underestimate how essential it is for our learners at all levels to be engaged in practice communities where professionals exhibit the moral foundation and associated responsibilities of their professional practice and are committed to imparting that to the learners. Evident in this case is the depth of commitment these clinicians express for having a role in preparing the next generation of physical therapists. Their enthusiasm for and willingness to take on this role is intertwined with a central and collective belief that learning never stops for members of this community. In this setting, therapists are intentionally engaging in learning experiences in which professional formation becomes a way of being as well as knowing and doing. There was also a strong presence of the importance of active participation in the profession and its association. What was absent in our observations at this site was evidence of a visible connection to the external community and the broader social responsibility of professionals. It might be that the opportunity to discuss this aspect of professional formation did not arise in our interviews or appear in the focused field observations we completed.

Envisioned Future for the Profession of Physical Therapy

Physical therapists continue to develop a strong sense of patient-centered care, with recognition of their moral obligation to place patient and client needs ahead of personal needs, thereby demonstrating an understanding of the meaning of being part of a profession in the realm of providing direct physical therapy services. This conviction can help physical therapists cope with the stresses that can be experienced when these obligations clash with the reality of practice. In the envisioned future, physical therapists also recognize their individual and collective responsibilities to society. This is demonstrated by continued involvement in professional organizations and by increased engagement with community groups and others to support and strengthen initiatives that promote the health of populations.

Academic institutions take leadership in extending the role of physical therapists in improving health across society and globally. This commitment to an expanded view of professional responsibility and moral obligation is reflected in the content of physical therapist education curricula, by intensified efforts of physical therapy programs to improve diversity in faculty and student body, and through the presence of programs that provide direct support to the community and society to enhance health. The power of the learning that occurs in the community of practice cannot be underestimated for the next generation of therapists. The strong temptation for the learner will be to focus on knowledge and skill with less attention given to the complexities of acting as a moral agent in uncertain situations.

The ethical obligations of individual practitioners to their patients has been a continual source of inquiry and focus in the health professions.[21] This focus is also reflected in physical therapy, through the Code of Ethics,[28,29] and the professional literature.[20,21,23,24] The professions have paid less attention to their obligations to society. Sullivan[21] speaks to this quite powerfully as he describes civic professionalization and the obligation of the professions to use their knowledge and skills to help those most in need and address social inequalities that lead to health disparities. We must remember and act upon the notion that professional schools are portals to professional life and that professional formation must be an intentional and shared commitment across academic and clinical environments.[20] Physical therapy's vision, "Transforming society by optimizing movement to improve the human experience,"[4] has the potential for the profession to fulfill that social responsibility.

Based on our study findings and drawing on literature, we developed recommendations and action items for the profession that address ways to advance the learning and the learning sciences in the profession across academic and clinical environments. Our recommendations and action items are discussed in depth in Part III (Chapters 8 to 11).

REFERENCES

1. Shulman L. Signature pedagogies in the professions. *Daedelus*. 2005;134:42-51.
2. Sullivan W, Colby A, Wegner JW, Bond L, Shulman L. *Educating Lawyers: Preparation for the Profession of Law*. San Francisco, CA: Jossey-Bass; 2007.
3. Shulman L. Excellence in education in the health professions: a critique. Session presentation. American Physical Therapy Association Combined Sections Meeting. Anaheim, CA, February 18, 2016.
4. American Physical Therapy Association. Physical therapist practice and the movement System. http://www.apta.org/MovementSystem/WhitePaper. Published August 2015. Accessed February 1, 2017.
5. Cooke M, Irby D, O'Brien B. *Educating Physicians: A Call for Reform of Medical School and Residency*. San Francisco, CA: Jossey-Bass; 2010.
6. Hafler JP, ed. *Extraordinary Learning in the Workplace*. New York, NY: Springer; 2011.

7. Schumacher D, Englander R, Carraccio C. Developing the master learner: applying learning theory to the learner, the teacher, and the learning environment. *Acad Med.* 2013;88:1635-1645.

8. Ambrose S, Bridges M, DiPietro M, Lovett M, Norman M. *How Learning Works: 7 Smart Research-Based Principles for Smart Teaching.* San Francisco, CA: Jossey-Bass; 2010.

9. Cutrer WB, Miller B, Pusic M, et al. Fostering the development of master adaptive learners: a conceptual model to guide skill acquisition in medical education. *Acad Med.* 2017;92:70-75.

10. Lave J, Wenger E. *Situated Learning: Legitimate Peripheral Participation.* Cambridge, UK: Cambridge University Press; 1991.

11. Wenger E. *Communities of Practice: Learning, Meaning and Identity.* Cambridge, UK: Cambridge University Press; 1998.

12. Wenger E, McDermott RA, Snyder W. *Cultivating Communities of Practice: A Guide to Managing Knowledge.* Boston, MA: Harvard Business Press; 2002.

13. Webster-Wright A. Reframing professional development through understanding authentic professional learning. *Rev Educ Res.* 2009;79:702-739.

14. Higgs J, Barnett R, Billett S, Hutchings M, Trede F, eds. *Practice-Based Education: Perspectives and Strategies.* Rotterdam, Netherlands: Sense Publishers; 2012.

15. Billett S. Situated learning-a workplace experience. *Australian Journal of Adult and Community Education.* 1994;34:112-130.

16. Shulman L. *The Wisdom of Practice: Essays on Teaching, Learning, and Learning to Teach.* San Francisco, CA: Jossey-Bass; 2004.

17. Bereiter C, Scardamalia M. *Surpassing Ourselves: An Inquiry Into the Nature and Implications of Expertise.* Peru, IL: Open Court Publishing Co; 1993.

18. Jensen GM, Gwyer J, Hack L, Shepard K. *Expertise in Physical Therapy Practice.* 2nd ed. St. Louis, MO: Elsevier; 2007.

19. Jensen GM, Nordstrom T, Segal R, McCullum C, Graham C, Greenfield B. Education research: visions of the possible, *Phys Ther.* 2016;96:1874-1884

20. Colby A, Sullivan W. Formation of professionalism and purpose: perspectives from the preparation for professions program. *University of St. Thomas Law Journal.* 2008;5:404-426.

21. Sullivan WM. *Work and Integrity: The Crisis and Promise of Professionalism in America.* 2nd ed. San Francisco, CA: Jossey-Bass; 2005.

22. Purtilo R. Moral courage in times of change: visions for the future. *J Phys Ther Educ.* 2000;14:4-6.

23. Purtilo R, Jensen GM, Royeen C, eds. *Educating for Moral Action: A Sourcebook in Health and Rehabilitation Ethics.* Philadelphia, PA: FA Davis; 2005.

24. Benner P, Sutphen M, Leonard-Kahn V, Day L. Formation and everyday ethical comportment. *Am J of Crit Care.* 2008;17:473-476.

25. Benner P. Formation in professional education: an examination of the relationship between theories of meaning and theories of self. *J Med Philos.* 2011;36:342-353.

26. Stone J. Saving and ignoring lives: physicians' obligations to address root social influences on health-moral justifications and educational implications. *Cambridge Quarterly of Health Care Ethics.* 2010;19:497-509.

27. Frenk J, Chen L, Bhutta ZA, et al. Health professionals for a new century: transforming education to strengthen health systems in an interdependent world. *Lancet.* 2010;376:1923-1958.

28. APTA. Code of Ethics for the Physical Therapist. https://www.apta.org/uploadedFiles/APTAorg/About_Us/Policies/Ethics/CodeofEthics.pdf. Published 2013. Accessed October 28, 2017.

29. APTA. Professionalism in Physical Therapy: Core Values. http://www.apta.org/uploadedFiles/APTAorg/About_Us/Policies/Judicial_Legal/ProfessionalismCoreValues.pdf. Updated May 8, 2018. Accessed October 28, 2018.

Organizational Context
Essential for Supporting Excellence

The final dimension of our model is developed from our observations of the organizational settings and the features in them that support excellence. It is seen as a base, representing the environment in which the other elements of the model are situated. This dimension of the model does not have individual elements, but it does address the critical structures and models and the resources in the environment that are foundational for transformation in both academic and clinical programs for physical therapist education (Figure 7-1).

FINDINGS ABOUT ACADEMIC PROGRAMS

As we described in Chapter 3, we selected a sample of academic programs based on pre-established criteria around the concept of excellence, but that also provided us with a range of program types that represents the breadth of physical therapist education programs.

Structures and Models

These programs were situated across the United States, with 3 in the Northeast, 1 in the Southeast, 1 in the Midwest, and 1 on the West Coast. They were based in a private institution focused on health professions education, a private institution with a liberal arts focus, large public institutions with research focus, and large private institutions with research focus (Table 7-1). Among the academic sites, there were as many models of how the physical therapist education program was organized within the institution as there were academic sites in our study. In addition to this structural variability, we observed curricular variability, including curricular type and the length and placement of clinical education (CE) experiences.

Jensen GM, Mostrom E, Hack LM, Nordstrom T, Gwyer J.
Educating Physical Therapists (pp 95-110).
© 2019 Taylor & Francis Group.

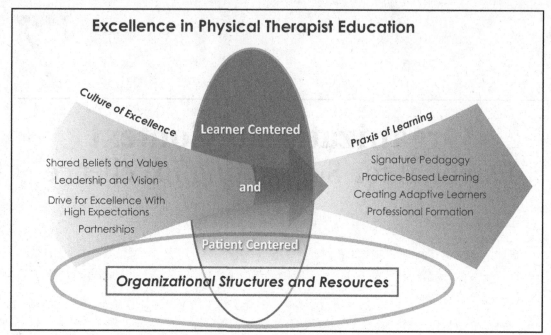

Figure 7-1. The organizational structures and resources dimension from the Model of Excellence in Physical Therapist Education.

While each structure brought unique challenges, the program's leadership provided skilled vision, leadership, and management that facilitated excellent, sustainable, and thriving programs. As we discussed in Chapter 4, shared leadership was one of the important values that was part of the Culture of Excellence. Academic faculty recognized that they played a role in leadership and that this role was respected and sought after by the leader. Within this shared leadership for the program, the formal leader took the prime role in securing the necessary resources to allow the program to flourish. As one administrative team member said:

> Supporting, advocating, including, informing, to helping us develop as faculty. I think that leadership provided lots of that incubator or nurturing, as well as a strength to move forward to higher administration and say, "Here's what we need." Or to be a voice out in the profession or a face at the table with directors from some of our clinical partners, large departments. It is a leadership that presents for us, but very much includes everybody.

The academic paradigm case in Chapter 5 illustrated the ways in which this leader navigated the institution's priorities and garnered resources for the program. We found some common factors in this leadership.

Acquisition and Management of Resources

The class sizes across our academic programs, which ranged from 55 to 94 students, were larger than the national average.[1] These larger class sizes provided the program with the finances necessary to acquire the intellectual resources needed to support faculty roles of research, teaching, service, and clinical care. As one faculty member said:

> I believe strongly that size matters and it didn't matter 40 years ago…would have 4 or 5 or 6 faculty who could teach physical therapy because physical therapy was a reduced discipline. Nowadays, it's a complex discipline. I don't think you can teach physical therapy with a faculty of 6 people…You can't just add more faculty and that automatically gives you better quality, but I think the reverse—I don't think you can have a quality program and have a small faculty. I don't think it's possible anymore.

TABLE 7-1

DEMOGRAPHIC DATA FOR ACADEMIC SITES AS OF VISIT DATE

ACADEMIC PROGRAM/ REGION	VISIT DATE	START DATE	CLASS SIZE	CORE FACULTY SIZE	RESIDENCIES	PHD PROGRAMS	INSTITUTION TYPE	LOCATION	CURRICULAR TYPE	CE TIMING/ PLACEMENT
1 Eastern	Mar 2013	1976	60	18 full-time 12 part-time	Orthopedics Sports Geriatrics	Biomechanics and Movement Science	Public, large, research intensive	Department of Physical Therapy College of Health Sciences	Traditional Systems-based	3 ICE experiences 7.5 months post-didactic work
2 Eastern	Feb 2013	1997	65 to 70	17 full-time 5 part-time	Orthopedics	Rehabilitation Sciences	Private, special-ized health sciences	Department of Physical Therapy School of Health and Rehabilitation Sciences	Case-based Systems-based	2 ICE experiences 5 months in 2 blocks within didactic work Year-long internship, 6 months after graduation
3 Eastern	Dec 2013	1984	60	14 full-time	Orthopedics	None	Private, masters	Department of Physical Therapy School of Medicine	Case-based using integrat-ed modules	8 weeks within didactic work 6 months post-didactic work

(continued)

TABLE 7-1 (CONTINUED)

DEMOGRAPHIC DATA FOR ACADEMIC SITES AS OF VISIT DATE

ACADEMIC PROGRAM/ REGION	VISIT DATE	START DATE	CLASS SIZE	CORE FACULTY SIZE	RESIDENCIES	PHD PROGRAMS	INSTITUTION TYPE	LOCATION	CURRICULAR TYPE	CE TIMING/ PLACEMENT
4 Midwestern	Jan 2014	1942	83	22 full-time 3 part-time	Women's Health Fellowship in Movement Science	Movement Science	Private, large, research intensive	Program of Physical Therapy School of Medicine	Traditional, systems-based	38 weeks in 4 blocks within didactic work
5 Western	Mar 2014	1946	94	25 full-time	Sports Orthopedics Neurology Pediatrics	Biokinesiology	Private, large, research intensive	Division of Biokinesiology and Physical Therapy School of Dentistry	Traditional, systems-based	Three 2-week blocks and one 6-week block within didactic work 32 weeks post-didactic work
6 Southern	April 2014	1960	55 (grow-ing to 75)	20 full-time	Orthopedics Sports Geriatrics	Rehabilitation Science	Public, large, research intensive	Deptartment of Physical Therapy College of Public Health and Health Professions	Traditional, systems-based	96 hours ICE 32 weeks within didactic work

ICE = Institute of Clinical Experience

Based on the categories used by the Commission on Accreditation of Physical Therapy Education.[1]

The larger class sizes also provided access to monetary resources to fund the programs' multiple needs. Increasing program size was an effective method used to ensure the program has the necessary resources to improve the quality of the program while also achieving economies of scale. The programs also sought other sources of revenue, such as grants and patient care services; these resources also complemented the mission of the program. A member of an administrative team commented:

And we've created revenue sources so that we could do new things. So, for example, raising to 60 students created a revenue stream that would pay for a portion of what the resources needed to train 60, and to allow us to have bigger space. It's not like we wait for someone to say, "Here you go," and then good for us. It's like we are fully engaged in designing the things that will allow us to have what it is that we really want. And the clinic is another example—you know, we have a hybrid system where some are on departmental funds, and some funded by treatments. So, if we created a new and innovative program that brought in more revenue, that money would be available to spend on whatever program that is.

Financial Autonomy

Another essential element found in these academic sites was financial autonomy over their own revenues and expenses, within the institution's overall financial system, whether a private or public institution. The institution in the previous quote, a public university, directly benefited from its increase in class size and knew that the financial benefits from innovative programs would, to some extent, accrue to the program. Another site, a private university, also proposed changes in revenue management, as described by the program director:

We actually proposed a budget with tuition which is no longer bound to [the] standard tuition rate of the university's graduate level and professional level tuition. We build in everything, so it has to be a self-sustaining program...

Negotiation

This financial autonomy did not occur automatically. Excellent programs sought necessary resources and negotiated access to these revenues to achieve their goals. Leaders were willing to negotiate for resources. These leaders saw negotiation as a better option than capitulating to demands for expansion without concomitant resources or than refusing to consider opportunities for growth. Successful negotiation occurred when the program was well positioned, recognized through faculty participation and integration across the institution, when institutional leaders understood the value of the program, and when the program leaders were respected. As a program chair explained:

Certainly, I think, as an administrator, it might be hard for the faculty to see always is the tenacity. You have to hang in there, right...You have to go back to the negotiation table until...You cannot leave money on the table...You have a deal, you go back on that deal until you got it all. I think you have to go for what...I always think that at the end of the day, I represent the department. If the department was promised money, then I'm going to fight for that with everything I got until that money is in. Being a Chair is a very...I see it as a privilege and an honor that you really representing a unit. I take that role very serious. I probably would be more willing to accept things if it was me, but, I think, as a department it's my duty. It's my responsibility to bring things back to department that belong there. I think that's my job. I was hired for that. That's my job.

Focus on Patient-Centered Care and Learner-Centered Education

While we did not identify a primary model for either the didactic or CE portions of the curriculum, we did see a focus on the critical ingredient of intentional, early, and continuous learning focused on patient care. We also saw a focus on learner-centered teaching. As another program director commented:

Another thing about the culture in the program is, I think, the soul of physical therapy remains central to us all. We have some non-physical therapist and we have some people who are staff or professional staff market-ing and all of those people have the soul of physical therapy in whatever way they can have it and I think what we've not done is embrace anyone who doesn't have the soul of physical therapy regardless of whether they're physical therapist or not. That makes for a much more cohesive organization. It makes for a commitment to the education students. It makes for a commitment to patients if they walk in the door.

Chapter 5 details our findings and interpretations of patient-centered care and learner-centered education.

Paradigm Case: The Value of Distributed Leadership

Each of the academic sites we visited displayed the characteristics described here. This case uses the organiza-tional dimensions that we encountered at one of the sites, Academic Site 1, to demonstrate the depth and breadth of our findings. This is a large public institution, with an emphasis on research. The Physical Therapy Department is 1 of 6 units in the College of Health Sciences, 1 of 7 colleges in the university. There are 17 core faculty, with 12 associated faculty. There is a management team consisting of the department chair, Director of the Doctor of Physical Therapy (DPT) Program, Associate Director of the DPT Program, Director of Clinical Education, Co-Director of Clinical Education, and Director of Clinical Services. The faculty use this structure to expand the roles of key leadership to assume responsibilities as the demands on the program change. The positions on the team change as the department changes, but the purpose of the group is to support shared decision making. Several faculty members referred to this leadership structure in our opening interview with the full faculty:

I do think there's a difference—and it really has to do with the decisions that get made, and the benefit—we have bigger negotiations and bigger things are coming down our plate, and I do think that's one of the reasons why we decided we wanted this structure, was so that everyone could speak from the value of something, and everyone didn't have to try to look at it from all sides all the time.

And the idea is that smart people all come together to one place to say, "Is this good for us?" And then we can debate it, talk about it, go back and check on some things—come back again. That's really the purpose, I think, of why we think this is important. And we've done some of that, we just haven't—we're doing it even from space, even from money. What if we get this money, where should we best spend it? Like, literally all those things are things we talk about as a group now, what's best for everybody.

The Department has been able to leverage its resources to meet its goals. Since its inception the Department has been housed in essentially the same space, but through creative management of the space, the faculty have been able to meet their goals, including growth in research activities and development of an onsite clinic. Again, from the introductory group interview:

How do you do all of that research in things that used to be a closet. How does that happen? The talk about [if] we broke down this wall in a bathroom, we can get another 2 feet for this office. It's amazing to me, the creativity that goes on to make excellence happen.

The Department has a long-standing history of federally funded research and has been able to negotiate that, in addition to direct monies to pay for researcher time, space, and equipment, funds have accrued back to the Department to support faculty release time, allowing expansion of the faculty.

But the faculty also recognized that more resources were necessary. Their current space limited their class size, so they negotiated with the university to increase from 36 to 60 students. The new revenues are to be used to support a move into much larger teaching, clinical, and research space, that is also collaborative space with other University departments. The faculty clearly see this as a negotiation, that gaining space may come at the price of changing the curriculum, and that they need to be deliberate about those changes to preserve excellence:

Remember, the reason we're going to 60...let's be clear...is yes, we want to produce the products, but now we've mortgaged ourselves.

The program director added:

I think the delivery model is going to have to be modified, as we get to these larger numbers. What we do now that we know works, and it's all of those secondary objectives that you don't realize you're getting the good stuff from, these presentation that you really don't want to lose, how are you going to get that otherwise...How are we going to really make sure that...and again, not just integrating acute care or musculoskeletal across the curriculum, that's just the one way, is that everything that comes together, and how do we pull it together, and look at all of the different threads and integration that we want, and make sure that at the end of the day, that they do have it all. We don't have all of that oversight, to be able to check all those boxes and say, in all these different curricular areas, we're positive that this is there.

Department leadership was able to read the broader organizational context and build support up and down the organization to advance its mission and gain support for its strategies. Importantly, Department leadership built trust throughout the University, but particularly with University leadership and that trust, coupled with tangible outcomes, has led them to be able to negotiate successfully to grow their programs. As one example, leadership anticipated how it could build respect for the program and thus have adequate resources distributed to it with a singular focus on building externally funded research. They did this while maintaining their focus on learning for clinical excellence, thus demonstrating program graduates were highly successful and serving their community. As another example, the Department leadership and faculty members also built strong relationships with other programs within the College of Health Sciences, particularly kinesiology and applied physiology and with the School of Nursing. The chair of one of the departments in the College provided good insight to the perspective about the Department in the University:

It seems to me as a non-physical therapist that the faculty have the appropriate stature in the field and I think that's important; it speaks well to the overall department and overall program.

I could guess why it's a strong program here. At least on campus I think how they stand out is not only do they run a very successful DPT program, but I really think the individual faculty and the strength of their research programs I think really stands out...That's a nice 1-2 punch with moving forward with a strong DPT and research program.

The one thing that I think they've also been able to do, and this is a little bit more of an outsider looking in, is my sense that they've really been able to leverage the PT clinic to be very successful. I think the PT clinic, I can only...I'm not involved in the DPT stuff but I'm sure that serves and helps that educational area. As well though, kind of the unique part I think it really supports, as best I can tell, their research agenda as well. I think they've done a real nice job, again outsider looking in of really (I'm not sure if leveraging is the right word) using the PT clinic to basically support the overall mission of the department. That mission I think could be broken into kind of the educational side and the research side.

Again, I don't know if it's unique across the country but here on campus having a clinic like that and a research program linked with the clinical program all kind of married together seems to me a very strong way of advancing the department and advancing departmental excellence.

I think there are few departments on campus that have a research-intensive culture as intensive as it is in physical therapy. I think this is really a live and breathe research intensive culture which I think is fantastic, which I think is great. I think other units are trying to...I wouldn't say catch up but I mean I think PT is really...I think that the faculty in particular and the program...and not just that they're kind of ranked number two but just in terms of the research culture here and the culture of getting grants and getting papers; it's very, very strong. I think there are a lot of units that look to PT as kind of a model.

Finally, this program demonstrates the patient- and learner-centeredness that we saw across all our sites. One way they demonstrated this was the presence of a highly integrated clinical practice within the department. The practice was managed by clinical faculty and provided early CE and residency programs. The practice also provided a revenue stream for the department. The concern of the faculty for keeping patient care and learning centermost was evident in their teaching, their clinical care, and their research, but particularly in their recognition of the value of integration of all 3 of these endeavors. A member of the administrative team said:

Because we would still have an excellent program, I would hope, and an excellent clinic, and excellent research. So, we'd be excellent in parts, but collectively excellent without the cohesion of leadership or being professionally excellent? Like, where is our spot within the bigger profession? And I think that that's the ultimate impetus for us is, we think we're good as a group, but where [are] we in the bigger whole, and what is our research contributing to the profession? And what is our education doing to patient care and our clinical practice? And so, we look beyond ourselves to [be] bigger.

This case is illustrative of the leadership and creativity that we found at all 6 academic sites that we visited. The leaders, and all faculty, at all sites demonstrated an understanding of the important place their programs hold in the profession and in their institutions. This was reflected in their commitment and the energy they displayed in describing the organizational characteristics of their programs.

FINDINGS ABOUT CLINICAL PROGRAMS

As with the academic programs, we selected a sample of clinical programs based on pre-established criteria around the concept of excellence, but that also provided us with a range of program types that represents the breadth of CE institutions participating in physical therapist education programs.

Structures and Models

These programs were situated across the United States, with 1 in the Northeast, 1 in the Southeast, 1 in the Midwest, and 2 on the West Coast. They were based in large rehabilitation hospitals with multiple outpatient centers, an orthopedic outpatient practice that is part of a large acute care hospital, a large practice providing multiple levels of care within a large urban medical center, and a physical therapist owned practice with multiple small practice sites. These sites represented variability in location, type of care, and size of practice (Table 7-2).

We persistently questioned how clinical organizations assessed and managed the cost of CE and whether the participants saw any barriers to participation in CE. What we found is a mission-driven commitment to CE founded on a deep commitment to preparing the next generation of physical therapists. The most common cost-benefit analysis of CE was more qualitative than quantitative and considered a range of tangible and intangible benefits, such as recruitment, development, and retention. As one clinic administrator commented:

It's been years since we've had any issues with staffing and recruitment because of our strong student program...We talked earlier that many of our students become our employees. Right there you have the benefit of not spending lots of time and energy on recruitment, on orientation. We feel like we have this built in flow of employees coming from students to becoming our employees. That's a huge cost savings.

The clinical agencies did focus on their financial status but, without exception, they did not have evidence suggesting the CE program negatively affected their financial performance. One clinical site developed a financial model for the cost of their CE and residency programs. When they tested that model, they found that these programs had a neutral to positive effect on their financial performance. Because clinical programs saw CE as central to their mission, they integrated the cost of CE into their core operation. They were sufficiently satisfied that the CE program did not have a negative effect on their financial performance, and they did not need to examine the cost in precise detail.

The clinical agencies most often used team-based methods to manage the cost of CE and therapist productivity. Commonly, they considered the student and clinical instructor (CI) as one unit for measuring productivity and they examined the productivity of the larger physical therapy team, of which the student and CI were members, as the other unit of analysis. They monitored productivity over longer periods of time vs daily. Another clinical administrator stated:

TABLE 7-2

DEMOGRAPHIC DATA FOR CLINICAL SITES AS OF VISIT DATE

CLINICAL PROGRAM/ REGION	VISIT DATE	TYPE OF SETTING	# OF SCHOOLS	STUDENTS PER YEAR	RESIDENTS	FELLOWS	# OF THERAPISTS AND CLINICAL SPECIALISTS
1 Eastern	Oct 2012	Inpatient Outpatient academic medical center (~2500 beds)	27	30	2	N/A	300 physical therapists 104 specialists
2 Midwestern	Nov 2012	Inpatient rehabilitation (96 beds) Outpatient rehabilitation	36	36	2	N/A	69 physical therapists 16 specialists
3 Southern	April 2014	Inpatient rehabilitation Outpatient rehabilitation Institute of higher learning (157 beds)	25	110	16	4	136 physical therpists 31 specialists
4 Western	Mar 2014	Outpatient Part of a 515-bed community hospital system	7	30	2	N/A	18 physical therapists 14 specialists
5 Northwestern	Aug 2014	Outpatient (80 clinics) Private practice (visited 2)	83	150	3 to 6	0 to 4	8 physical therapists 5 specialists (at sites visited)

From an administrative perspective, because we have such excellent clinicians, the productivity dip that may occur in the initial phase of having someone who is taking more time to understand what's going on is really not so apparent, because the excellence that comes out of that in the end is really so worthwhile that it's compensated for in a lot of different ways.

Paradigm Case: Clinical Education Culture, Costs, and Complexities

Each of the clinical sites demonstrated the characteristics described previously. We will use one of the sites, Clinical Site 3, as a case that exemplifies these characteristics. This institution is a non-profit organization with multiple types of rehabilitation services: a 157-bed rehabilitation hospital, 27 outpatient facilities, home health care, assisted living, and a skilled nursing facility. The institution has created an education division offering continuing education in all areas of rehabilitation for its employees as well as the outside professional community, residency education, fellowship education, and CE experiences for students from all disciplines within the system. The institution offered American Board of Physical Therapy Residencies and Fellowships credentialed residency programs in orthopedics, women's health, neurology, and geriatrics at the time of our visit and has since added pediatrics and sports residency programs. They also offer an American Board of Physical Therapy Residencies and Fellowships credentialed fellowship in orthopedic manual therapy in collaboration with a nearby university with a physical therapist education program. In addition, the organization has a clinical research center, begun in 1999 in collaboration with the leading physical therapist education program in the state. The research center has an array of active clinical trials and other research studies focused in stroke, traumatic brain injury, spinal cord injury, orthopedics, Parkinson's disease, chronic pain, musculoskeletal conditions, and aging.

This institution has CE for the professionals practicing there at the very center of its mission. For example, their values statement is, "Excellence in Care, as demonstrated through innovation, integrity, service, compassion, teamwork, accountability, and continuous learning." One of the 5 goals in their strategic plan was, "To attract, develop, and engage the highest caliber workforce who choose to dedicate themselves to providing and supporting world class rehabilitation."

The CE mission is:

The [institution's] intern program will create an excellent clinical learning experience for the students that perform clinical internships within [institution name].

The CE philosophy is:

All health professions are founded in response to the health care needs of individuals and society. Attitudes and beliefs about the quality of life, the nature of health and illness, and man's right to reach life's full potential are implicit in its philosophical tenets. As a practitioner in a health care profession, we seek to maintain, improve, or restore dignity and health through the delivery of quality clinical services. A pursuit of excellence, as well as a commitment to service and the helping process enables the clinician to function as an integral part of the health care team. In addition, it is the expectation of [institution] for all of its clinical staff to embrace and commit to lifelong learning and professional/career development.

With this intent, the focus of the [institution] student intern program becomes dynamic and diverse. The educational process involves active, responsible participation by both clinical instructor mentors and students. Through an exemplary quest for professional skill in educational and professional practice, the clinical instructor mentors become role models and guides. The student must also accept responsibility to develop and grow professionally to the full extent possible. We believe the combination of experience, scholarship, and opportunity embedded in the [institution] student intern program will enable the students to assume responsibility for the health care needs of individuals and society. For these reasons, the [institution] student intern program is committed to promoting a respect for human dignity and a quest for excellence. The curriculum is designed to impart to the student the requisite knowledge, skills, and attitudes necessary to function as a clinical and professional leader within health care.

The decision to create the education division is an example of a tangible commitment to education. The director of the education division described the process:

...through conversations with PLO as well as my boss, who is the vice president and administrator of the hospital, we talked about the opportunity of what we could do beyond this Clinical Education Department by turning it into what we call the [education division]. Philosophically, there's a big, big difference, so logistically, everything that was in clinical education just shifted over into the institute...That didn't take anything. But philosophically how the institute is now viewed, instead of being a department underneath the corporate structure of [institution], now the [education division] is another division of [institution]...[There] are 4 clinical operational divisions and then we have the [education division], which is the division of [institution], dedicated to clinical learning and professional development.

By creating this activity explicitly as a division, with status equal to the 4 clinical divisions, there is an explicit message of education's centrality to the mission of the institution. Leadership's vision, willingness to change, and an emphasis on teams and shared leadership play important roles in developing the education program at this institution. That leadership considers the multiple benefits to a myriad of stakeholders. That culture of looking not only at the benefits to the individual, particularly as it relates to learning, practice, and advancing excellence, but also at the benefits for the system is promulgated by the institution's leadership, as described by the director of the division:

We look for opportunities to learn and we look for that concept of continuous lifelong learning. Everybody's on that quest to continue learning, to continue to try and make themselves better as individuals but make the system better. It's not trying to make any one person better. It's really how can we make everything better. We spend a lot of time, a lot of my time is spent on professional mentoring and helping people move along their path and a lot of that is working on trying to get people to come back in and do more things. A lot of programs that we have are being performed by past residents and fellows.

All of these core documents reflect both patient- and learner-centeredness as the focus of the institution and its programs, with a clear recognition of how they are linked. A clinical administrator said:

So, there's really a need to build a culture that is the same across all our settings and that there are standards on how we approach treatment. So, it's through the institute of higher learning and the next evolution is we're building system clinical advisory panels (SCAPS), that are going to be facilitated through the institute... Members of every setting will be at those councils with the whole idea of using what we've learned in the demonstration projects and how successful and how much better the outcomes are when we look and transfer our care approach, our treatment, so that there's some core standardization among our different conditions.

The leadership also creates a culture in which they are focused on tangible outcomes, such as building and improving residencies or CE, while also having the purpose of simultaneously building and creating teams. Once again, as the director of the division describes, there is a culture in which what occurs, and the outcome is something bigger than any individual:

It's the culture that we have created of going back to the very, very beginning, the very first residencies, people understood that this was a group effort, and this was a team we were building...We weren't doing one class and, unlike medicine and maybe some of the other programs where the residents come in and they are there for a year and then they go off and go someplace else...Those [residents] that did come in from the outside, by the end of the year, they all want to stay...They get it that it's not about just being here for a year. It's about developing something, creating something that's bigger of any of us individually and the teamwork and the camaraderie that any of them can call me at any time.

A clinic administrator adds:

To work here, there is a citizenship or a stewardship or a contribution that you owe the organization that you're working in. It's not just 9 to 5...it's that you're part of the [institution] system. You are going to contribute...They don't have to all be leaders, but they have to have passion.

The leadership of the education division has a clear idea about how to continuously grow and improve the program through developing the people in the organization:

I think that early on, as we're building our system—Because again, we're still in our infancy. We're not where we need to be, and we're not where we're going to be 5 or 10 years from now. But for today, as we're building the system, and building the infrastructure, and building...probably most importantly the people. And getting them to have the expertise to be able to manage students...There's going to come a point when people start developing and acquiring more skill, where then the next step to...the CIs' professional development, is start having some weaker students...That will help them, quite frankly, obviously...That I start off and we're going to train them and get people to a certain level. Then when we get the critical mass of people to that level, then we can change the rules a little bit and we can bring on a bigger variety of students. And when we get comfortable with that, then...acquire the skill to work at that level, then we can continue widening that group so that at some point in the future there won't be restrictions on the students that we take. And we'll be willing and able to handle virtually any student that comes here.

There is recognition that the institution's commitment to CE, residency education, and research means resources are available for these functions. As part of planning for expansion of CE programs, the director of the education division prepared a series of detailed cost and income scenarios. These scenarios were used to design a program that was able to maximize both quality and revenue.

At the same time, the clinical educators are aware of their obligations to the patient care enterprise. As the residency director said:

I personally feel like we live in a vacuum and what we do is special because we have resources, we have a budget and we have [the education division director]...How do you take this type of program and move it into a large hospital system that doesn't have the same amount of resources...You really have to show that what you do assist with operations whether it's outcomes or filling positions...I am very much aware that there are settings that don't have these kinds of resources that we do. I think that's the first answer to the question is how can you make a program facilitate operations. Because the bottom line is we provide patient care, that's really what we do in this organization...I think that's one piece to this is that if you're going to do clinical education you have to make sure that you're allied with, in alliance and in line with the operators.

Within this context of having abundant resources, there is an eye to the overall institution's financial performance and a clear statement of the net revenue margin they can achieve. With that margin comes a realization of how critical it is to manage well, as the director of the education division stated:

We're a not-for-profit. We're not looking to generate excessive revenue, but we have to keep the doors open. We have to deal with a limited reimbursement world. For us, because of trying to be realistic and reasonable with our patient management on the outpatient side, I think our productivity requirements are really soft, compared to the industry standard. Our average PT in outpatient, orthopedic outpatient, will see between 12 and 14 patients a day, that's their productivity requirement. I talk to friends around the country and, depending where they're at, it might be 17, 18, or more a day that they're seeing. That's fine. Whatever it is, it is, for those different groups. Ours is 12 or 14, and so our margin for outpatient is somewhere between 1% and 3%. We don't have any room for error. We want to promote and provide a learning environment for everybody here, whether it's students or clinicians, but we have to be realistic, given the financial situation right now. When I hear that in 6 months the productivity level of the student is a break-even point, then that excites me. From turning around, at that point, I see it as a win-win for everybody. I'm just sharing that from a clinical or from an algorithm standpoint how we're making decisions about who we're going to partner with, that's one of the questions that we ask...One of the questions is, how long are your clinicals, and if they say it's 8 weeks then we probably don't go much further. I'll ask a follow-up, "Do you have any intention or plans of expanding that and going further?" If they say no, we're really happy with our long term being 8 or 10 weeks, then we're not going to move forward and develop a relationship with them. That's just one of the criteria we're using right now.

This is further documented in the student handbook:

There are clear norms for student productivity throughout the internship. The CI and student share a caseload and the student's responsibility for that caseload progresses to full responsibility for the case load over the clinical experience. On an inpatient rotation, the shared caseload does not exceed 100% of the physical therapists' case load whereas in outpatient, the shared team will reach 150% of the PT case load by the end of the internship.

This last quote demonstrates the role that clinical sites can play in shaping the form of CE. As the people at the actual site, directly observing the impact of education on patients, staff, students, and the institution, they are in the best position to determine the appropriate pattern and structure of CE.

The staff at this institution realizes that the financial gain to the institution is in long-term issues such as recruitment and retention. They are also strategic about the academic institutions with which they partner; these partnerships must be directly related to their goals for developing their clinical programs, including their residencies. The Residency Director commented:

I think you have to look at the long term, I mean I really think in the beginning it does affect operations but once you get a good CI in entry level education, once you get those higher level academic institutions knocking on your door to send students, then all of a sudden you get a great group of students that you're working with. Then those great group of students want to stick around because they want to be in your residency and then those residents want to stay. In the long term, 3, 5 years later you're in a really sweet spot as an operator and I feel like we're finally there. There's always attrition, always people have babies, people move, you know, those types of things but we just don't have the promise filling positions like we did even 3 years ago, 4 years ago.

It is a long-term investment in that, you can't sell it right away, there's going to be some up front cost to it. It's been interesting to watch it grow because when we started we weren't excellent, we weren't excellent and so how we got more excellent I don't know—maybe you can help me figure it out.

Yeah, no. I'm sure we spend a lot of money but what we have seen in the last ten years is a rate of attrition decline within our clinicians. We don't have open positions like we did 4 years ago. We have people clamoring because in my resident's case at the end of the year they are out of their job. They basically are here for a year and then they are done and every year I have the problem of trying to find places for these highly trained, wonderful people. Then of course I have the crew who wants to get a job with [Clinic] so that they can get into the residency. I always look at it from an operator's kind of hat because I was operator for many years—is I think what we've done and strive to do as a residency is assist operations.

Not only are there specific strategies for the types of clinical experiences and the academic institutions, but they engage in strategies that minimize the impact a student has on productivity and clinical practice. As an administrator describes it:

...at one of our clinics where the staff is residency and fellowship trained, they're running a 2 students per 1one clinician model. Like (PT) [Physical Therapist] said, it's had quite the opposite effect [not a revenue loss]. We're only taking a particular level of student in our final clinical internship. These fellows, they have such a quick and precise decisions process that they can manage two students and work through them and still be able to have that student work 1-on-1 with a particular patient, but they're going back and forth between each patient, performing hands on and education. Then they are bouncing back and forth between the two students, it's definitely had quite the opposite effect for us. Now we've had it before in the past when we've taken first year or first clinical, and that's gone the opposite way. They're not grasping basic concepts and the therapist has to take all this time out to educate them on the process...We're taking them from specific institutes as well. So, it's not just a shotgun approach. It's definitely had the opposite. We know of other organizations in the community that utilize students purely based on the impact that it has on their clinic, in the wrong manner. So, they can staff it very, very well with students, but we prefer to have that well balance of education as well as productivity. That productivity is a plus for us, a bonus.

An important element of the institution's CE program is their relationship with the academic institutions. This institution demonstrates the best of the partnership between a CE site and academic education site. The director of the education division commented:

I guess a strong program, a better word might be more a better partner in terms of who we are and how we can cooperate with each other. Our philosophy here is that we don't want to be a dumping ground for universities to take on their clinical education. We want to be a partner with the universities, to carry out clinical education, which means that when curriculum development comes around, we want to be, at some point, at the table. Being an equal partner with them for the education of those students. Some programs don't really see that as a model, and don't have that as something they want to work towards, and some programs do. I think those are the programs, that would be a better way of saying it in terms of strong programs would be strong, meaning that we have a similar philosophy, core values, and desires of what we want to accomplish as a result of this relationship. I guess that's how I would address that. The closest we're getting to that right now, and this is long term expectation, is what we have with [a local physical therapist education program] moving towards being a partner where we have representation at the table when it comes to curriculum review, development, and assessment. Not that we're there yet, but I think we're moving in that direction. That's really what we're looking for.

The therapists at this institution have reflected on the needs of the profession, our patients, and the current state of CE:

Like probably a lot of people, we think that clinical education has lots of opportunity for improvement. This is my personal bias and perspective, I don't believe that the system is working right now. That there's a disconnect between what the universities are teaching, and what the clinical entities are providing, and that gap has to be closed. The way, at least from my perspective, is that we're going to close that gap by bringing the groups together. We started off with whatever that end was, that's what it was. Then we said, let's cast a bigger net, let's work with more people, more universities. Part of the decision making with that, part of our decision making to who was going to even work with at all was, we would put those out there and say, "Is this something that sounds feasible and reasonable to you?" If they said yes, then we can move forward.

That's where I think there needs to be a joint partnership between the clinical and academic environments. If there's not, then we pretty much continue to perpetuate this dysfunctional arrangement, where students are going out and being dumped into clinical arrangements. Regardless of how good the preparation at the academic institution is, it's always going to be limited by what happens out in the clinic.

Between the programs and the clinical entities where the students are doing their clinical education. It's a black hole. Universities do such a great job of developing syllabi with beautiful objectives. They have beautiful curriculum, and everything is sequenced, and they tie everything together. Then, all of a sudden, clinical education comes. And it's just like—Be gone, be gone! Good luck, little birdies! They all just go out, and they fly around, and they flutter. Some of them do really, really well because they were going to do well anyway, regardless of where you put them. Some of them struggle, not because there was inherently wrong with them, but it was just a bad fit and it didn't work. Some of them maybe aren't such great students because of lots of reasons. Nobody did anything about picking that up, trying to match them, and doing good things with them.

I think the disconnect in my mind, visually, is so strong. This disconnect between what's taking place in the clinical education sites and what's happening in the university. Being having worked on both sides, actively, and I've learned that not from being on this side, I learned it from being in the academic side. We would send our students out and do beautiful training. We'd teach them what we felt was the best evidence, and the best things, and they'd go out into clinics and the horror stories we'd hear back about what they were learning and how they were trying to integrate information. The worst part about it was, they looked at those guys and said, "They're the ones doing it, so they must know what the hell they're doing," and they would go down and become the lowest common denominator. They would end up doing what they learned in their clinical education part. It was like, "You're killing me here! Here I am, I spent, do you know how much blood, and sweat, and tears I put into this to teach you that stuff and train you up? Then you go out and you work with this knucklehead, and you start doing what they're doing? You're killing me here!" I've seen that every year, over and over again. From my standpoint, that's the biggest problem that we have. That the academic institutions have no...I don't think it should be a control issue, because I don't think that's correct. It's not the opportunity for it to even be that. That's why I really think that it's got to be a partnership. There's got to be a strong collaborative relationship between the clinical entities where the students are doing their rotations, and the academic institutions. Where the two of them have a mutual agreement. This is what we're trying to create, this is how we're going to go about doing it, and this is the effort that we're equally going to put into this.

This case serves as an exemplar for all the clinical sites we visited. We found clinicians who recognized CE as central to their mission as patient care is, perhaps because they saw the inextricable link between CE and patient care. They understood that CE improved patient care and enhanced recruitment and retention in ways that made CE economically successful. And they recognized their role as equal partners with academic sites in making educational decisions about curriculum and students.

Envisioned Future for Physical Therapist Education

The organizational structure of academic and CE provides the base on which the Culture of Excellence, focusing on patient- and learner-centeredness, leads to development of the Praxis of Learning. As we saw in our research, excellence is supported by an organizational environment characterized by shared leadership that is mission driven, with a commitment to maintaining adequate resources. Programs were willing and able to think creatively about revenue generation. There was a prevailing recognition that developing strong relationships within and without the institution is essential to achieving excellence. At academic centers this was focused on relationships with other units in the university; at clinical sites, internal relationships were important, but there was also the recognition of the importance of the partnership with academic sites.

For physical therapist education to thrive and excel, the academic and CE programs engaged in physical therapist education, while displaying a diversity of curricular models and organizational structures, need to adopt collective recommendations that arise from our research. There is no substitute for highly skilled leaders who can navigate the complex organizational structures and dynamic environments of professional education in every setting in which physical therapist education occurs. These leaders must also maintain a sustained commitment within their program and from their institution to fulfill the profession's public purpose and core aims. These leaders must surround themselves with engaged, dynamic professional colleagues in a vibrant community of practice focused on learning and excellence. In addition to using economic models for revenue generation through multiple means (eg, tuition, development, grants, clinical revenues), the programs must be respected, valued partners within their organizations and have influence over their resources. These leaders and educational researchers must have access to a national data set that includes essential metrics of performance outcomes, structures, and processes of physical therapist education that can be used for meaningful research and to guide evidence-based improvement in physical therapist education. We spoke with many academic leaders outside of physical therapy during our site visits. They confirmed that the programs in our studies were in institutions with reasonable and high expectations of the program. Generally, we also heard that there was effective leadership at the school or college level. We recognize that not all programs experience effective leadership at the school, college, or institutional level, yet the program must find a way to flourish and prepare physical therapists who can contribute to the profession's vision.

The profession has been too focused in dialogue and debate about seeking a single best educational model and in defending personal perceptions of the best models. There are physical therapist educators who are implicitly engaging in educational practices that are not supported by evidence, admittedly because often there is none, and thus, are often tradition or trial and error or empirically based. Many physical therapist education programs are under-resourced; when coupled with a belief that small classes are in some way better, programs are not able to achieve important goals for excellence. Other physical therapist education programs are being used to financially support the academic institution's financial position, thus siphoning a greater percentage of the program's revenue to the institution. Control of the program's resources often does not lie with the program's leadership and too often the ability to advocate for and accrue additional resources is limited by the abilities and the will of the leadership within the program or at the institution. Often clinical sites use arbitrary and sometimes unduly high productivity standards in assessing the economic impact of CE, without considering the benefits to the organization and the profession.

Our recommendations for this dimension will be discussed in depth in Chapter 10. In addition, we have developed action items for the profession related to the organizational dimension, discussed in Chapter 11.

REFERENCE

1. Commission on Accreditation of Physical Therapy Education. aggregate program data, 2016–2017 Physical Therapist Education Programs fact sheets, CAPTE, 2017. http://www.capteonline.org/uploadedFiles/CAPTEorg/About_CAPTE/Resources/Aggregate_Program_Data/AggregateProgramData_PTPrograms.pdf. Published 2017. Accessed September 4, 2018.

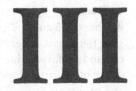

Transforming Physical Therapist Education
Accelerating Positive Change

In Part II, we presented the Conceptual Model of Excellence in Physical Therapist Education and the findings from our study that led to and support that model. In Part III, we delve deeper into the meaning and implications of our findings for the future of physical therapist education. We do so by considering our findings in light of literature and evidence from other health professions and disciplines; this expanded perspective can enrich our understandings of how we might further promote excellence in physical therapist education in the 21st century. Working from our model, study findings, and the insights provided by the investigations and experiences of others, we formulated 30 recommendations that we believe have great promise for facilitating positive change in physical therapist education.

Collectively, Chapters 8, 9, and 10 present the 30 recommendations that we believe have the potential to transform physical therapist education. The recommendations discussed in these 3 chapters can be acted on largely at the level of individual academic and clinical faculty and physical therapist professional and post-professional education programs in both academic and clinical settings. Each of the chapters shines a light on one of the 3 major dimensions of our model: the Culture of Excellence, the Praxis of Learning, and Organizational Structures and Resources. The recommendations discussed in each of the chapters are directly linked to the model dimension and the elements that comprise it.

Chapter 8, "Creating a Culture of Excellence", builds on the evidence presented in Chapter 4 where we described the beliefs, values, and behaviors that contributed to cultures of excellence in physical therapist education. The 4 elements we observed, shared beliefs and values, distributed leadership and a clear vision, a drive for excellence with high expectations, and vital partnerships, are discussed in relation to the need for changes in each of these elements. In Chapter 8, 8 recommendations for enhancing physical therapist education are presented in addition to a series of reflective questions. The reflective questions are raised to help individuals and programs thoughtfully examine their current practices and imagine (or re-imagine) how they might facilitate positive change within themselves and their organizations.

Chapter 9, "Advancing Learning and the Learning Sciences", builds on the evidence described in Chapters 5 and 6. The focus in this chapter is on the 4 elements in the conceptual model dimension, the Praxis of Learning: signature pedagogy, practice-based learning, creating adaptive learners, and professional formation. In this chapter, a total of 15 recommendations are presented and distributed across these 4 elements. Once again, reflective questions are included to urge faculty and programs to consider how teaching and learning might be enhanced in their own settings so that they might realize the important components of excellence that constitute the Praxis of Learning.

Chapter 10, "Organizational Imperatives", focuses on the third and final dimension of the conceptual model. In this chapter, there are 7 recommendations put forth related to important structures and resources that are essential to support physical therapist education. Reflective questions are again provided to encourage readers to engage in deliberative inquiry and consideration of change that may be necessary within their organizations to ensure excellence in physical therapist education.

The final chapter in Part III, Chapter 11, "Systems-Based Reform", urges—and hopefully impels—the reader to look beyond needed change at the individual, programmatic, or organizational/institutional level to achieve excellence in physical therapist education. All the former levels are nested in a larger societal or system-based realm of influence and control. These realms are often populated by a variety of external stakeholders and shaped by policy, regulation, and legislation, in addition to societal and cultural norms. For significant and substantive change to occur, action needs to occur at all these levels. The calls for reform presented in Chapter 11 are directed toward change that needs to take place at the systems level; this includes professional organizations and components, the health care system, and higher education. The actions we encourage in this chapter can succeed only when approached from a system-wide perspective, involving multiple stakeholders. Here, we present calls for reform in 5 key areas or broad categories: leadership, partnership, professional preparation, and participation in society, all of which are supported by education research.

Creating a Culture of Excellence

Organizational cultures are characterized by the important, commonly held values and beliefs that are expressed by the individual and collective behaviors of the people in that organization. Those values and behaviors are evident internally, in how people relate to one another, and externally, in how the people and organization relate to their partners and to the broader community.[1,2] While changing culture can be difficult, studies in higher education provide evidence of the successful relationship between leadership and culture and how cultural change can occur.[1-3]

In Chapter 4, we described the values and behaviors that contributed to cultures of excellence in physical therapist education. The 4 elements we observed were shared beliefs and values, shared leadership with a clear vision, a drive for excellence with high expectations, and vital partnerships. In this chapter, we will discuss recommendations that can create a Culture of Excellence related to each of these 4 elements.

SHARED BELIEFS AND VALUES

The importance of beliefs and values that are explicit among members of the team, that are evident in team members' behaviors, and recognize the contributions of all members of the team were central features of our findings related to culture. The 2 recommendations here highlight findings of how organizational culture can contribute to creating a climate for excellence.

- **Cultivate and make explicit the shared values within the learning community that will create a drive for excellence in education. Do so by strengthening the mutual trust, respect, and collaboration for all members of the community, particularly the learners.**

- **Demonstrate the dual values of:**
  - **Learner-centered teaching, focusing on the needs, skills, and interests of the engaged learner**
  - **Patient-centered care, focusing on the needs, interests, and goals of the patient, across all educational venues, whether in academic or clinical settings**

Jensen GM, Mostrom E, Hack LM, Nordstrom T, Gwyer J.
Educating Physical Therapists (pp 113-124).
© 2019 Taylor & Francis Group.

These recommendations reflect the literature of management sciences and health care. While the artifacts of mission statements and values that are imprinted on employee's name badges, plaques on walls, and inspirational photographs help impart culture, what is more important is the way those values are lived and expressed throughout the organization.[1] The first recommendation gets to the heart of the key values that, when evident among the behaviors of all members of the team, can create the culture in which learning is paramount.

Collaboration can occur between a teacher and student, or between a practitioner and administrator, but neither individual nor team collaborations can significantly impact the organization's outcomes without a culture of mutual trust. The culture of an organization has long been known to have a large impact on the ability of the organization to meet its goals.[4] More recent research has confirmed that those organizations characterized by a culture of giving and sharing are more successful on almost all organizational parameters.[5] In this research, giving cultures were characterized by people oriented toward helping, sharing knowledge, mentoring, and making connections without expecting anything in return. The emphasis in this recommendation, to develop the learners' ability to collaborate with more senior personnel with trust and respect, is a crucial component of understanding a culture of excellence.

Higher education and health care can be characterized by cultures that are hierarchical, siloed, and power-laden.[6,7] In clinical settings where these cultural characteristics are present, patient safety is threatened and the chance of positive outcomes is diminished.[8-10] In higher education, cultures where those characteristics predominate would threaten learning and collaboration, both antithetical to the very core of higher education.[11] In cultures characterized by hierarchies, power, and autonomy without collaboration, people who can astutely manage using a political framework would likely be successful;[2] however, collaborative, productive team work would not be easily achieved in that culture.[12]

Instead, when the culture is characterized by trust, respect, and collaboration among all members of the community, there are mutually reinforcing benefits that create the environment in which other elements important to a culture of excellence, such as shared leadership, a drive for excellence, and partnerships, can flourish.[12]

While the profession has developed a set of core professional values,[13] the members of the learning community in each organization need to fully engage in the process of identifying and inculcating the shared beliefs and values that represent excellence in education, research, and practice in physical therapy. These strongly shared beliefs and values of mutual trust, respect, and collaboration are crucial if faculty and clinicians are to work together to pursue excellence, and if learners are to adopt the beliefs and values of excellence modeled for them. These values are also essential for effective, collaborative teams who have clear purposes within the institution.[12]

In Chapter 5 we describe the importance of the Nexus of our model of excellence, which focuses on the coming together of learner-centered teaching and patient-centered practice. Patient- and learner-centeredness were 2 commonly held values we observed within the academic and clinical environments. Efforts to reduce errors and improve outcomes and quality has led patient-centered care to become a widely accepted, important concept in 21st century health care that has permeated all health professions, including physical therapy.[8-10,14-20] Learner-centered education is also a widely-adopted concept employed in education at all levels, including health professions education.[21-23] We found there were reciprocal values of patient- and learner-centeredness in academic and clinical settings. In clinical settings, where patient-centered care was foremost, there was also an emphasis on learner-centered teaching. In academic environments, where learner-centered teaching was foremost, faculty consistently framed learning experiences in such a way that placed an emphasis on patient-centered care.

These findings were similar to those found in the Carnegie study of nursing[24] in which effective learning experiences were contextualized to practice in order to create a sense of salience for the learners. Patient-centeredness, when extended to populations, also has importance from a systems perspective. *The Lancet Commission*[25] proposed a systems model in which the interdependence of the health professions education and health care was paramount and driven by the health needs of the diverse population that drives the education and health care systems, and that also produces the health care professionals who meet the needs of the population. This systems model extends the concept of patient-centeredness to that of community-centeredness.

In physical therapy, educational researchers and leaders have repeatedly identified being learner centered as an important element in professional education.[26,27] Given that physical therapist education is where the Nexus of learning and practice occurs, educators, practitioners and learners can create cultures that equally value and genuinely express these two concepts. These shared values form the foundation for the nexus for the translation of a Culture of Excellence into the Praxis of Learning.

REFLECTIVE QUESTIONS: SHARED BELIEFS AND VALUES

- Do I and my colleagues have a commitment to making the 7 core values that define professionalism in physical therapy[13] explicit in our academic and clinical programs so that they provide an enacted set of shared beliefs and values?
- Do I and my colleagues have a deep understanding of the profession's Code of Ethics[7] such that we have integrated the implications of the Code in how we relate with one another, students, patients, clients, our partners, and the community and larger society in which we function?
- Do I and my colleagues promote and experience a culture of trust and respect characterized by our collaboration throughout the academic enterprise regardless of each person's role as clinician, researcher, or teacher in the academic and clinical setting?
- Do I and my colleagues have a shared, explicit understanding of patient-centeredness through all practice and learning environments? Do we value and enact patient-centered care in all of these environments and in all of the ways we interact among ourselves, with learners, and with the patients/clients with whom we provide physical therapy?
- Do I and my colleagues have a shared, explicit understanding of learner-centeredness through all learning environments? Do we value and enact learner-centered teaching in all learning and practice environments and in all of the ways we interact among ourselves and with learners?

SHARED LEADERSHIP WITH A SHARED VISION

Our findings show that shared leadership among effective teams was the norm and these teams valued innovation to promote a Culture of Excellence. In addition, leaders leveraged the institutional mission to advance the profession's goals and responsibilities to society. Leaders were attentive to internal and external forces influencing physical therapist education, practice, and research. These leaders expressed a clear vision and worked to facilitate team-based collaborations toward this greater goal. There are 3 recommendations that emerged relative to leadership that can drive transformative change in physical therapist education.

- **Provide leadership for academic and clinical faculties to prepare practitioners who can thrive in a dynamic, rapidly changing health care system that focuses on the health outcomes for individuals and populations through leveraging technology, addressing the social determinants of health, reducing costs, and improving access to care.**
- **Develop stronger leaders in academic and clinical settings leaders who share a compelling vision in which practice, education, and research mutually reinforce and advance each of these components of professional preparation.**

- **Institute leadership development that reinforces the value of shared leadership, effective teams, innovation, and culture of excellence. This development must begin in professional education and continue across a professional's career.**

In each of these recommendations a theme emerges for both knowledgeable and skilled leaders. We recommend that leaders in both academic and clinical settings educate themselves in the complex and connected institutions of health care and higher education. Examples of trends in both these institutions highlight the importance of knowledge to enable our professional leaders to envision innovation and excellence.

The trend in the US health care system over the past 30 years has been toward an increasing importance of population health, preventive care, a shift to value-based care predicated on outcomes, bundled payments for services, and increasingly available, useful data about the costs and outcomes of care at the individual practitioner, health system, and population levels.[28] While there have been reversals in the trends for any one of these components, the overall trend has been toward the primacy of the outcomes of care at the population level, and this is not likely to change.[28] Over this same period of time there has been continued progress in genomics, regenerative medicine, and bioengineering that are radically altering health care outcomes that directly affect the care given by physical therapists.[29] Alternative health care delivery models that include telehealth and e-communication are altering the nature of the interaction between practitioners and patients and the accessibility of health care.

Despite improvements in care and technology, threats to patient safety and quality continue to be problematic in the health care system in the 17 years since publication of *To Err is Human: Building a Safer Health System*,[30] which highlighted the crises of human and systems-caused errors in health care. In 2008, Berwick et al,[9] through the Institute of Healthcare Improvement, promulgated the Triple Aim, a conceptual model to improve health care quality by improving the experience of care, improving the health of populations, and reducing the per capita costs of health care. The Institute of Healthcare Improvement has continued to provide means to improve quality and safety in the health care system, including curricula, learning materials, and ways for health care professionals and health professions students to engage in improving quality and safety of the health care system.[9] The Triple Aim was altered to the Quadruple Aim in order to include the importance of health care providers' work life to ensure they are prepared for the rigors of clinical practice by developing resilience to avoid burnout.[31] The Agency for Healthcare Quality and Research developed the TeamSTEPPS (Strategies and Tools to Enhance Performance and Patient Safety) curriculum that emphasizes development of communication and teamwork skills among health care professionals.[10] The TeamSTEPPS curriculum is being adopted in health systems and health professions education in the United States. Large-scale adoption of this curriculum, coupled with attention to patient safety, the Quadruple Aim, and quality improvement elements in physical therapist professional education within an interprofessional learning environment has the potential to have a positive effect on health system safety and quality. Accreditation criteria in the health professions, including the Commission on Accreditation for Physical Therapy Education (CAPTE), are increasing the requirements that health profession educators prepare graduates for interprofessional, collaborative care, who are able to address safety and quality improvement at the systems level as well as at the level of the individual patient. These criteria also reinforce the importance of systems-level safety and quality, and can facilitate curricular change and have the potential to support health professions education that advances the Quadruple Aim.[32]

In 2010, *the Lancet Commission* on Education of Health Professionals for the 21st Century identified global challenges of health inequities, uneven advances in health and health care among countries, and risks from new infectious, environmental, and behavioral sources.[25] In a global health system, the United States is not immune from those challenges. The incidence of non-communicable diseases, including drug addiction, have reached epidemic proportions and the health of people is declining in the United States and the world. These diseases not only lead to increasing rates of morbidity and mortality, but they are rending the social fabric of families and communities.[33-37] While these diseases occur within all socioeconomic strata and across all races and ethnicities, there are social determinants of health that result in health disparities that disproportionately affect people at lower socioeconomic levels and in communities of color. Political and social structures at the local, state, and national levels create and perpetuate these disparities and inequities. Thus, while individual choice may appear to play an important role in these disease trends, the practitioner will not be effective if he or she does not attend to the societal contributions to illness and disease at the individual level as well as the population level. As a profession, we shirk our moral responsibility to society and the people we serve if we ignore these trends. In 2016, the National Academies of Sciences, Engineering, and Medicine published a conceptual framework for educating health professionals to address the social determinants of health.[38] The purpose was to raise awareness of the problems associated with the social determinants of health and to develop a model that would guide health professions educators to address them. That model was based on the interdependence of education, communities, and organizations to address the social determinants of health, including the structural mechanisms that cause them. One of the 3 recommendations in their report was to prepare health professionals who are able to take action in concert with members of the community, health care, education, and government to address the social determinants of health. Curricular models in which students learn to address the structural inequalities in health care will enhance learner preparation for practice.[39]

Higher education in the United States is being buffeted by forces as equally powerful as those that are occurring in health care.[40] Decreasing levels of financial support for public education from states is a contributor to increased tuition costs. Similar financial constraints at the federal level are effecting funding for research and grant support in higher education. Throughout higher education, including health professions education, there are increasing concerns over rising student indebtedness, the role that the government plays in financial aid and the incentives that influence student indebtedness and how that affects choices in employment. Technology, including virtual reality, simulation, and online learning modalities, is playing an increasingly important role in higher education, even though there are questions about effectiveness, scalability, and cost structures of some of these modalities.[41,42] There will be fewer people of college age through the next decade in the United States, and those students will be increasingly racially and ethnically diverse.[43,44] This demographic shift will place increasing pressure on undergraduate institutions to enroll adequate numbers of students to ensure their financial viability and likely increase competition for well-qualified students throughout all of graduate education, and physical therapy will be a part of that competition.

The growth in physical therapist education programs is of concern to the profession, as resources throughout higher education tighten, including space, qualified academic faculty, and clinical education (CE) faculty. Clinical sites that provide learning resources for physical therapist students is an extraordinarily important component of professional education, and demands on this resource are compounded by the need for physical therapist assistant students who need the same learning opportunities. Concerns about CE resulted in several actions in the profession, including a summit on CE and actions from the American Physical Therapy Association (APTA) House of Delegates.[45,46] While the outcomes from these initiatives are unknown, the crisis must bring health care and education leaders together in order to prepare knowledgeable leaders who can envision new options.

This confluence of events in health care and higher education, when coupled with societal expectations of the health professions, requires that the profession adopts a comprehensive approach to leadership development from professional through post-professional education and ongoing professional development. That approach must be based on theoretically sound research evidence on leadership, innovation, teams, and other areas of effective business practice. Students, clinicians, faculty and leaders will fail if they hold on to outdated leadership practices, linear thinking about curricular design, curriculum content that does not consider the realities of practice now and in the near future, discipline-specific silos, and individualistic thinking about learning, practice, research, or leadership. Kezar et al[3] described a revolution in our understanding of leadership over the past 20 years with a shift away from a leader-centered orientation that attempts to ascribe traits or characteristics of effective leaders in hierarchical systems where leaders have power over followers. The revolution in the evidence supporting current thinking about leadership is primarily based in social constructivist and critical and postmodern paradigms. These paradigms lead to leadership that is contextual, relational, collective, and non-hierarchical. The emphasis is on mutual power and influence among all of the participants in the organization and promoting learning, empowerment, and change are foremost elements. When one considers the environment of physical therapist professional education and clinical practice, then these leadership models become even more important and lead to the importance of effective teams. Education and practice require people to integrate perspectives from different disciplines across dispersed locations with high demand for effective communication and coordination. People in both environments must gather, synthesize, and apply complex information; however, the variability in the nature of work makes such coordination challenging. Research by Edmondson[12] suggests that these contextual characteristics of work make effective teams even more essential for success. Too often, health professionals in clinical practice and higher education view conflict as negative and disruptive. However, evidence suggests that conflict can be a source of innovation and learning if effectively managed within high functioning teams.[47] The complexities of leading organizations in complex systems suggests that the profession and organizations would benefit from physical therapists who pursue advanced education in business administration and leadership.

The APTA vision, "transforming society by optimizing movement to improve the human experience"[48] provides a unifying core purpose for the profession's future that can unite education, practice, and research. At the institutional level, the faculty and clinicians must translate that vision into their particular context, but in doing so they have to assure that the profession's commitment to society expressed in that vision is retained when it is translated at the institutional level. Kouzes and Posner[49] speak to the power of an inspirational vision that is brought to life throughout the people in the organization and that is connected to their hopes and aspirations.

If we are to prepare physical therapists who can make positive contributions as integral members of teams within the health care system, in community-centered public health programs, and as advocates in the public policy arena, then we must develop a cadre of academic and clinical leaders who have a deep understanding of complex systems in health care and higher education.[7,40] That preparation must start during professional education. *The Lancet Commission* report posited that health professions education must be focused on transformative learning experiences that develops "enlightened change agents"[25(p1924)] who are developing leadership attributes.

Transformative learning involves 3 fundamental shifts: from fact memorization to searching, analysis, and synthesis of information for decision making; from seeking professional credentials to achieving core competencies for effective teamwork in health systems; and from non-critical adoption of educational models to creative adaptation of global resources to address local priorities.[p1924]

For post-professional learning, the Education Leadership Institute fellowship program[50] and the Health Policy and Administration Section Catalyst's LAMP Institute for Leadership in Physical Therapy,[51] both offered under the umbrella of the APTA, are preparing leaders for physical therapy education and clinical practice. However, those programs are not sufficient when one considers the demands for effective leadership at all levels of the profession, particularly when one considers the sheer volume of clinical practice settings and the number of physical therapist and physical therapist assistant education programs. Leadership development in the profession must start through curriculum and cocurricular learning in professional education and must go beyond minimal curricular content standards set by the CAPTE.[52,53] Ongoing post-professional development of faculty and clinicians can occur informally through mentorship and community volunteer experiences, advocacy roles, peer mentorship and learning networks.[54] Post-professional leadership development programs need to be scalable so that they can reach hundreds, if not thousands, of practitioners if the leadership needs of the profession are to be met. Local or regional partnerships among current and developing leaders of education programs and key clinical sites could foster collaborative, creative means to solve pressing problems that affect practice and education and development of the leadership abilities required in both settings.

REFLECTIVE QUESTIONS: SHARED LEADERSHIP WITH A SHARED VISION

- Is the leadership in my organization based on shared leadership in which we function as members of a collaborative team or is it more hierarchical or autocratic in nature? Are the team norms and behaviors of leaders characterized by a view of failures as learning opportunity, accountability, open, direct communication, and approachability?[12]
- Does my organization have a clear vision and mission for the future that guides leadership? Do our vision and mission address key issues confronting health care in the United States, locally and nationally, today and into the future, such as the Triple Aim[9] reducing health disparities and addressing the social determinants of health[38] and how to improve the health outcomes at the individual and population level? How well do we enact that vision and mission in all of our work?
- How do leaders express their understanding of the internal and external environment that shapes my organization, such as changing priorities and opportunities for partnerships, and that influence our institution and the profession, such as advances in practice and research?
- Where do we stand on having visionary, qualified leaders who can lead our academic and CE programs toward excellence?
- Are physical therapy academic and clinical leaders sufficiently engaged in policy development that strengthens the roles of physical therapists in helping to meet significant issues that affect the health of our society?

DRIVE FOR EXCELLENCE

We found communities of faculty, learners, and clinicians who had a thirst for learning, a commitment to excellence through setting of high expectations, and a willingness to hold each other accountable in meeting those high expectations. There is one recommendation that is germane to this area:

- **Continually innovate and take risks to drive the shared vision for practice and education forward. This means that the CAPTE standards should have the flexibility to recognize innovation in physical therapy education. The current CAPTE accreditation program standards also need to better reflect the resources and processes needed to achieve excellence.**

The willingness to take risk has been shown to be a valuable trait for managers across many businesses.[55] Drucker,[56] in an early description of strategic planning, defined it as a process of making risk-taking decisions in an organized fashion, based on a good assessment of the current and future situation, and measuring the outcomes. He stressed that taking risk is essential for innovation and growth of the enterprise.[57] One of the 5 components of effective leadership in Kouzes and Posner's model[49] is the leaders' search for ways to change the status quo and a willingness to experiment and take risks that lead to innovation. These leaders are willing to take risks and make mistakes that could lead to failure but, importantly, learn from those mistakes. The inter-relatedness of the elements in a culture of excellence becomes important to consider. A culture of trust and mutual respect, combined with teams of people who are committed to learning and who are functioning in successful teams with clear vision and purpose, establish a foundation in which innovation and risk taking is more likely to occur.[12]

The Lancet Commission report[25] hypothesized that information technology, driven by people with understanding of learning and technology, would be the biggest driver of transformative learning. They cited 2 technologies in particular, the open education source movement and the ability of technology to create global and regional learning communities and shared resources. As early as 2008, Tufts University had placed 50% of its health sciences education courses online using OpenCourseWare with one of its goals to distribute course materials globally, particularly in under resourced countries.[25] The ubiquity of mobile phones that can serve as digital content delivery devices and learning platforms provides the opportunity for distribution to learners without regard to geographical boundaries. As only one example of an application of innovations in this domain, if one considers the increasing knowledge that underlies physical therapy education and the shortage of qualified faculty who can address the breadth of knowledge in the profession, there is the potential to meet learners' needs using innovative technologies among consortia of physical therapist education programs or to learners in remote areas.

Accreditation, with its emphasis on compliance with standards, processes, and outcomes, and operating within strict confines imposed through government regulation, is not viewed as supporting innovation.[57] Accreditors do not necessarily view their purpose to support the ability of the profession to meet its responsibilities entrusted to it by society. *The Lancet Commission* specifically addressed the need for accreditors to adopt a social accountability approach that aligns their function while ensuring societal needs for health care are met by the profession, including equity, efficiency, and quality.[25] Making social accountability an important component of accreditation could unleash innovative approaches in curriculum, interprofessional learning, community-based health care, and means to increase the diversity of the physical therapist workforce.

The types of innovations that could be spurred through application of technology and other sources and means could, at the least, not be discouraged by the accreditation processes. We would look forward to accreditation processes that focused on outcomes, achievement of competencies adopted by the profession, and that demonstrated alignment with social needs of the health care system. The threat of non-compliance with accreditation standards, whether perceived or actual, could hypothetically be used by risk-averse leaders to adopt risk-avoidance behaviors, including the pursuit of innovative approaches to physical therapist education. The current siloes among accrediting agencies in the health professions do not serve the health system priority of interprofessional collaborative practice, particularly in communities in which there are health inequities.[57] Collaborative forums or agencies composed of key stakeholders in accreditation from the spectrum of health professions education, including governmental regulators, would be a first step in crossing that divide. They could break down the current siloes and direct attention to how these agencies can unleash innovations to solve the pressing problems in health care and health professions education facing society.

REFLECTIVE QUESTIONS: DRIVE FOR EXCELLENCE

- How willing are we to take risks and innovate, particularly when that leads us to excel and exceed our own parochial interests that protect the status quo? When we engage in efforts to improve, how are members of the organization held accountable for actions or inactions?

- Do we as a faculty recognize that meeting CAPTE criteria, having acceptable licensure pass rates or satisfied students and faculty/staff are the baseline, and that excellence requires setting high standards that cause us to stretch our capacity that we might not always attain?

PARTNERSHIP

Intentional, equal partnerships among clinical sites and academic programs in which faculty, clinicians, students, and residents shared and used information to guide learning and practice were a prominent feature of our findings. There are 2 recommendations related to partnerships.

- **Create, develop, and support fair, creative, and responsible partnerships between academic and clinical organizations in both clinical and classroom teaching; educational programs cannot exist in isolation and be excellent.**
- **Move from an uneven model for clinical learning, where there are not true partnerships, to a fully integrated, practice-based learning model with the clinical faculty as full partners with the academic program. The practice-based learning model requires clinical faculty to become full partners in the academic program, and fully integrated clinical learning spaces must be accessible to students and faculty.**

In a 2002 editorial in *Physical Therapy*, Rothstein[58] criticized the lack of a common understanding of the role and function of CE among the many stakeholders and the failure to pursue partnerships among those stakeholders despite its importance to the preparation of future professionals.

Without a proper ongoing partnership between faculties in schools and people in practice, clinical education will never prepare our new graduates to the level necessary, to the level described by our Association's vision statement, and to the level that justifies the professional doctorate.(p127)

Ten years later, at the 2012 Combined Section Meeting, the American Council of Academic Physical Therapy, the APTA, the Academy of Physical Therapy Education, the Federation of State Boards of Physical Therapy, and the CAPTE began work on a CE summit that would develop a process for a shared vision for CE. As Kelly[59] described in that editorial in preparation for the summit:

From this first meeting, it was recognized that a "shared vision" is one that recognizes and strengthens partnerships across the entire spectrum of physical therapist education, from entry-level through post-professional, clinical through academic.(p3)

Leading up to that summit, a special supplement of the *Journal of Physical Therapy Education* was devoted to articles that established the context for the discussions at the summit. Among those articles, 2 provided frameworks for CE partnerships,[60,61] 1 argued for the importance for a national collaboration among clinical and academic partners to come to agreement over structures, processes and outcomes to improve quality,[62] and 1 suggested that practice-education partnerships were essential if professional education is to respond to changes in the health care system and the nature of health care.[63] The Clinical Education Summit was held in October 2014, bringing together hundreds of stakeholders in physical therapy CE. The final report, a synthesis of the work of those stakeholders, emphasized the role of partnerships to achieve a common shared vision that would prepare physical therapists for clinical practice.[64] The report emphasized that all of the stakeholders, including students and patients, in CE engage in education and communication to reach a national consensus of shared values and common goals for CE in which they are held accountable for achieving results. There were 11 "harmonizing recommendations," all of which require collaborative, mutual, equal partnerships among academic and clinical partners if the results are to be achieved. Chief among those that will require partnerships were: (1) achieving shared values for CE; (2) preparing and developing clinical educators; (3) achieving a commonly agreed upon clinical curriculum; (4) offering diverse integrated clinical experiences; (5) developing terminal internships that prepare graduates for commonly encountered practice opportunities; (6) developing a required set of knowledge, skills, attitudes, and professional behaviors to progress through CE experiences; and (7) establishing core performance competencies for entry to practice. While these activities of the profession are in the early stages of development,[64] they align well with the 2 recommendations from our study.

REFLECTIVE QUESTIONS: PARTNERSHIP

- What is the nature of the relationship between the academic and clinical entities in my organization? Do these relationships demonstrate equity? In what ways are we true partners across all aspects of education?
- If in an academic program, how much do we focus on clinical sites as slots for our students and how well do we know the abilities of clinical instructors?
- If in a clinic, why do we have students and how do we collaborate with the academic program to achieve the optimal learning outcomes for each student?

Recent management literature has focused on collaborative work for success in the workplace with the desire to benefit others, including the consideration of others' perspectives, as an antecedent to collaborative behavior.[65-67] Positive interpersonal interaction increases emphasis on collaboration, leading to businesses success,[12,68] including in academic health centers.[7] The culture in which collaboration and positive interaction can occur through creation of environments characterized by personal safety in which people are able to take risks and where conflict and disagreements are constructively viewed as a source for innovation, improvement, and learning.[69]

Developing a culture of mutual respect and trust with a shared vision underlies all of the recommendations related to creating a culture of excellence in physical therapist education. Similar to our findings about the importance of mutual respect, trust, and a shared vision, the American Association of the Colleges of Nursing identified the core values of mutual respect and trust and possession of a shared vision as cornerstones for academic-practice partnerships and has chosen to feature such collaborations explicitly by giving an annual award for academic-practice partnership.[70] Collaboration is one of the guiding principles to implement the Vision for the APTA.[48] However, the profession's description of collaboration does not explicitly recognize the importance of collaboration across clinical and academic environments as a component of how collaboration will contribute to the profession achieving its vision. The profession's vision, "transforming society by optimizing movement to improve the human experience" provides the foundation for a shared vision within and amongst all education and practice settings. As the profession's "nurseries," the future of physical therapy and its ability to achieve its vision will require that every practice and learning environment are characterized by values of mutual respect and trust and the enacted values of patient- and learner-centeredness. Those shared values must be promulgated through shared leadership models and effective teams that are laser-focused on achieving institutional mission and vision that are attuned to the emerging health needs of society and that are relentlessly seeking excellence.

REFERENCES

1. Schein E. *Organizational Culture and Leadership.* 4th ed. San Francisco, CA: Jossey-Bass; 2010.
2. Bolman LG, Deal TE. *Reframing Organizations: Artistry, Choice and Leadership.* 4th ed. San Francisco, CA: Jossey-Bass; 2008.
3. Kezar A, Carducci R, Contreras-McGavin M. Rethinking the "L" word in higher education: the revolution of research on leadership. *ASHE Higher Education Report.* 2006;31(6).
4. O'Reilley C. Corporations, culture, and commitment: motivation and social control in organizations. *California Management Review.* 1989;31(4):9-25.

5. Grant A. Givers take all: the hidden dimension of corporate culture. *McKinsey Quarterly*. http://www.mckinsey.com/business-functions/organization/our insights/givers-take-all-the-hidden-dimension-of-corporate-culture. Published April 2013. Accessed Februry 1, 2017.

6. Grogan M, ed. *Educational Leadership*. 3rd ed. San Francisco, CA: Jossey-Bass; 2013.

7. Wartman S, ed. *The Transformation of Academic Health Centers: Meeting the Challenges of Healthcare's Changing Landscape*. Boston, MA: Elsevier Publishing; 2015.

8. US Department of Health and Human Services. Agency for Healthcare Research and Quality. National Healthcare Quality and Disparities Reports. https://www.ahrq.gov/research/findings/nhqrdr/index.html. Published 2013. Accessed November 25, 2017.

9. Berwick DM, Nolan TW, Whittington J. The Triple Aim: care, health, and cost. *Health Affairs*. 2008;27(3):759-769.

10. US Department of Health and Human Services. Agency for Healthcare Research and Quality. TeamSTEPPS training. https://www.ahrq.gov/teamstepps/index.html. Accessed November 25, 2017.

11. Ashkansay N, Wildersom C, Peterson M, eds. *Handbook of Organizational Culture and Climate*. 2nd ed. Thousand Oaks, CA: Sage Publishing; 2011.

12. Edmondson A. *Teaming: How Organizations Learn, Innovate, and Compete in the Knowledge Economy*. San Francisco, CA: Jossey-Bass; 2012.

13. American Physical Therapy Association. Professionalism in physical therapy: core values. https://www.apta.org/uploadedFiles/APTAorg/About_Us/Policies/BOD/Judicial/ProfessionalisminPT.pdf. Accessed November 25, 2017.

14. Salas E, Rosen MA, Building high reliability teams: progress and some reflections on teamwork training. *BMJ Qual Saf*. 2013;22:369-373.

15. Valentine M, Edmonson A. Improving on-the-fly teamwork in healthcare. *Harvard Business Review*. 2016.

16. Institute of Medicine. *Crossing the Quality Chasm: A New Health System for the 21st Century*. Washington, DC: National Academy Press; 2001.

17. Epstein RM, Street RL. The values and value of patient-centered care. *Ann Fam Med*. 2011;9(2):100-103.

18. Barry MJ, Edgman-Levitan S. Shared decision making—the pinnacle of patient-centered care. *N Engl J Med*. 2012;366:780-781.

19. Wolf DM, Lehman L, Quinlin R, Zullo T, Hoffman L. Effect of patient centered care on patient satisfaction and quality of care. *J Nursing Care Quality*. 2008;23(4):316-321.

20. APTA. Code of Ethics. https://www.apta.org/uploadedFiles/APTAorg/About_Us/Policies/Ethics/CodeofEthics.pdf. Published 2013. Accessed February 7, 2017.

21. Ambrose SA, Bridges MW, DiPietro M, Lovett MC, Norma MK. *How Learning Works: Seven Research-Based Principles for Smart Teaching*. San Francisco, CA: Jossey-Bass; 2010.

22. Ludmerer K. Learner-centered medical education. *N Engl J Med* 2004;351:1163-1164.

23. Halfer J, ed. *Extraordinary Learning in the Workplace*. New York, NY: Springer; 2011.

24. Benner P, Sutphen M, Leonard C, Day L. *Educating Nurses: A Call for Radical Transformation*. San Francisco, CA: Jossey-Bass; 2010.

25. Frenk J, Chen L, Bhutta Z, et al. Health professional for a new century: transforming education to strengthen health systems in an interdependent world. *Lancet*. 2010;376:1923-1958.

26. Hakim EW, Moffat M, Becker E, et al. Application of educational theory and evidence in support of an integrated model of clinical education. *J Phys Ther Educ*. 2014;28(suppl 1):13-21.

27. Jensen GM, Mostrom EM. *Handbook of Teaching and Learning for Physical Therapists*. 3rd ed. St. Louis, MO: Elsevier Publishing; 2013.

28. Bodenheimer T, Grumbach, K. *Understanding Health Policy: A Clinical Approach*. 7th ed. New York, NY: Lange Medical Books/McGraw-Hill; 2016.

29. American Physical Therapy Association. Frontiers in Research, Science and Technology (FiRST) council. http://www.apta.org/FiRST/. Accessed December 29, 2017.

30. Kohn L, Corrigan J, Donaldson M, eds. *To Err is Human: Building a Safer Health System*. Institute of Medicine: Committee on Quality of Health Care in America; 2000.

31. Bodenheimer T, Sinsky C. From Triple to Quadruple Aim: care of the patient requires care of the provider. *Ann of Fam Med*. 2017:12(6);573-576.

32. Cox M, Blouin A, Cuff P, Paniagua M, Phillips S, Vlasses P. The role of accreditation in achieving the Quadruple Aim. *Nat Acad of Med*. 2017; October 2.

33. Kaiser Family Foundation. The US Government and global NCD efforts. https://www.kff.org/global-health-policy/fact-sheet/the-u-s-government-and-global-non-communicable-diseases/. Accessed November 25, 2017.

34. Kalache A. The greying world: a challenge for the 21st century. *Science Progress*. 2000:83;33-54.

35. Carter S, Rychetnik L. A public health ethics approach to NCD. *Bioethical Inquiry*. 2013;10:17-18.

36. Chetty R, Stepner M, Abraham S, et al. The association between income and life expectancy in the United States, 2001-2014. *JAMA*. 2016;315(16):1750-1766

37. World Health Organization. Social determinants of Health. http://www.who.int/social_determinants/en/. Accessed November 25, 2017.

38. National Academies of Sciences, Engineering, and Medicine. A framework for educating health professional to address social determinants of health. https://www.nap.edu/catalog/21923/a-framework-for-educating-health-professionals-to-address-the-social-determinants-of-health. Accessed November 25, 2017.

39. Metzl JM, Perry J. Integrating and assessing structural competency in an innovative prehealth curriculum at Vanderbilt University. *Acad Med*. 2017;92:354-359. doi: 10.1097/ACM.0000000000001477.

40. Ruben BD, De Lisi R, Gigliotti RA. *A Guide for Leaders in Higher Education: Core Concepts, Competencies and Tools*. Sterling, VA: Stylus Publishing LLC; 2017.

41. Zemsky R. *Checklist for Change: Making Higher Education a Sustainable Enterprise*. New Brunswick, NJ: Rutgers University Press; 2013.

42. Macy Foundation. Enhancing health professions education through technology: building a continuous learning health system. http://macyfoundation.org/publications/publication/enhancing-health-professions-education-technology. Accessed November 25, 2017.

43. Selingo J. *2026, The Decade Ahead: The Seismic Shifts Transforming the Future of Higher Education*. Washington, DC: Chronicle of Higher Education; 2017.

44. US Department of Education. National Center for Education Statistics. https://nces.ed.gov/fastfacts/display.asp?id=98. Accessed November 25, 2017.

45. American Council of Academic Physical Therapy. Clinical Education Summit report and recommendations. http://acapt.org/docs/default-source/reports/post-summit-report-sept-2015.pdf?sfvrsn=2. Published 2015. Accessed December 29, 2017.

46. American Physical Therapy Association. Best practices for physical therapy clinical education. In 2017 reports to the House of Delegates. http://communities.apta.org/p/do/sd/sid=3940. Published 2017. Accessed December 29, 2017.

47. Eichbaum Q. Collaboration and teamwork in the health professions: rethinking the role of conflict. *Acad Med.* 2017;93:4:574-580(7) doi: 10.1097/ACM.0000000000002015.

48. American Physical Therapy Association. Vision Statement for the Profession of Physical Therapy and Guiding Principles. http://www.apta.org/Vision/. Accessed December 29, 2017.

49. Kouzes J, Posner B. *The Leadership Challenge: How to Make Extraordinary Things Happen in Organizations*. 6th ed. San Francisco, CA: Jossey-Bass; 2017.

50. American Physical Therapy Association. Education Leadership Institute (ELI) fellowship. http://www.apta.org/ELI/. Accessed January 2, 2018.

51. HPA the Catalyst. LAMP Leadership Development Certificate Program. http://www.aptahpa.org/page/LAMP. Accessed January 2, 2018.

52. Gabel S. Expanding the scope of leadership training in medicine. *Acad Med.* 2014;89:848-852.

53. Varkey P, Peloquin J, Reed D, Lindor K, Harris I. Leadership curriculum in undergraduate medical education: a study of student and faculty perspectives. *Med Teach.* 2009;31:244-250.

54. Steinart Y, ed. *Faculty Development in the Health Professions: A Focus on Research and Practice*. New York, NY: Springer; 2014.

55. Damodaran A. *Strategic Risk Taking: A Framework for Risk Management*. Upper Saddle River, NJ. FT Press; 2007.

56. Drucker P. *Management: Tasks, Responsibilities, Practices*. New York, NY: Harper & Row; 1974.

57. National Academies of Sciences, Engineering, and Medicine. Exploring the role of accreditation in enhancing quality and innovation in health professions education: proceedings of a workshop. Washington, DC: The National Academies Press; 2017.

58. Rothstein JM. "Clinical education" versus clinical education. *Phys Ther.* 2002:82(2);126-127.

59. Kelly S. On the summit. *J Phys Ther Edu.* 2014:28(suppl);3.

60. Applebaum D, Portney L, Kolosky L, et al. Building physical therapist education networks. *J Phys Ther Edu.* 2014:28(suppl);30-38.

61. McCallum CA, Mosher PD, Homan J, Englehard C, Euype S, Cook CE. Development of regional core networks for the development of physical therapist clinical education. *J Phys Ther Edu.* 2014:28(suppl);39-47.

62. Jette DU, Nelson L, Palaima M, Wetherbee E. How do we improve clinical education? Examination of structures, processes and outcomes. *J Phys Ther Edu.* 2014:28(suppl);6-12.

63. Deusinger SS, Crowner BE, Burliss TL, Stith JS. Meeting contemporary expectations for physical therapists: imperatives, challenges and proposed solutions for professional education. *J Phys Ther Edu.* 2014;28(suppl);56-61.

64. American Council of Academic Physical Therapy. *Clinical Education Summit. Summit Report and Recommendations*. Washington, DC: American Council of Academic Physical Therapy; 2017.

65. Grant AM, Berry JW. The necessity of others is the mother of invention: intrinsic and prosocial motivations, perspective-taking, and creativity. *Acad Manage J;* 2011:(54);73-96.

66. Grant AM. *Give and Take: Why Helping Others Drives Our Success*. New York, NY. Penguin Books; 2013.

67. Grant AM, Berg JM, Prosocial motivation at work: how making a difference makes a difference. In: Cameron K, Spreitzer G, eds. *Handbook of Positive Organizational Scholarship*. Oxford, United Kingdom: Oxford University Press; 2011.

68. Gratton L, Erickson T. 8 ways to build collaborative teams. *Harvard Business Review.* 2007;85:100-109.

69. Eichbaum Q. Collaboration and teamwork in the health professions: rethinking the role of conflict. *Acad Med;* 2017; November 14. doi: 10.1097/ACM.0000000000002015.

70. American Association of Colleges of Nursing. Guiding principles to academic-practice partnerships. http://www.aacnnursing.org/Academic-Practice-Partnerships/The-Guiding-Principles. Published January 2012. Accessed December 29, 2017.

9

Advancing Learning and the Learning Sciences

Part I

INFUSING THE LEARNING SCIENCES INTO PHYSICAL THERAPIST EDUCATION, PRACTICE, AND RESEARCH

An important assumption in this chapter is the critical importance of understanding more deeply the 3 apprenticeships of professional education from the Carnegie Preparation for Professions Program studies—apprenticeships that develop habits of head, hand, and heart—applied and interpreted for us in physical therapist education. This is not a simple application of teaching concepts or skills but must be connected to a deeper understanding of the role of the learning sciences in professional education. Shulman argues that pedagogies for professional education must continue to "forge connections between key ideas and effective practice."[1(p18)]

> [I]t is insufficient to claim that a combination of theory, practice, and ethics defines a professional's work; it is also characterized by conditions of inherent and unavoidable uncertainty professional education is about developing pedagogies to link ideas, practices, and values under conditions of inherent uncertainty that necessitate not only judgment in order to act, but cognizance of the consequences of one's action...In the presence of uncertainty, one is obligated to learning from experience.[1(p19)]

We found many examples of excellence in a variety of teaching and learning environments across our academic and clinical sites. Even so, the faculty at these sites often lacked a deep understanding of the learning sciences and, thus, a consistent language for discussing the science of teaching and learning that is critical for advancing and transforming physical therapist education. Three core elements in the learning dimension (Praxis of Learning) of our model, signature

Jensen GM, Mostrom E, Hack LM, Nordstrom T, Gwyer J.
Educating Physical Therapists (pp 125-145).
© 2019 Taylor & Francis Group.

pedagogy, practice-based learning, and creating adaptive learners, have associated recommendations that we believe, if enacted, have the potential to truly transform physical therapist education through advancing learning and infusing the learning sciences into all that we do. Learning sciences are an essential component in the development of domain-specific pedagogies. For physical therapists, a domain-specific pedagogy attends to the use of one's own body in demonstrating movement and learning to be observant in assessing patients' needs for facilitation and improvement of movement so that implementation of interventions for patients to improve movement are highly individualized.[1]

Signature Pedagogy

We have identified that the signature pedagogy for physical therapy is the human body as teacher. These 3 recommendations provide us with insights into how we can use the concept of signature pedagogy as an important multidimensional lens for further understanding and developing the unique and fundamental way we educate physical therapists.[2]

- **Adopt the profession's signature pedagogy, the human body as teacher, as it is foundational to achieve excellence in physical therapist education.**
- **Require early authentic clinical experiences, which are essential for teaching and learning through our signature pedagogy in the context of practice and make this signature pedagogy more evidence-based, explicit, and visible in all learning environments.**
- **Develop consistent, shared language on the role of movement and what is meant by the movement system that can be implemented across academic and clinical settings. Intentionally integrate sociocultural factors in improving human movement into all curricula.**

Physical therapy has long identified the centrality of movement and the analysis and improvement of movement as foundational to the profession. The profession continues to emphasize the analysis and understanding of movement through establishing and growing our knowledge base in movement science, motor learning, and motor control theory, as well as putting in place curricular requirements, practice guidelines, accreditation standards, and expected learner outcomes related to the observation, analysis and enhancement of human movement.[3] We have not been fully intentional about exploring and seeking to understand the role of the *human body as teacher* about movement; perhaps it is so much a part of our work that we often take it for granted. Teaching and learning about the human body as teacher can be enriched through further exploration, development, and articulation of physical therapy's domain-specific pedagogy so that we can better understand how different learners come to know how to use their own bodies effectively in teaching and learning about movement. The recognition and consideration of psychosocial and cultural factors that influence a patient's illness experience and movement is essential in clinical practice, yet these critical dimensions are often addressed in the curriculum through a separate course or module and can seem disconnected from how we facilitate the improvement of human movement and function with diverse patients.[2-5] In the study of expert practice in physical therapy, skilled facilitation of movement was identified as a core dimension of the practice of experts through their examination and data gathering process, hands-on skills, and astute assessment of movement through observation, palpation, and touch.[6] Using a method of qualitative situational analysis, Covington and Barcinas[7] examined how physical therapist clinical instructors (CIs) perceive and facilitate students' emerging integration of movement into practice and identified 5 core behaviors of CIs that facilitate this integration—adapt, prepare, enhance, connect, and develop.

Part of every physical therapist's journey in school is developing those skills of observation, palpation, and use of his or her body. Most of us can name colleagues or mentors who have great hands and are therapists that we would seek out for treatment of certain conditions or refer our family members to them. How we develop the use of our bodies and our body as instrument is part of our invisible tradition—our tacit taken-for granted knowledge of how to enhance movement with individual patients. While the use of our bodies and the bodies of others in our work may be taken for granted and thus, invisible to us, that is not so to others. Mike Rose,[8] a well-known anthropologist/sociologist, published a classic paper, describing teaching and learning in a physical therapy musculoskeletal laboratory,

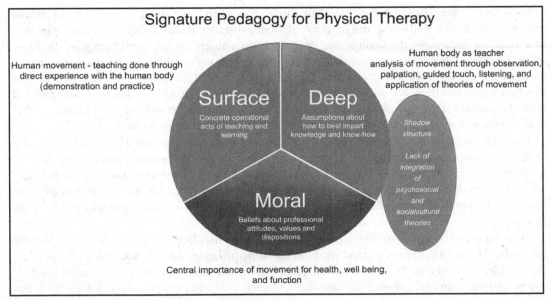

Figure 9-1. Signature pedagogy for physical therapy.[1,9,10]

which he investigated using a situated cognition framework. His insights provide us with a window on how much more we need to do to fully understand what we learn through our body and that of our patients, how we use our bodies in therapy, and our connection to movement. In the excerpt below, Rose[8] shares his observations about how students learned to use their bodies as instruments:

> The body becomes the physical therapist's instrument in several metaphoric senses of the word. It is, first of all, the means by which physical therapists perform a technique, whether for diagnostic or for treatment purposes...novice therapists have to learn how to position their bodies in order to perform the technique most effectively...There is another reason for this care in the positioning of the body: to protect oneself from fatigue or injury...There is a second sense in which the body is the physical therapist's instrument: it is the primary means by which they get "good information" about a patient's condition—through feeling and seeing and listening to a patient's response the therapist's body becomes both tool and gauge.(p139,140)

We introduced the structural dimensions (ie, surface, deep, implicit/moral, shadow) of signature pedagogy in Chapter 6. Here, we apply these dimensions to physical therapy (Figure 9-1).

The teaching and learning of physical therapy cannot take place without fully understanding one's own body and how it works and moves. This understanding then provides a scaffold for learning through working with another's body (eg, peer, faculty member, patient) to observe structure and movement and for applying and facilitating skilled movement. This surface structure of our signature pedagogy is readily apparent when observing the amount of teaching and learning done through observation of the human body and movement and repeated demonstration and practice, often in laboratory classrooms early-on in physical therapist curricula. The deeper structure of our signature pedagogy is the assumption that close attention to the human body is the best teacher for honing the skills of analysis of movement using a variety of senses (vision, what can be observed; touch, what can be palpated or felt; hearing, what the patient says). Furthermore, our signature pedagogy assumes that the best way to learn about improving movement is through direct experience with the human body—learning the skills of guided touch, how to apply theories of movement in practice, how to listen sensitively for information about what the patient is experiencing and how he or she needs to move to fulfill social roles. The implicit or moral structure is our deep belief about the centrality of human movement for health, well-being and function. Shulman also identifies a fourth structural dimension of a signature pedagogy—the shadow side or that which is absent or only weakly engaged (hidden) in our pedagogy.[9] We would propose that our often lack of strong attention to and integration of the psychosocial and sociocultural factors so critical for improving and facilitating human movement and experience may constitute a shadow side of our signature pedagogy. Relational skills required to learn from the patient's styles of embodiment, postures, function, and movement are often hidden in that shadow and have not been a strong focus of physical therapy education or research.

Investigations into our signature pedagogy also need to take place across the learner continuum from entry into professional preparation programs to post-professional learning experiences and professional development activities.[10] Such cross-sectional and longitudinal investigations will not only uncover the multidimensional ways in which we educate and advance the development of physical therapists, it may also expose where we have rigidity, gaps, or a limited range of teaching and learning strategies.

Two examples from other studies of professional education may help to illustrate how these investigations could help to better understand what our signature pedagogy does, or does not do, for physical therapist learners. In a study of professional education for the clergy, teaching, and clinical psychology by Grossman and colleagues,[11] the investigators uncovered 3 key teaching concepts and activities that were used across the learner continuum to prepare these learners for practice. These included (1) various *representations* of practice (these allow novices to see and learn about practice through direct observation, videos, and cases), (2) *decompositions* of practice into component parts (breaking down complex practice activities so students can name, see and enact the component parts of practice), and (3) *approximations* of practice that were more or less closely aligned with actual practice over time across the curriculum (allowing learners to move from learning opportunities, such as role playing or simulation, where there is the freedom to experiment and reflect as they gain skills before moving into real practice). As one participant in the Grossman[11] study put it, these approximations are like "learning to kayak";[11(p2076)] novices learn to paddle first in calm waters before taking on rapids. Of interest was that this investigation was directed toward better understanding preparation for relational practices (ie, clergy, teaching, clinical psychology). Physical therapy is most certainly a relational practice.[11,12]

Education research focused on our signature pedagogy is an important opportunity to make what has long been implicit and tacit—the human body as teacher[13] and make it explicit and intentional. There is much investigative work to be done in our profession that can help us develop a deeper understanding of our signature pedagogy and what it teaches our learners about what it means to be a physical therapist. In addition, investigation of our signature pedagogy should be continuous and ongoing because this pedagogy must be responsive to changes in professional practice, requisite competencies for practice, and constantly evolving societal expectations for professional education and practice. Like clinical practice itself, our signature pedagogy cannot be static.

REFLECTIVE QUESTIONS

When concurrently examining the 3 apprenticeships (head, hand, and heart) and our signature pedagogy, several questions emerged that would be important in physical therapy for further reflection and investigation:

- What does the signature pedagogy of human body as teacher teach (or not teach) about habits of head? Habits of hand? Habits of heart?
- Does the signature pedagogy of the profession privilege one or more of the 3 apprenticeships (head, hand and heart) while neglecting or diminishing the importance of another?
- To what extent are the 3 apprenticeships integrated when teaching practice-based skills?
- How and what does the signature pedagogy teach about movement and the movement system?
- Is there a shadow side to our signature pedagogy? If so, what is it?
- What are the implications of a shadow dimension of the signature pedagogy for learning and future practice? How might this be changed?
- What does it mean to learn a practice? What does that mean in physical therapy?

Practice-Based Learning

A consistent hallmark of excellence across our programs was a strong integration of academic and clinical partnerships that facilitated learning experiences grounded in practice—what we refer to here as *practice-based learning*. While we found ample evidence of practice-based learning occurring in both academic and clinical sites, we did not find that most faculty in these sites had a broad and deep understanding of this central concept. Our recommendations highlight the need to connect faculty development efforts to the learning sciences and foster recognition of how to take advantage of essential elements in the structure and nature of the practice environment to advance learning.[2,13]

- **Implement faculty development programs/activities focused on teaching and learning strategies grounded in the learning sciences, as the profession must develop a shared language, understanding of and competence in the pedagogy of learning for practice. The learning that occurs in the context of practice (situated learning) is powerful and critically important in the development of professionals and should be a central focus of faculty development.**
- **Develop models of learning environments across academic and clinical settings centered on practice-based learning with clear visibility of active clinical teaching, classroom/lab teaching, research, and practice. The situated learning that is central to practice-based learning needs to be intentionally structured and sequenced and occur early, often, and continuously.**
- **Require academic programs to participate in residency education as it provides essential opportunities for interaction, mutual reflection, and reciprocal teaching and learning between professional and post-professional learners in communities of practice.**

All programs in physical therapist education would rightfully claim that they are intentional about making connections between knowledge and skills and clinical application including integration of concepts of evidence-based practice. An essential concept here is a full understanding of situated cognition in the practice environment. Situated cognition is not just the application of knowledge or skills in a practice environment; it must also include productive thinking about how to use the knowledge-in-practice. For example, physical therapy students are taught to take vital signs as a basic skill (knowing that it is important and knowing how to assess heart rate), but it is the interpretation of those vital signs in a clinical situation that constitutes the productive thinking that enables them to know if, how, and when it is appropriate to engage the patient in exercise.

Given the strong reputation that our academic programs had for research, we fully expected to observe an intense focus on research and the use of evidence in classroom and laboratory teaching. We did find this to be true, and we also observed that these programs intentionally created powerful situated learning environments that connect academic and clinical communities in various ways so that learning was centered on and around practice. While this focus on practice was an essential goal, there was little evidence of exploration or real understanding of why practice-based learning is so robust. In education, we have long placed most of our emphasis on structures (eg, learning objectives, outcomes, goals) often aimed at producing measurable behaviors. The work of well-known educational leaders like Ralph Tyler,[14] Benjamin Bloom,[15] and Robert Mager[16] provided us descriptions of these important structures in ways that are strongly grounded in behaviorism and fit well with traditional assessment of knowledge and skills. Unfortunately, such structures are not well suited for designing or capturing the power of authentic situated activities and learning that occurs in the context and complexity of practice. Our most important outcomes for preparing professionals have to do with promoting higher-order thinking, conceptual understanding, and the ability to adapt to and successfully navigate the uncertainty of practice.[1,17-19] Situated cognition requires knowing how and when, in addition to knowing that and about, as well as being skillful in relating to the patient's motivation, concerns, and dominant styles of movement. We need to shift our attention from conceptions of learning that view learning as primarily an internal and individual process or phenomenon to those that view learning as a much broader phenomenon that is embedded in and supported by social engagement in meaningful and distributed activity. Students' practice imagination needs to embrace entering a dialogue and inquiry into theories, instead of just applying theories to practice. There is a large body of theory and research in a variety of professions that encourages such a view.[5,20-24] Once we adopt this expanded view of learning, a critical question becomes: "How is learning shaped by participation in practice?" How do students and faculty observe, articulate, foster, and enhance situated cognition, skilled know-how, and practice imagination and creativity through their encounters with patients?

Academic faculty know well that students often return from clinical experiences enthusiastically reporting on how much they learned in the clinic. The explanation for this is not simply that they got to practice what they had learned previously in classrooms and laboratories; it is far more than mere application of prior learning. Practice is a way of knowing, and students must learn to problematize and question what they are learning in practice in relation to the theories that they are learning in classrooms. Situated learning or learning that occurs through interaction in a community of practice has these common components:[25-28]

- *Communities of practice*: A community of people who share common goals and/or concerns/problems and who are involved in the learning activities
- *Legitimate peripheral participation*: A starting point for novices as they become part of the more experienced community through engagement in genuine and progressive activities, knowledge acquisition and co-construction, and transformation of their identity within the community
- *Cognitive apprenticeships*: Guided participation and learning by working closely with mentors and others in a social/cultural context

The key concept here is that thinking and learning are situated or located within the larger physical, social, and cultural context of the learning environment (Figure 9-2).

In our sites, we also found communities of practice with many different levels of learners (professional and post-professional). For example, in several sites there were entry-level students, residents, fellows, other graduate students, academic and clinical faculty, and other professionals interacting with each other. This diverse community of learners creates a distinctive affordance and provides an important and rich context for learning and knowledge transformation in that environment. The integration of learners at various levels provides a unique layering of teachers and learners and fosters opportunities for modeling and reciprocal teaching/learning within the community.

Our recommendations point to the need for intentional faculty development that helps faculty understand the deeper meaning of practice-based learning. Finding ways to create learning environments that have this community of practice element is essential for facilitating and realizing the full potential of situated learning.

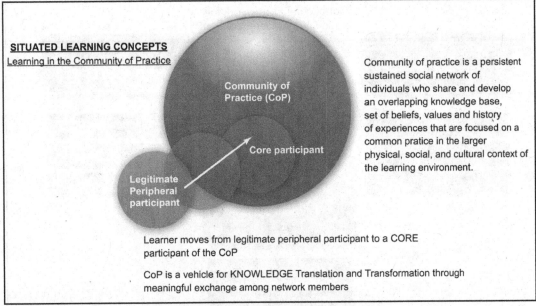

Figure 9-2. Situated learning concepts that are part of all communities of practice.[25]

We found that access to and involvement in clinical practice was a non-negotiable factor in creating optimal practice-based learning experiences and environments. We also found that the academic programs we studied worked to ensure that practice-based experiences occurred early in the curricula and were integrated across the curricula. Programs had various ways of creating academic-clinical partnerships that supported a variety of forms of practice-based learning. There was no one way to create and sustain partnerships or no one type of practice-based learning experience that was predominant. What was important, however, was that they were intentionally structured, occurred relatively early in the learners' professional program, and were sequential. We need every physical therapist program to have this commitment to creating robust and sustainable practice-based learning environments and providing learners with early, frequent, and progressively integrated practice-based learning experiences. Our findings and recommendations in this regard are consonant with some of the recommendations that emerged from a 2014 Clinical Education Summit organized by the American Council on Academic Physical Therapy.[29]

The profession has much to gain by exploring different approaches and innovative models that make optimal practice-based learning not only a reality but a constant in physical therapist professional education. We cannot underestimate the critical importance of practice-based learning as it is robust, authentic, and long lasting. Practice-based learning, also referred to as *workplace learning*, is a social process where the learning is influenced by relationships, interactions, and the opportunities and support provided to learners. Learning is not just a 1:1 relationship with a CI or mentor but occurs all the time in this community of practice.

Billett,[17,18,30] well known for his research on workplace learning, is highly critical of those who claim there is no curricular structure in workplace settings.

> Learning in workplace settings is often referred to as informal, ad hoc and non-formal forms of learning or education. Yet such a set of descriptors is neither helpful, accurate nor likely to provide the bases for effective educational provisions that would utilize and integrate these experiences to help students become able to practice their occupation in particular settings beyond graduation.[30(p106)]

O'Brien's adaptation[19] and expansion of Billett's key concepts provides a good working model for us to consider as we pose important reflective questions about practice-based or workplace learning for our consideration (Figure 9-3).[17-19]

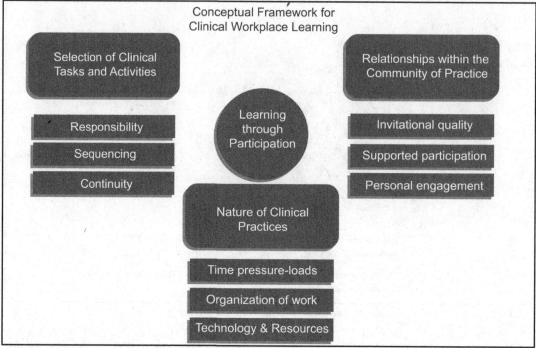

Figure 9-3. Conceptual model for elements central in workplace learning. (Adapted from Billet S. *Learning in the Workplace: Strategies for Effective Practice.* Austrailia: Allen and Unwin; 2001. and O'Brien B. Envisioning the future. In: Hafler J, ed. *Extraordinary Learning in the Workplace.* New York, NY: Springer; 2011:165-194.)

REFLECTIVE QUESTIONS

- What are the practice-based learning experiences in your curriculum? Where and when do they occur in the curriculum?
- In what ways can we make practice-based learning experiences more authentic, robust and frequent? What theories and research can inform our efforts to strengthen practice-based learning experiences?
- How might practice-based learning experiences influence change in classroom practices? The professional curriculum?
- What practice-based learning experiences and environments are most powerful in shaping learners for entry into the profession and future practice? What are the features of those experiences that make them so meaningful and powerful?
- To what extent are students guided in reflecting on and interpreting what they have learned experientially in practice?
- Is there a sequence or hierarchy of practice-based learning experiences that create successive approximations of practice that make them most effective in preparing learners for practice?
- What are the unique affordances of faculty practices vs other types of practice settings for early clinical experiences?
- What are the best ways to create an invitational quality with supported participation and personal engagement of learners in practice-based learning experiences in academic and clinical settings?
- How do we acknowledge and address the constraints of the workplace (eg, time, resources, productivity demands) in ways that still prepare learners to optimally respond to the reality and uncertainties inherent in practice?

Creating Adaptive Learners

Just as we found faculty engaged in learning environments where situated learning was centered around patients (practice-based learning), we also observed faculty facilitating many of the skills, attributes, and dispositions that characterize the adaptive learner as described in Chapter 6. Our observations and interviews also suggested that these faculty were doing this almost intuitively by placing students in situations where they could safely struggle with some of the complexity and uncertainty inherent in clinical practice. An alternative to an intuitive approach, however, is an intentional approach to the development of adaptive learners that is grounded in learning theory and educational research.[31-33] If we are to be more intentional in the development of adaptive learners,[32] then we need faculty to understand exactly what an adaptive learner is and what they can do in complex clinical situations so that our teaching and learning goals are clear. Furthermore, we need faculty to engage in education research to explore what teaching and learning strategies work best and how they work if we wish to create master adaptive learners.

The following are recommendations for physical therapist education relevant to creating adaptive learners:[2]

- **Establish a comprehensive, longitudinal approach for standardization of performance-based learning outcomes across the learner continuum that is grounded in foundational domains of professional competence. These learning outcomes will require development of performance-based assessment measures aligned with standardization of learning outcomes that are integrated and cumulative.**
- **Consistent with the profession's commitment to evidence-based practice, teaching and learning also needs to be evidence-based. The profession needs intentional development of physical therapist educational researchers who can provide such evidence for the profession and address urgent problems of learning in the profession. Researchers need to understand and explore the teaching and learning strategies that prepare adaptive learners who can assume responsibility for their learning through openness to feedback, self, and situational awareness grounded in strong self-monitoring skills, and a lifelong commitment to learning.**
- **Create a national data set that includes essential metrics of performance outcomes, structures, and processes that can be used for meaningful research to guide future evidence-based change.**

The continued development of physical therapy as a profession has resulted in the creation of the clinical doctoral degree as the first professional degree, several clinical specialties and descriptions of advanced practice for clinical specialization, along with rapid growth in post-professional residency and fellowship programs. One might call this an organic approach to a career trajectory and the development of the profession. To date, there has not been a specific focus on how we develop a framework that would identify and set expectations for performance across a career. We believe there must be significant effort directed toward the establishment of a comprehensive, longitudinal approach to describing and facilitating the development of the learner across a career that is intentional, integrative and cumulative if we are to create adaptive learners.[29,30]

Other health professions are doing work along these lines. Medicine, in response to a call for greater accountability and patient safety, has been engaged in an extensive process focused on the establishment of performance expectations across the learner continuum. The framework they have used to guide this process is grounded in entrustable professional activities (EPAs). EPAs are observable and measurable units of work (tasks or responsibilities associated with practice), that can be mapped to specific competencies and developmental milestones.[34-37] An EPA requires multiple domains of competencies simultaneously (eg, content knowledge, communication, clinical skills, values, attitudes). The student must be able to demonstrate that they are entrustable (trustworthy) to perform an activity competently and safely without supervision to proceed. Milestones have been

TABLE 9-1			
AN EXAMPLE OF AN ENTRUSTABLE PROFESSIONAL ACTIVITY AND CONNECTIONS ACROSS COMPETENCY DOMAINS, COMPETENCIES, AND MILESTONES[35,38,49]			
ENTRUSTABLE PROFESSIONAL ACTIVITY	DOMAINS OF COMPETENCE FOR PHYSICAL THERAPY	COMPETENCIES	MILESTONES
Unit of essential professional activity	Key dimensions critical to profession	Observable ability to integrate knowledge, skills, attitudes, values, and habits	Behavioral descriptor indicates level of performance for a given competency
Collaborate as a member of an interprofessional team	Knowledge for practice Communication* Professionalism* Clinical reasoning Inquiry skills Clinical skills Systems-based practice* *involved domains	Listen attentively to team members Establish and maintain a climate of mutual respect Help team members in need	Novice: Identify roles of others, communication may be unidirectional Advanced beginner: Listen actively, demonstrate respectful interactions, elicit ideas from others Competent: Support other members of the team, keep team members informed, articulate unique contributions of others on the team

identified for residency education and provide narrative descriptions of expected behaviors across a developmental sequence (novice, advanced beginner, and competent) (Table 9-1).

In medicine, the development of core EPAs for entering residency has now spawned other efforts to examine and develop additional EPAs for the undergraduate medical student, practicing physicians, and specialists. The EPA work in medical education is grounded in a model of learning and assessment that is well aligned with ongoing education research. The Core EPAs pilot project began in 2014 and pilot workgroups were established to address concepts connected to EPAs (curriculum development, learner assessment, faculty development, and entrustment decisions). These pilot efforts continue to encourage and support ongoing education research including explorations of what constitutes trustworthiness and the development of guiding principles for entrustment decisions.[38]

The pharmacy profession is also engaged in a process of defining and assessing pharmacy practice skills through EPAs.[39] While, the application of the framework of EPAs, competency domains, competencies, and milestones may not be a direct fit with physical therapy, engaging in intentional dialogue and a process that defines a developmental trajectory for therapists across their career is needed. Development of this kind of foundation for learner outcomes is clearly necessary, but may not be sufficient, as we work to fully understand and capture the dynamic use of knowledge with patients and their capacities for movement in particular situations. This is where development of paradigm cases and exemplars of adaptive strategies used in practice will be important and help us move beyond competencies. Such representations will help us to better portray and understand the social context of physical therapist practice that is so essential in the therapeutic relationship.

Current medical education research on learning and assessment has an intentional focus on the following question: What makes a good learner who can function in a rapidly changing and complex health care environment? Inquiry around this question has led to a robust and generative discussion about the knowledge, attributes, and skills of a master adaptive learner and how best to prepare such a learner.[31,32] We have a shared understanding in professional education that professionals must be prepared to not only apply their knowledge and skills but also manage uncertainty and think productively and creatively in actual clinical situations. As Schon[40] notes, "professionals practice in the swampy complexity of practice" and as Shulman[41] eloquently reminds us:

> ...the universal features that are traditionally associated with the idea of a profession are...the exercise of judgment under conditions of unavoidable uncertainty, the need for learning from experience as theory and practice interact.[(p530)]

Shulman paints a picture of productive thinking and learning directly from practice. Practice has much to teach every physical therapy student. Practice needs to be seen not as multiple sources of deficits but also as multiple sources of situated possibilities. It is these features of professions that demand the creation of adaptive learners.

We observed faculty in a variety of teaching and learning environments promoting developmental skills, attributes, and dispositions that we believe represent the characteristics of an adaptive learner. Current conceptions of adaptive learners come from work and dialogue that continues to emerge regarding the nature of adaptive expertise. Adaptive expertise has a grounding concept that "individuals will learn and innovate in response to practice challenges."[32] Adaptive expertise requires (1) openness to reflecting on practice, (2) metacognitive and reasoning skills, (3) critical thinking and willingness to challenge current assumptions, and 4) the ability to reconstruct the problem space.[32] A central component of adaptive expertise is metacognition, the ability to monitor one's current level of understanding and decide when it is or is not adequate for defining or solving a problem as it arises.[42] Furthermore, adaptive expertise highlights the critical importance of engaging in progressive problem solving and learning through that process. How do we best develop this kind of learner?

The American Medical Association supported a project, the Accelerating Change in Education program,[43] which had as one of its outcomes the creation of a conceptual model for developing a learner that could effectively manage uncertainty. This model draws on the literature in medical education and the learning sciences.[32] Adaptive learners are those learners who possess the following characteristics:

- Recognize gaps in their knowledge or skills and seek out opportunities or resources for learning
- Engage in continuous learning
- Have strong self-monitoring skills and can accurately self-assess
- Seek out and embrace feedback
- Reflect on, take action, and learn from their experience
- Incorporate new learning into practice so that they can function in complex, uncertain, and novel situations

To what extent are we incorporating concepts on developing master adaptive learners in physical therapy education and how can we strengthen learner development throughout the continuum of learning?[31,32] A starting point for the profession should be to develop targeted and far-reaching efforts to help the physical therapy education community develop a broader and deeper understanding of learning theories, critical learning concepts, and educational research that can inform and advance our work as educators.

The development of a comprehensive, longitudinal standardization of performance-based learning outcomes across the learner continuum is an important foundation for generating a shared national data set. The development of such a shared structure and consistent metrics for assessment of learner performance would also facilitate meaningful education research.[13,44]

We began this discussion about creating adaptive learners by asserting that the profession needs to take a longitudinal approach for the development of performance-based learning outcomes across the learner continuum and across a physical therapist's career. An area that continues to deserve and receive our attention in the profession is exploration of how we can foster the development of sound clinical reasoning abilities.[45-47] This is an area where we have great opportunity and an urgent need.

- **The profession must establish a comprehensive, longitudinal approach for the explicit develop-ment of learners' clinical reasoning skills that spans entry-level through clinical residencies and continues across the therapist's career. This comprehensive approach to clinical reasoning will require that academic and clinical faculty develop robust teaching, learning, and assess-ment strategies.**

While we observed faculty facilitating the development of learners' clinical reasoning in many learning environments, there was little evidence of (1) a shared language around clinical reasoning, (2) the ability to clearly articulate explicit teaching strategies for advancing clinical reasoning, or (3) standard tools for assessment of clinical reasoning. These are all areas that can be improved through the establishment of the comprehensive, longitudinal approach to advancing clinical reasoning skills that we recommend.

On a positive note, the growth of clinical residency programs in physical therapy has led to an increase in an intentional focus on the development of clinical reasoning skills.[48] When interviewing the resident mentors who participated in our study, we found that these clinical mentors were very focused on, and committed to, the development of residents' clinical reasoning abilities; they reported that they had learned a great deal about how to foster such abilities through their everyday work as a mentor. As a result, they now saw themselves as better teachers when working with entry-level physical therapist students in clinical and classroom environments. These mentors reported that they were now more intentional in facilitating clinical reasoning with learners in professional education in ways like those they used with post-professional learners.

We are not alone here in our need to further define, describe, and investigate clinical reasoning because it is a complex and multifaceted concept. Gruppen[49] says it well:

> Like the fable of the blind men and the elephant, each of whom, feeling a different part of the elephant, described it in very different ways, clinical reasoning is a vast, complex construct that is described and used in different ways by different people. A skeptic may ask "What is not clini-cal reasoning?"[(p4)]

While clinical reasoning is an area that continues to receive more attention in the profession through a variety of small, often single institution studies, it remains an area of education research that needs serious, immediate attention.[45,48] Christensen et al found in a survey of physical therapist programs that while clinical reasoning was explicitly integrated into these programs, there was wide variation as to the definition of clinical reasoning, how to best teach clinical reasoning, and how to best assess student learning of clinical reasoning.[46] The profession can certainly build on emerging theories and concepts from medical education, but physical therapy has much to gain by uncovering the unique dimensions of clinical reasoning that are central to the work of physical therapists. Clinical reasoning in any practice discipline calls for reasoning across time about the in relation to the general.

The current interest in the importance of context, affect, and distinguishing diagnostic reasoning from therapeutic reasoning has great potential for physical therapy. From past research in physical therapy, we know that collaboration with the patient is an important element in the clinical reasoning of expert therapists.[50-52] The research by Edwards et al[51] on clinical reasoning strategies in physical therapy identified clinical reasoning strategies focused on interaction, procedure, teaching, collabora-tion, prediction, and ethics, integrated in their dialectic model of clinical reasoning. In this dialectic model, the therapist moves among a more instrumental or hypothetico-deductive approach, to reason-ing and action, to a narrative approach of reasoning and action as the therapist works to understand the patient's lived experience and the assumptions underlying a patient's values and beliefs. Physical thera-py, as a profession where patient outcome often depends on the patient engaging with the therapist and participating in the interventions, relies heavily on our interaction and relationship with patients.[47,52]

We know that collaboration with the patient is an important element in the clinical reasoning of expert therapists,[6,50,51] but there is much more to be learned. While critical thinking continues to be a strong focus in higher education, others advocate for an expanded understanding of the reasoning processes that are essential in clinical practice environments.[53,54] These environments require clinical reasoning across time and through changes in the patient's status as well as changes in the clinician's understanding of the situation. Critical thinking is necessary but not sufficient in practice disciplines. For physical therapy, this means that practice is grounded in established scientific evidence and our knowledge about physical movement, but our clinical (practical) reasoning helps us to make sense of movement as it is embodied in our patients and their ability to understand their own movement at a given point in time. Physical therapists need to think productively, engage in progressive problem solving, and act in clinical situations that are constantly evolving; such practice demands mean we must move well beyond narrower conceptions of critical thinking in classrooms.

If we were to identify a shadow side (neglected area) of teaching and learning strategies currently in use to facilitate in clinical reasoning, it is likely to be how we fully integrate our understanding of movement, the movement system, the skills of engagement and relational skills between therapist and patient, and the psychosocial and cultural aspects of the human experience into our clinical reasoning and decision making.

Reflective Questions

- What are the characteristics of a master adaptive learner in physical therapy? How are these similar to or different from those described in other professions? Are there any unique features that distinguish adaptive expertise in physical therapy?
- What knowledge, skills, and attitudes are most critical for facilitating the development of an adaptive learner and adaptive expertise?
- What teaching and learning strategies are most effective in helping learners to engage in critical self-appraisal?
- How do we define, describe, and assess clinical reasoning in physical therapy? What more do we need to know? How can we improve?
- How might we develop a learner continuum for the development and refinement of clinical reasoning abilities in our learners?
- How do we broaden our understanding and teaching of clinical reasoning that is explicitly inclusive of the psychological and sociocultural aspects of human movement?

In Part I of this chapter, we have provided and elaborated on recommendations related to the first 3 elements in the *Praxis of Learning* dimension of our model of excellence in physical therapist education. These recommendations emanate from our observations of excellence and innovation in our participant sites, and from non-observations; that is, things that we were not seeing that might further promote excellence in those educational environments and across the physical therapist education community in general. A theme that runs through all our recommendations related to the elements of *Signature Pedagogy, Practice-Based Learning,* and *Creating Adaptive Learners,* is the urgent need for infusing learning theory and the learning sciences into all that we do in physical therapist education in academic and clinical settings. A corollary to this, and no less urgent, is the need for academicians and clinicians alike to engage in rigorous, systematic, and broadly-based education research in physical therapy so that our teaching and learning practices are grounded in evidence. The time to do this is now if we are to truly transform physical therapist education so we are optimally preparing the practitioners of the future practitioners equipped to not only navigate the complexity of a constantly changing health care environment, but to thrive in it.

Part II

Understanding and Enacting
Our Social Contract

The underlying framework for the Carnegie studies includes the 3 apprenticeships that are well established in professional education: knowledge (habits of head), skill development (habits of hand) and development of a professional identity or formation (habits of heart).[55-59] We observed many examples of professional identify formation across academic and clinical settings where academic and clinical organizations held a strong commitment to quality patient care as well as authentic engagement in their communities to meet health care needs. Similar to the Carnegie studies,[56-59] we found far more emphasis across our sites in these first 2 apprenticeships (habits of head and hand) with less intentional emphasis on the third apprenticeship (habit of heart). Colby and Sullivan[59] encourage all professions to develop a stronger and integrative function for professional formation that they believe is essential for a profession to assume its fundamental purpose to meet societal needs. Not surprisingly, this element in our conceptual model generated the most recommendations. These first 2 recommendations highlight how critical the professional curriculum is in the professional formation of learners. Intentional development of learners' moral foundation and understanding of their professional obligations should be a non-negotiable and explicit component in the curriculum.[2]

Professional Formation

- **Develop a strong sense of the moral foundations that underpin and are inseparable from practice in all physical therapists so that they demonstrate a full understanding of the meaning of being part of a profession, including their obligations as advocates in organizational and policy arenas for patients, clients, and the health needs of society. Physical therapists must develop the moral courage and ability to respond to substandard practice. The moral dimensions of patient-centered care permeate practice and, thus, must be explicit and deeply embedded in the professional curriculum. There must be faculty who have expertise in the moral foundations and who collaborate with other faculty members to integrate the moral foundation of practice into learning throughout the curriculum.**

- **Develop the moral courage and ability to respond to substandard practice in all physical therapists. Teaching and learning activities must help physical therapists resist the stresses that can be experienced with meeting these obligations in the reality of practice, and lead to reduction in the level of stress as practice changes to more clearly reflect these obligations. Just as learning in clinical courses must be practice based, so too should the learning experience in these areas be grounded in actual practice, leading to learners who have strong self-monitoring skills, able to function as moral agents in complex and uncertain situations.**

Physical therapy has long struggled with the question "are we a profession?" We would argue, along with many of the colleagues upon whose shoulders we stand, that we do indeed believe we are profession.[60-63] Professional status is not something we claim through our claim for a doctor of physical therapy as the degree for entry into the profession or asserting our own autonomy, but it is in how the profession, individually and collectively, is demonstrating deep engagement in our public purposes to meet societal needs and how our contributions are valued by society.[64,65] The advent of the Doctor of Physical Therapy as the first professional degree for physical therapists has produced many activities and rituals focused on developing students' professional identity as a doctoring profession (eg, professionalism, white coat ceremonies), but professionalism must be more than teaching about accepted professional standards.

This third apprenticeship has a deeper purpose that goes well beyond understanding a code of ethics, standards of practice, and regulatory requirements. Nor is professional formation just obtained implicitly through professional socialization or role modeling. The third apprenticeship, professional formation, means learners must develop, internalize, and sustain their commitment to professionalism. Socialization focuses on the influence of mentors and other professionals on the development of professional identity and role functions within the social context of practice. Professional formation moves beyond this and includes the student's agency in participating in their own formation and their aspirations to change themselves to become an excellent physical therapist. In addition, students must learn to embody moral foundations in their everyday practice. Professionalism that incorporates all these characteristics and commitments, will often be challenged through regulatory, fiscal, and political pressures in their workplace.[64] Learners need to embrace the profession's core values as well as develop deliberate habits or dispositions that demonstrate skills, practices, and a predictable way of being and acting as a professional.[65,66]

Benner et al[57] describe formation well here:

Formation...denotes the development of perceptual abilities, the ability to draw on knowledge and skilled know-how, and a way of being and acting in practice and in the world...Students are formed by all they do, all they read, all they perceive and interpret, and in all models of practice, not only in the context of what they think or know intellectually, but also in terms of their taken-for-granted assumptions and expectations.[(p166)]

The classroom and the clinic are not separate entities. We found that the partnership between the academic and clinical worlds is a necessary factor contributing to excellence. The learning that occurs in the community of practice is often the most powerful and long lasting. Our challenge is to find ways that fully integrate classroom and clinical learning across the 3 apprenticeships (habits of head, hand, heart) in a seamless manner. Professional formation as a focus in physical therapist education must go well beyond teaching the code of ethics or application of biomedical ethical principles to clinical cases. While teaching basic ethics concepts provide important fundamental knowledge for students, professional formation occurs as the result of the integration of knowledge, skilled know-how, and ethical comportment that is learned in situations over time and requires the learner to transform his or her ways of perceiving and acting.[67] Learners engage in a transformation process of perceiving and acting through "metacognition" or a process of reflection.[41] The resolution of difficult ethical dilemmas is not done merely through application of ethical principles or standards but requires strong self-monitoring skills (metacognition) and the ability of the learner to demonstrate moral courage in taking necessary actions.

As Triezenberg and Davis[68] eloquently state, "No matter how thorough and refined our educational process, a huge gap exists between knowing what is good or right and doing it."[(p53)] They made a plea for the profession to think beyond the code of ethics and educate for moral agency in their 2001 article.[68] Since that time, we have had continued commentary in our literature about how critical it is for the profession to educate for moral action, yet we have more work to do.[68-72] As the Carnegie studies demonstrate, it is this integration of the third apprenticeship that is most challenging.

Benner has long advocated for the central importance of ethical comportment in everyday clinical practice. Benner et al[67] found these ethical themes present in the formative learning experiences that they believe are part of the everyday ethical comportment of nurses:

- Meeting the patient as a person, not a diagnosis or an object
- Preserving the dignity and personhood of patients and awareness of when the dignity of a patient is not honored
- Ability to respond to substandard practice even though students are challenged because of their status
- Patient advocacy by giving the patient a voice and advocating on the patient's behalf

- Students and faculty engaged in good practice through a pervasive concern for ongoing improvement of their practice
- Learning how to be present with patient and family suffering

Formation is a process that moves beyond knowledge and must identify the moral content of practices that includes the obligations and demands that are imposed. The Carnegie studies identify necessary shifts in how educators think about their teaching.[68]

- Move from curricular threads/competencies to the integration of the 3 apprenticeships (cognitive knowledge, practice know-how, and ethical comportment/formation)
- Expand our focus beyond critical thinking to clinical reasoning and multiple ways of thinking and acting as a moral agent
- Partnerships between academic and clinical settings that are focused on integration of teaching, moving beyond socialization to formation

In the nursing book, Benner et al[73] use Margaret Mohrmann's metaphor of dance to describe formation.

> ...having and displaying integrity is more a matter of being able to move in ways that are consistent with the originating and developing themes of our lives. Teachers, guides, and practice make us better dancers because they help us listen more carefully and follow the music we hear more confidently. We learn which movements fit the rhythms and which do not.[(p87)]

Our recommendations also span the need for our professional community to understand and find ways to address the social problems that underlie health of individuals and communities. This requires engagement of physical therapists as citizens in their communities and the profession finding an important collective voice in advocating for the health needs of society (our public purpose).[69-71] Physical therapists are on the frontline in terms of confronting the impact of social policies on health, and health care policies on designing and implementing best care for clients. Students need to learn how to move from their first-hand experience of the specific individual cases to the implications at the population and health care policy levels.

- **Act on our individual and collective responsibilities to society, or we jeopardize our status as a profession. Individual therapists and the profession must fully commit to eliminate health disparities, address the social determinants of health, and improve the health care, health, and well-being of our communities and promote the health of populations. The profession must be integral partners within the health care community, public health, community agencies, and governments to achieve this commitment.**
- **Recognize the unique responsibility as academic programs to partner with the community in developing and implementing programs that place positive health outcomes to the community as their primary focus.**

This broader conception of professionalism that centers on the profession recognizing and acting as a moral community is a crucial area for transformative growth. We must remember that health is all about people. The strongest influences on health are social influences or social determinants where people live, and their level of education, social supports, and economic status.[69-71,74-76]

How can the profession both individually and collectively be change agents in addressing these social influences on health? We can begin by ensuring that we have a dynamic curriculum that is both patient-centered and population based in preparing students with the professional competencies to meet the societal, demographic challenges. Students need to learn to aggregate the everyday consequences of unjust and ineffective social health policies, and health care inequities that they find in their practice. The level of discourse must not remain at the individual level, students need to see and imagine the broader implications of lack of good health and social policies that they encounter in their practice that influence the health of society and populations.

In the United States, from 2015 to 2030 the population 65 and over will increase by 55%, and this greying of the population will be accompanied by a shift from communicable diseases to non-communicable diseases. By 2040, the United States will have a majority minority population (racial and ethnic diversity being the majority group) and by 2060, the number of Americans ages 65 and older will double and represent nearly 25% of all Americans.[77,78] The profession needs to ensure that our students and faculty not only fully understand the social determinants of health but also the deeper meanings of poverty and oppression that they have less to do with individual responsibility than social structural forces such as education and opportunity, often called upstream factors.

We did observe examples of programs providing physical therapy care through community-based activities, yet most were focused on immediate curricular needs and not developed nor implemented in such a way that students and faculty investigated any root social influences on health and demonstrated any professional obligation to work toward elimination of social inequities. Sharma et al[79] argue that the current approach to teaching the social determinants of health has too much emphasis on facts to be known rather than a challenging of the conditions of power and privilege that lead to inequities. Students would benefit from developing critical consciousness where they can reflect on these conditions and develop an active commitment to social justice. Berwick,[80] in an editorial addressing moral choices for today's physicians, states:

> Silence is now political. Either engage or assist the harm. There is no third choice. Ethics cannot be taken for granted, not when the interests to be served as those of society. Professional silence in the face of social injustice is wrong.(p282)

Colby and Sullivan[59] assert that professional schools serve as important portals to professional life and need to attend to these 5 key qualities to ensure sustainable, lifelong growth of professional competence and commitment:

1. Deep engagement with the profession's public purposes
2. A strong sense of professional identity that includes integrity as an essential feature
3. Habits of salience which allows the professional to frame and understand complex situations in moral terms
4. Habitual patterns of behavior with patients and others that are well aligned with the profession's standards and ideals and not overriding self-interest
5. Sense of moral agency in relation to questionable aspects of institutional context and the moral courage to create more constructive structures and practices

Our team has one final recommendation, which is the need for the profession to engage in a critical self-reflective process and assume responsibility for creating more diverse and inclusive communities across academic and practice environments.

- **Academic institutions must take a leadership role to create more diverse and inclusive learning and practice environments for the profession to have a positive impact on addressing the social determinants of health. Physical therapy programs must recruit and retain faculty and students who represent the racial, and ethnic, cultural, and socioeconomic diversity of our country, particularly for people who are from unrepresented minorities in health care and from socioeconomically disadvantaged backgrounds. There must be an active rejection of the assumption that lack of diversity is a problem that cannot be solved. Curricular content, admissions and retention policies, and hiring policies, among other topics, all must be addressed.**

Several of our colleagues have highlighted the need for the profession to address our lack of diversity. Ruth Purtilo, in the 31st McMillan Lecture,[63] passionately argued that cultural competence needed to be as non-negotiable a graduation requirement and tested rigorously as our expectations for competence in pathokinesiology. She went on to say that we are diversity-challenged in our profession, "Just look at how pale this audience is! Ninety-three percent of the physical therapists in the American Physical Therapy Association list themselves as White."63(p1119) The 2013 APTA membership profile[81] shows that 91.7% list themselves as White, not much of a change from 2000 to 2013[72] and the 2015 APTA membership, statistics for physical therapists show that 2.3% are Black, 3.0% are Hispanic/Latino 3.0%, and 85.6% are White.[82]

Domholdt,[83] in the 2007 Cerasoli lecture, identified "excessive elitism in admissions decisions" as one of our professional sins. Jette[84] reminded us in her 2016 Cerasoli lecture that while the demographics of the country are shifting in terms of race and ethnicity, this is not true in higher education:

> Physical Therapy Centralized Appication Service data for 2013 to 2014 show that students enrolled in our programs are not reflective of the racial/ethnic diversity represented by the college undergraduate population in the United States. We often are looking for student fit in a program, which translates to just like us.[(p6)]

We can no longer claim that our challenges with developing a more racially and ethnically diverse profession remain because we cannot compete with other health professions such as medicine, dentistry, or pharmacy or the geographic locations of our programs. We have a professional responsibility and a commitment to a higher social purpose in meeting the needs of an increasingly diverse society. If we truly want to enhance the diversity of our profession, we must leverage critical points in the preparation of pipeline stages that include recruitment and selection of students, and recruitment and selection of faculty.[63,64]

REFLECTIVE QUESTIONS

- What are we doing explicitly for the professional formation of our learners that moves beyond professional identity though common rituals such as white coat ceremonies? What are we doing to prepare students as moral agents?
- Does the profession of physical therapy have a responsibility to work toward elimination of these social inequities that affect health? If so, then what are the educational implications?
- How well are our curricula aligned with population health and what society needs from health care professionals? Do we have curriculum and learning experiences that prepare students to manage the challenges of an aging population?
- How should we prepare students so they that the profession has a fundamental commitment to social justice, or do we?
- Do our learners develop critical consciousness so they understand the social, cultural, and historical context that underlies social problems? If not, how might we facilitate this?

Part II of this chapter focused on the recommendations specific to the element *Professional Formation*. This element generated 5 recommendations, the largest number of recommendations for any of the elements in the Praxis of Learning dimension of our model of excellence in physical therapist education. Not unlike the Carnegie Preparation for the Professions Program studies, the third apprenticeship (habits of heart or professional formation) is often the weakest apprenticeship in professional education with the predominant focus on knowledge and clinical skills. As a profession that is still in the phase of adoption of a clinical doctoral degree for entry into the profession, we have challenges along with great opportunities in demonstrating how we can better prepare our graduates for professional responsibility giving them the skills of taking individual health and clinical issues and raising them to a public policy level of analysis. A pervasive theme in our recommendations is the urgent need for preparing learners to have the moral courage and agency in challenging questionable aspects in our work environments that undermine the profession's fundamental purposes and quality education and practice. Just as we argued across the elements in our model of excellence, collaboration between professional schools and the clinical practice communities is essential in the professional formation of physical therapists.

ACKNOWLEDGEMENTS

We acknowledge Dr. Patricia Benner's insightful and wise comments that have been incorporated into this chapter.

REFERENCES

1. Shulman L. Pedagogies of uncertainty. *Liberal Education.* 2005;91(2):18-25.
2. Jensen GM, Hack L, Nordstrom T, Gwyer J, Mostrom E. National study of excellence and innovation in physical therapist education: part 2: call for reform. *Phys Ther.* 2017;97:875-888.
3. American Physical Therapy Association. Vision statement. http://www.apta.org/Vision/. Updated March 20, 2018. Accessed December 28, 2017.
4. Shepard KF. 34th Mary McMillan Lecture. Are you waving or drowning? *Phys Ther.* 2007;87:1543-1554.
5. Jensen GM. 42nd Mary McMillan Lecture. Learning: what matters most. *Phys Ther.* 2011;91:1674-1689.
6. Jensen GM, Gwyer J, Hack L, Shepard KF. *Expertise in Physical Therapy Practice.* 2nd ed. St. Louis, MO: Elsevier; 2007.
7. Covington K, Barcinas SJ. Situational analysis of physical therapist clinical instructors' facilitation of students' emerging embodiment of movement in practice. *Phys Ther.* 2017;97:603-614.
8. Rose M. Our hands will know: the development of tactile diagnostic skill-teaching, learning, and situated cognition in a physical therapy program. *Anthropology and Education Quarterly.* 1999;30:133-160.
9. Shulman LS. Signature pedagogies in the professions. *Daedelus.* 2005;134:52-59.
10. Sullivan W, Colby A, Wegner JW, Bond L, Shulman LS. *Educating Lawyers: Preparation for the Profession of Law.* San Francisco, CA: Jossey Bass; 2007.
11. Grossman P, Compton C, Igra D, Ronfeldt M, Shahan E, Williamson P. Teaching practice: a cross-professional perspective. *Teachers College Record.* 2009;111:2055-2100.
12. Cohen D. Professions of human improvement: predicaments of teaching. In: Nisan M, Schremer O, eds. *Educational Deliberations.* Jerusalem, Isreal: Keter Publishers; 2005:278-294.
13. Jensen GM, Nordstrom T, Mostrom EM, Hack LM, Gwyer J. A national study of excellence and innovation in physical therapist education: part 1–design, methods, and results. *Phys Ther.* 2017;97:857-874.
14. Tyler R. *Basic Principles of Curriculum and Instruction.* Chicago, IL: University of Chicago Press; 1949.
15. Bloom B, ed. *Taxonomy of Educational Objectives, Handbook I: Cognitive Domain.* New York, NY: David McKay; 1956.
16. Mager R. *Preparing Instructional Objectives: A Critical Tool in the Development of Effective Instruction.* 3rd ed. Atlanta, GA: Center for Effective Performance; 1997.
17. Billet S. *Learning in the Workplace: Strategies for Effective Practice.* Crows Nest, Australia: Allen and Unwin; 2001.
18. Billet S. Workplace participatory practices: conceptualizing workplaces as learning environments. *J Workplace Learn.* 2004;16(6):312-324.
19. O'Brien B. Envisioning the future. In: Hafler J, ed. *Extraordinary Learning in the Workplace.* New York, NY: Springer; 2011:165-194.
20. Bleakley A, Bligh J. Students learning from patients: let's get real in medical education. *Adv in the Health Sci Edu.* 2008;13:89-107.
21. Mostrom EM. 16th Pauline Cerasoli Lecture. Life lessons: teaching for learning that lasts. *J Phys Ther Educ.* 2013;27:4-11.
22. Halfer J, ed. *Extraordinary Learning in the Workplace.* New York, NY; Springer; 2011.
23. Higgs J, Sheehan D, Currens J, Letts W, Jensen G, eds. *Realising Exemplary Practice-Based Education.* Rotterdam, Netherlands: Sense Publishers; 2013.
24. Murphy PK, Knight S. Exploring a century of advancements in the science of learning. *Review of Research in Education.* 2016;40:402-456.
25. Lave J, Wenger E. *Situated Learning: Legitimate Peripheral Participation.* Cambridge, UK: Cambridge University Press; 1991.
26. Brown JS, Collins A, Duguid P. Situated cognition and the culture of learning. *Educ Res.* 1989;18:32-42.
27. Rogoff B. *Apprenticeship in Thinking: Cognitive Development in Social Context.* New York, NY: Oxford University Press; 1990.
28. Wenger E, McDermott R, Snyder WM. *Cultivating Communities of Practice.* Boston, MA: Harvard Business School Press; 2002.
29. American Council of Academic Physical Therapy. Clinical Education Summit, Final Report. http://www.acapt.org/docs/default-source/pdfs/clinical-education-summit-2014-final-report-1.pdf. Published December 2014. Accessed February 1, 2017.

30. Billet S. Practice-based learning and professional education. In: Higgs J, BarnettR, Billett S, Hutchings M, Trede F, eds. *Practice-Based Education*. Boston, MA: Sense Publishing; 2012:101-112.

31. Schumacher D, Englander R, Carraccio C. Developing the master learner: applying learning theory to the learner, the teacher, and the learning environment. *Acad Med*. 2013;88:1635-1645.

32. Cutrer WB, Miller B, Pusic M, et al. Fostering the development of master adaptive learners: a conceptual model to guide skill acquisition in medical education. *Acad Med*. 2017;92:70-75.

33. Mann K. Theoretical perspectives in medical education: past experience and future possibilities. *Med Ed*. 2011;45:60-68.

34. Association of American Medical Colleges. *Core Entrustable Activities for Entering Residency: Curriculum Developers Guide*. https://members.aamc.org/eweb/upload/Core%20EPA%20Curriculum%20Dev%20Guide.pdf. Published 2014. Accessed July 14, 2017.

35. Ten Cate O, Chen HC, Hoff RG, Peters H, Bok H, van der Schaaf M. Curriculum development for the workplace using Entrustable Professional Activities (EPAs). AMEE Guide No. 99. *Med Teach*. 2015;37(11):983-1002.

36. Carracio C, Englander R, Gilhooly J, et al. Building a framework of entrustable professional activities, supported by competencies and milestones, to bridge the education continuum. *Acad Med*. 2017;92:324-330.

37. Chesbro S, Jensen GM, Boissonnault W. Entrustable professional activities as a framework for continued professional competence: is now the time? *Phys Ther*. 2018;98:3-7.

38. Brown D, Warren J, Hyderi A, et al. Finding a path to entrustment in undergraduate medical education: a progress report from the AAMC core entrustable professional activities for entering residency entrustment concept group. *Acad Med*. 2017;92(6):774-779.

39. Pittenger AL, Chapman SA, Frail CK, et al. Entrustable professional activities for pharmacy practice. *Am J Pharm Educ*. 2016;80(4):1-4.

40. Schon D. *Educating the Reflective Practitioner*. San Francisco, CA: Jossey-Bass; 1987.

41. Shulman L. *The Wisdom of Practice: Essays on Teaching, Learning, and Learning to Teach*. San Francisco, CA: Jossey-Bass; 2004.

42. Bransford J, Brown A, Cocking R, eds. *How People Learn*. Washington, DC: National Academy Press; 2000.

43. American Medical Association. Accelerating change in medical education: creating a community of innovation. https://www.ama-assn.org/education/creating-medical-school-future. Accessed November 26, 2017.

44. Jensen GM, Nordstrom T, Segal R, McCallum C, Graham C, Greenfield B. Education research in physical therapy: visions of the possible. *Phys Ther*. 2016;96:1874-1884.

45. Christensen N, Nordstrom T. Facilitating the teaching and learning of clinical reasoning. In: Jensen GM, Mostrom E. *Handbook of Teaching and Learning for Physical Therapists*. 3rd ed. Boston, MA: Elsevier; 2013:183-199.

46. Christensen N, Black L, Furze J, Hun K, Vendrely A, Wainwright S. Clinical reasoning: survey of teaching methods, integration, and assessment in entry-level physical therapist academic education. *Phys Ther*. 2017;97:175-186.

47. Gilliland S, Wainwright S. Patterns of clinical reasoning in physical therapist students. *Phys Ther*. 2017;97:499-511.

48. Furze J, Tichenor C, Fisher B, Jensen G, Rapport M. Physical therapy residency and fellowship education: reflections on the past, present, and future. *Phys Ther*. 2016;96(7):949-960.

49. Gruppen L. Clinical reasoning: defining it, teaching it, assessing it, studying it. Editorial. *J Emerg Med*. 2017;18:4-7.

50. Edwards I, Jones M. Clinical reasoning and expertise. In: Jensen GM, Gwyer J, Hack L, Shepard K, eds. *Expertise in Physical Therapy Practice*. 2nd ed. Boston, MA: Elsevier; 2007:192-213.

51. Edwards I, Jones M, Carr J, Braunack-Mayer A, Jensen GM. Clinical reasoning strategies in physical therapy. *Phys Ther*. 2004; 84:312-330.

52. Wainwright S, Shepard KF, Harman L, Stephens J. Factors that influence the clinical decision making of novice and experienced physical therapists. *Phys Ther*. 2011;91:87-101.

53. Benner P, Hooper-Kyriakidis P, Stannard D. *Clinical Wisdom and Interventions in Acute and Critical Care*. 2nd ed. New York, NY: Springer; 2011.

54. Sullivan W, Rosin M. *A New Agenda for Higher Education: Shaping a Life of the Mind for Practice*. San Francisco, CA: Jossey-Bass; 2008.

55. Foster C, Dahill L, Goleman L, Tolentino BW. *Educating Clergy: Teaching Practices and Pastoral Imagination*. San Francisco, CA: Jossey-Bass; 2006.

56. Sheppard S, Macatangay K, Colby A, Sullivan W. *Educating Engineers: Designing the Future of the Field*. San Francisco, CA: Jossey-Bass; 2009.

57. Benner P, Sutphen M, Leonard C, Day L. *Educating Nurses: A Call for Radical Transformation*. San Francisco, CA: Jossey-Bass; 2010.

58. Cooke M, Irby D, O'Brien B. *Educating Physicians: A Call for Reform of Medical School and Residency*. San Francisco, CA: Jossey-Bass; 2010.

59. Colby A, Sullivan W. Formation of professionalism and purpose: perspectives from the preparation for professions program. *University of St. Thomas Law Journal*. 2008;5:404-426.

60. Rothstein J. 32nd Mary McMillan Lecture. Journeys beyond the horizon. *Phys Ther*. 2001;81:1817-1829.

61. Worthingham C. Complementary functions and responsibilities in an emerging profession. *Phys Ther*. 1965;45:935-939.

62. Magistro C. 22nd Mary McMillan Lecture. *Phys Ther*. 1987;67:1726-1732.

63. Purtilo RB. 32nd Mary McMillan Lecture. A time to harvest, a time to sow; ethics for a shifting landscape. *Phys Ther.* 2000;80:112-119.

64. Mitchell DE, Ream R, eds. *Professional Responsibility: The Fundamental Issue in Education and Health Care Reform.* New York, NY: Springer Publishing; 2015.

65. Sullivan W. *Work and Integrity: The Crisis and Promise of Professionalism in America.* 2nd ed. San Francisco, CA: Jossey-Bass; 2005.

66. Benner P, Sutphen M. Learning across professions: the clergy, a case in point. *J Nursing Educ.* 2007;46:3c.

67. Benner P, Sutphen M, Leonard-Kahn V, Day L. Formation and everyday ethical comportment. *Am J Crit Care.* 2008;17:473-476.

68. Triezenberg H, Davis CM. Beyond the code of ethics: educating physical therapists for their role as moral agents. *J Phys Ther Educ.* 2001;14:48-58.

69. Purtilo R, Jensen GM, Royeen CB, eds. *Educating for Moral Action: A Sourcebook in Health and Rehabilitation Ethics.* Philadelphia, PA: FA Davis; 2005.

70. Edwards I, Delany C, Townsend A, Swisher L. New perspectives on the theory of justice: implications for physical therapy ethics and clinical practice. *Phys Ther.* 2011;91:1642-1652.

71. Edwards I, Delany C, Townsend A, Swisher L. Moral agency as enacted justice: a clinical and ethical decision making framework for responding to health inequities and social injustice. *Phys Ther.* 2011;91:1653-1663.

72. Delany C, Edwards I, Jensen GM, Skinner E. Closing the gap between ethics knowledge and practice through active engagement: an applied model of physical therapy ethics. *Phys Ther.* 2010;90:1068-1078.

73. Mohrmann M. In: Benner P, Sutphen M, Leonard C, Day L. *Educating Nurses: A Call for Radical Transformation.* San Francisco, CA: Jossey-Bass; 2010:93-95.

74. Stone J. Saving and ignoring lives: physicians' obligations to address root social influences on health—moral justifications and educational implications. *Cambridge Quarterly of Health Care Ethics.* 2010;19:497-509.

75. Frenk J, Chen L, Bhutta ZA, et al. Health professionals for a new century: transforming education to strengthen health systems in an interdependent world. *Lancet.* 2010;376:1923-1958.

76. Dean E, Greig A, Murphy S, et al. Raising the priority of lifestyle-related noncommunicable diseases in physical therapy curricula. *Phys Ther.* 2016;96:940-948.

77. Kalache A. The greying world: a challenge for the 21st century. *Science Progress.* 2000;83:33-54.

78. Population Reference Bureau. Fact sheet: aging in the United States. http://www.prb.org/Publications/Media-Guides/2016/aging-unitedstates-fact-sheet.aspx. Accessed November 28, 2017.

79. Sharma M, Pinto A, Kumagai A. Teaching the social determinants of health: a path to equity or a road to nowhere? *Acad Med.* 2018;93:25-30.

80. Berwick D. Moral choices for today's physician. *JAMA.* 2017;318:2081-282.

81. American Physical Therapy Association. 2013 Membership Profile. https://www.apta.org/WorkforceData/DemographicProfile/PTMember/. Accessed November 28, 2017.

82. ACAPT Diversity Report. http://www.aptaaz.org/docs/default-source/practice/house-of-delegates/2017-az-motion--professional-diversity-02-25-17.pdf?sfvrsn=4. Published February 2017. Accessed September 4, 2018.

83. Domholdt E. 2007 Polly Cerasoli Lecture: sins of the professional programs. *J Phys Ther Educ.* 2007;21:4-9.

84. Jette D. 19th Annual Polly Cerasoli Lecture: unflattening. *J Phys Ther Educ.* 2016;30:4-10.

10

Organizational Imperatives

Our observations of the academic and clinical sites in our study (described in Chapter 7) demonstrate that changes in organizational structures and resources can transform physical therapist education. We have developed 7 recommendations based on these observations and supporting literature. These recommendations can be accomplished by the individuals and institutions engaged in physical therapist education. Their enactment will lead to real, positive change in physical therapist education.

RECOMMENDATIONS RELATED TO ACADEMIC PROGRAMS

1. Ensure that academic programs have control of their financial resources, and that they develop economic models for revenue generation through multiple means, (eg, tuition, development, grants, clinical revenues). They must discard beliefs that small class sizes are inherently better and move towards larger programs to increase the range and depth of faculty expertise and other necessary resources.

2. Develop strategies so that academic programs become respected, valued partners within their organizations and have influence over their resources.

Almost since the beginning of physical therapist education, there have been efforts to improve the skills of educational leaders in the financial management of their programs. This takes a twofold approach. First, it is essential to understand financial management in higher education. There has been little emphasis on learning the skills of financial management as part of the preparation of academic leaders. The American Physical Therapy Association Educational Leadership Institute

Jensen GM, Mostrom E, Hack LM, Nordstrom T, Gwyer J.
Educating Physical Therapists (pp 147-154).
© 2019 Taylor & Francis Group.

program includes a module on financial management, but this program is available to only a small number of people each year.[1]

The second aspect is to ensure that physical therapist education programs have access to a reasonable share of the revenues that they produce in higher education. Many physical therapist education programs are under-resourced; when coupled with a belief that small classes are in some way better, these programs are not able to achieve important goals for excellence. Other physical therapist education programs are being used to financially support the academic institution's financial position, thus siphoning a greater percentage of the program's revenue to the institution. Control of the program's resources often does not lie with the program's leadership and too often the ability to advocate for and accrue additional resources is limited by the abilities, institutional awareness, and the will of the leadership within the program or at the institution.

There is a long tradition in much of higher education of conserving all revenues centrally.[2] Higher education is currently in a state of flux, with many institutions seriously concerned about finding adequate resources for survival. A business analysis of higher education predicts a negative picture for higher education based on these factors: growth will slow for most revenue streams; the rate of expense growth will outpace softening revenue growth; and uncertainty at the federal level continues; while solid financial reserves can add a stabilizing element.[3]

Forces such as these make it difficult for individual programs to have access to enough resources to re-invest and grow. The impact of these issues is compounded when physical therapist educational program directors are not sufficiently knowledgeable about the current state of finance in higher education in general and of finances at their institution in particular. If program directors are to make cogent arguments about financial support for the physical therapist program at their institution, they must have a thorough understanding of both. Within the institution, they must understand the relationship between undergraduate and graduate enrollment and trends in both, how tuition is derived throughout the institution, how tuition discounting is used at the institution, the relative financial contribution the institution receives from its undergraduate, graduate and professional programs, how institutional overhead costs are supported or allocated within the institution, and to what extent tuition revenue from professional programs accrues to the programs and to what extent it supports the institution's overall finances.[4]

The leaders at the academic programs we studied were able to garner such resources. They did this by pursuing multiple sources of funding. As we documented, a principal source of funding was tuition dollars from classes that were larger than the average for physical therapist educational programs by 10 to 50 students.[5] Increasing class size is, quite simply, the easiest way for academic programs to increase their resources. With these resources, programs can add faculty, increase space and equipment, update technology, support faculty research, and develop supplemental programs, such as pro bono practices. The accrued benefit from this approach occurred through the financial and management acumen of the program leadership who were able to garner the trust and support of institutional leaders. This is clearly a benefit to the individual program. Expanding all programs does present issues for physical therapist education collectively. The profession must be responsive to the needs of society in terms of the supply of physical therapists needed. The current workforce model provided by the American Physical Therapy Association, based on data from 2016, shows a range in in the relationship between demand and supply, based on varying assumptions regarding attrition rates. A lower attrition rate of 1.5% could result in a surplus of around 8500 physical therapists. An attrition rate of 3.5% could result in a shortage of over 25,000 therapists.[6] This range makes it difficult for there to be centralized planning for the right number of graduates. Despite this difficulty, addition of more programs with small class sizes does not seem to be in the best interest of the profession or society. Nor is it in the best interest of the profession or society to support current small programs that do not have the capability to develop necessary resources.

These issues are not confined to physical therapist education. A National Academies Press proceedings on the financial economics of health professions education[7] identified several principles that should be followed in building the financial aspects of health professions education (HPE):

- *Responsive to society*: Investments in HPE should be designed to encourage practitioners to choose to work in settings and geography that are responsive to population health needs.
- *Transparent*: HPE should make the economic value of various professions and various institutions in preparing for those occupations clear to potential students and other stakeholders.
- *Nimble*: HPE systems must be able to respond to the rapid changes in the needs of society, including shifting population health needs, changing technology, and new models of care.
- *Generate value to actors and the system*: Programs should be evaluated for their cost-effectiveness, benefit, or usefulness, but, there currently are no accepted ways to do this.
- *Lifelong*: Because the majority of a health professional's education takes place after graduation, there is a responsibility to support continued workforce development.
- *Ethical*: There are concerns when students accrue debt for their education and graduate with no job prospects, as well as with the growth in for-profit institutions.
- *Interconnected*: Educators must be aware of the needs for reform in practice, just as practitioners must be aware of the needed changes in education.

These principles would serve physical therapist education well and reflect many of the approaches used by the leaders in the programs we visited.

Most importantly, these leaders actively worked to place themselves and their programs in a position to successfully negotiate for a fair share of the revenue produced by their programs. Another feature of the programs we visited was their faculty size. Three programs had between 20 and 25 full-time faculty. Even the other 3, ranging from 14 to 18 full-time faculty, were larger than the average full-time faculty size of 10.6 reported in the Commission on Accreditation in Physical Therpay Education data.[5] This larger faculty size may well be related to the ability to acquire necessary resources. On the other hand, smaller faculties may well not have the time for the institutional engagement necessary to garner recognition of the program and the ability to negotiate for better resources.

These recommendations call on leaders and faculty to carefully consider their options in developing resources that produce revenues. They also speak to the need for all faculty to be actively engaged within their institutions, thereby making the value of the physical therapy program clearly known across the campus. This engagement also means that the physical therapy faculty will have a better understanding of the needs of the institution and of the leadership styles of the institution's administrators. These factors will contribute to improved ability to successfully negotiate in ways that meet the needs of the program and the institution.

Implementation of these recommendations is in the hands of individual faculty and academic leaders at the institutions that house physical therapist education. The box in this section asks a series of reflection questions that each member of the academy should ask themselves about their situation relative to organizational resources. If the faculty members cannot answer each of these questions positively, it is time to start a dialogue with colleagues to achieve the changes that are necessary to reach excellence.

REFLECTIVE QUESTIONS:
ACADEMIC PROGRAMS, ORGANIZATIONAL STRUCTURES AND RESOURCES

- How much budgetary authority does my program have over its resources and what financial incentives exist that recognize the program's initiatives to support and advance excellence in teaching, learning, scholarship, service, and practice?
- How well do I understand the relationship of the academic program budget to the budgets of the unit housing the program and institution?
- How well integrated is my program into the overall strategic plan, including enrollment management, academic planning, and master/building plans?
- How can my program leadership be better prepared to successfully negotiate for, advocate for, and accrue additional necessary resources?
- What would be the effect if my program increased its program size within the institution, (eg, as an effective method to ensure the program has the necessary resources to improve the quality of the program while achieving economies of scale) and on the external community?
- What is the reputation of my program and its faculty in the institution, based on what the institution considers value, including research or educational quality, and how well-integrated are we into institutional life?
- To what extent is my program considered to be under-resourced or one being used primarily to financially support the academic institution's financial position by siphoning a greater percentage of the program's revenue to the institution?

RECOMMENDATIONS RELATED
TO CLINICAL PROGRAMS

3. Use reasonable productivity standards in clinical education (CE) sites that recognize the contribution of the clinical instructor/student team to patient care with analysis over relatively longer time frames.

4. Include professional and post-professional education in the missions of CE sites. All clinicians at CE sites should recognize the need to contribute to CE, either by direct teaching, or by supporting the clinical instructor/student team.

5. Recognize and more clearly articulate the financial and other benefits from CE, including savings related to recruitment and retention, and by contributions of students and academic programs to professional development.

For at least the last 50 years, the physical therapist education community has discussed the cost of CE.[8-10] The nature of this discussion has taken many forms, but the essential questions asked are "what does it cost?" and "who should pay?" More nuanced questions included "what benefits are there?" and "who should accrue those benefits?" Several attempts have been made to identify the actual costs of CE, primarily asking the question from the perspective of the clinical site, and generally focused on specific aspects of cost, particularly productivity.[8-10] None of these analyses have been adopted as a standard format for assessing costs across CE. There do not appear to be analyses of costs from the perspective of the academic program, the student, or society in general, all important stakeholders in CE. Only one analysis looked at costs and benefits from the perspectives of the clinical site, the academic program, and the student. This analysis was done in the context of physical therapist education in developing countries in 1968.[8]

Our work has provided a different perspective by asking successful programs how they managed costs as they perceived them. They identified 2 important strategies related to concerns over productivity. One was to consider productivity in the context of teams of practitioners and students. The second was to take a long view of measuring productivity, recognizing the variance that occurs over time as the student moves from inexperienced to experienced. There is little documentation on typical productivity loads in various settings and less on what productivity loads are appropriate.[8] The sites we visited included inpatient acute care, inpatient rehabilitation, skilled nursing care, and outpatient care. All of them reported productivity levels that met the income demands for their institutions and saw themselves as having productivity levels that were neither extremely high nor low.

Another feature of the sites we visited was that CE was viewed as part of the essential mission of the institution. This was based on 2 factors: the recognition of the need to support the continuation of the profession and the recognition that good CE contributes to improved quality of patient care. This centrality of CE changed many things. For example, it was expected that all therapists in the practice would participate in CE activities in some way. Professional development was focused on knowledge and skills related to CE, in addition to knowledge and skills related to patient care. CE was a focus of therapists' conversations and there were mentoring activities among the therapists as they assisted each other to improve their skills. Clinical site coordinators thought about student placements primarily in curricular terms rather than in staffing terms. Placing CE, at both the entry-level and post-professional levels, as part of the institution's mission causes expectations to change.

Perhaps because of this centrality to their mission, these sites took a very broad view when determining the financial impact of CE on their institutions. They recognized that recruiting new practitioners from among graduating students and residents provides direct savings to the institution. At one institution, the savings was over $20,000 per position. Savings also were found in shorter orientation periods. Other positive effects included improved retention, often attributed to staff satisfaction related to participating in CE; improved patient care related to the contribution of students to new clinical knowledge and skills; and improved institutional reputation.

All these factors were identified by the therapists we met as a part of their reality for entry-level and post-professional CE. Setting reasonable expectations, placing value on CE, and thinking broadly about the benefits of CE to the institution, the profession, and society will all serve to improve physical therapist education. As we discuss later, it is also important that these observations be tested with sound research to determine their validity and generalizability across multiple institutions and to establish commonly agreed upon metrics for assessing the cost and benefits of CE at the institutional and societal levels. This research needs to account for the shift in focus from volume- to value-based measures in clinical practice. Additionally, how much progress can be made to improve CE by applying these recommendations?

Implementation of these recommendations is in the hands of individual clinicians and clinical leaders at the institutions that provide physical therapist CE and residencies. The box in this section asks a series of reflective questions that each member of the clinical community should ask themselves about their situation relative to organizational resources. Like the reflective questions for academic programs, if the clinicians cannot answer each of these questions positively, it is time to start a dialogue with colleagues to achieve the changes that are necessary to reach excellence.

REFLECTIVE QUESTIONS:
CLINICAL PROGRAMS, ORGANIZATIONAL STRUCTURES AND RESOURCES

- How fair and reasonable vs arbitrary and sometimes unduly high, are the productivity standards my institution uses to assess the economic impact of CE provided by student-clinician teams?
- How is the CI/student team accounted for in patient care assignments and volume-based productivity expectations and how does that team fit into larger groups of the physical therapy service?
- How do we balance short-term (eg, daily) compared with long-term assessment of productivity over time and across clinical teams to account for the impact as students enter, gain experience, and leave the clinical site?
- How is CE reflected as a priority in its mission, and how is that reflected in the institution's commitment to meeting the needs of the community and society for physical therapy?
- How does my institution reflect the totality of the benefits of CE to the organization, (eg, recruitment, retention, orientation, training, and development) and balance those with accurate assessment of the costs?

RECOMMENDATIONS RELATED TO
PHYSICAL THERAPIST EDUCATION

6. Stop expending resources of the profession, and of academic and clinical programs, in attempting to identify a narrow set of specific academic organizational structures or curricular models for physical therapist education. Rather, resources should be expended on using sound educational research to identify the best array of options that lead to success with the other characteristics identified here. This would result in academic and CE programs that display a diversity of models and organizational structures, all of which have been shown to lead to success in achieving excellence and innovation.

7. Focus attention across the profession on improved graduates' outcomes, the need to reduce the cost of education to students and society, and the acquisition of resources to support physical therapy education if the public's expectations for greater accountability throughout higher education are to be met.

For too long, there has been a focus in physical therapist education, both academic and clinical, on searching for the best structure or model. Is being in a college of health professions better than being in a medical school? Is being in a large public university better than being in a private liberal arts university? Is a year-long internship better than multiple shorter experiences? All 11 academic and clinical sites in our study used different curricular models. There were varied structures for how each of the academic programs were housed within the institution. While each structure brought different challenges, the program's leadership was able to provide skilled vision and administrative navigation that facilitated excellent, sustainable, and thriving programs. Thus, we cannot conclude that structure is a critical component of excellence. However, a high degree of financial control and incentives for improvement were critical, as discussed previously. There were varied patterns for the length and timing of CE experiences. A focus on the critical ingredient of intentional, early, and continuous learning focused on patient care, as described in detail in Chapters 6 and 9, rather than a defined model for CE was essential.

The variety of structures and models found in the academic and clinical sites we visited demonstrate that excellence can be found in many places. The focus needs to change to assess the characteristics that have been found to lead to excellence. In Chapters 8 and 9, we discussed many of these characteristics. We are not able to reach conclusions about the potential benefits and risks of standardization in CE, such as sequence, expected outcomes, and length of clinical experiences, as that was beyond the scope of the study; however, the profession would benefit from a deliberative, research-based consideration of the question.

Once we move the conversation away from trying to find the one best way, we can expend those same energies on developing a set of useful performance metrics that can be used in doing sound evidence-based research. This type of research will then allow us to focus at a much higher level. There are important societal issues to address and questions to answer. See Chapter 9 for a discussion of outcome assessment in physical therapy and other health professions.

While there needs to be concerted effort by the profession to address concerns regarding the cost of physical therapist education, individual programs also need to assess their curricula and their tuition policies to determine the most efficient way to provide physical therapist education. This is a difficult proposition for programs that often exist because of their ability to add to an institution's bottom line. Academic programs must find ways to improve their efficiency, reducing costs to allow a reduction in tuition without expecting institutions to absorb all reductions centrally. Clinical programs must also recognize the actual costs and benefits of CE and seek only the economic reward that is necessary to not add a financial burden to patient care.

Implementation of these recommendations is in the hands of individual faculty and academic leaders at the institutions that house physical therapist academic and CE. The box in this section asks a series of reflective questions that the members of these communities should ask themselves about their situation relative to physical therapist education. Like the previous reflective questions, if the academic and clinical program faculties cannot answer each of these questions positively, it is time to start a dialogue with colleagues to achieve the changes that are necessary to reach excellence.

REFLECTIVE QUESTIONS: PHYSICAL THERAPIST EDUCATION

- To what extent do my colleagues and I rely on the evidence about sound academic principles to design curricula rather than using our own perceptions about what we think is best?
- How deeply do my colleagues and I delve into the evidence to build excellent programs, rather than relying on the most recent wave of academic changes to remain competitive?
- How are my colleagues and I exploring all the options to make our program the most efficient and least costly that it can be?
- To what extent are my colleagues and I caught in the trap of defending personal perceptions of best models instead of engaging in a conversation and exploration of the attributes and practices that can help us achieve excellence?

These 7 recommendations all offer ways for individual educators and academic and clinical institutions to make real changes that will result in better physical therapist education. The sites we visited and the educators we met were able to position themselves and their physical therapist education programs in their institutions in a way that helped those programs meet their goals. The organizational structures and processes they created were able to provide the basis for the Culture of Excellence (Chapter 4) and the Praxis of Learning (Chapter 6) that we discovered in the sites we visited. Similarly, enacting these recommendations will provide the basis for the recommendations highlighted in Chapters 8 and 9.

REFERENCES

1. American Physical Therapy Association. Educational Leadership Institute. http://www.apta.org/ELI/. Updated May 13, 2018. Accessed September 4, 2018.
2. Soares L, Steele P, Wayt L. *Evolving Higher Education Business Models: Leading with Data to Deliver Results.* Washington DC: American Council on Education; 2016.
3. Moody's Investor Services. 2018 outlook for higher education. https://www.insidehighered.com/sites/default/server_files/media/2018%20Outlook%20for%20Higher%20Education%20Changed%20to%20Negative.pdf. Accessed January 7, 2018.
4. Ruben BD, DeLisi R, Gigliotti RA. *A Guide for Leaders in Higher Education.* Sterling, VA: Stylus Publishing; 2017.
5. Commission on Accreditation of Physical Therapy Education. Aggregate Program Data, 2016-2017 Physical Therapist Education Programs Fact Sheets, CAPTE. http://www.capteonline.org/uploadedFiles/CAPTEorg/About_CAPTE/Resources/Aggregate_Program_Data/AggregateProgramData_PTPrograms.pdf. Accessed September 4, 2018.
6. American Physical Therapy Association. A model to project the supply and demand of physical therapists 2010-2025. http://www.apta.org/WorkforceData/ModelDescriptionFigures/. Published 2017. Accessed September 4, 2018.
7. National Academies of Sciences, Engineering, and Medicine. *Future Financial Economics of Health Professional Education: Proceedings of a Workshop.* Washington, DC: The National Academies Press; 2017.
8. Watts NT. *Costs and Benefits of Training Health Personnel: Implications for Educational Planning in Developing Countries.* Unpublished dissertation, University of Chicago; 1968.
9. Lopopolo R. Financial model to determine the effect of clinical education programs on physical therapy departments. *Phys Ther.* 1984;64:1396-1402.
10. Pabian PS, Dyson J, Levine C. Physical therapist productivity using a collaborative clinical education model within an acute care setting: a longitudinal study. *J Phys Ther Educ.* 2017;31:11-17.

11

Systems-Based Reform

The Carnegie studies of the professions[1-5] demonstrated the profound changes that can be achieved in professional education when leaders in the field find compelling evidence of both the need for positive change and the means to achieve that change, as well as documentation of aspects of professional education that are not accomplishing desired aims or adequately addressing societal needs. This study was designed to identify positive change in the academic and clinical aspects of physical therapist education, and the reforms needed to achieve this change and to identify aspects of physical therapist education that are not as successful as we would prefer, also leading to the possibility of change and growth.

The focus of our research was to uncover and richly describe components of excellence and innovation. We consider the 30 recommendations discussed in Chapters 8 to 10 to be focused on actions that individuals and groups of faculty, clinicians, and students may undertake to enhance their teaching in academic or clinical settings. In this chapter, we discuss a broader perspective on the positive changes needed in physical therapist education. The calls for reform we discuss here will require the support of a variety of stakeholders and members of the profession or the health care system. These are actions that can succeed only when approached from a system-wide perspective, involving multiple stakeholders. The pursuit of excellence is foundational and a professional obligation for all professions. We believe there are critical action steps, that identify essential stakeholders, necessary to advance excellence and transform physical therapist education. Excellence in physical therapist education cannot be achieved without a clear commitment to identifying professional development paths for people who seek excellence in all their efforts. Leaders within educational programs, clinical settings, and professional organizations must set the tone and seek resources to partner with those who also value excellence.

Our proposed reforms are focused on these areas: leadership, partnership, professional preparation, and participation in society, all of which need to be explored, informed, and supported through educational research.

Jensen GM, Mostrom E, Hack LM, Nordstrom T, Gwyer J.
Educating Physical Therapists (pp 155-171).
© 2019 Taylor & Francis Group.

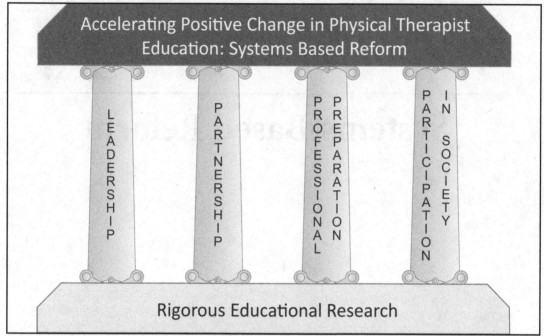

Figure 11-1. Areas for systems-based reform in physical therapist education.

In each area, we have identified specific actions that must be addressed by collaborative action by the major stakeholders in physical therapy. These stakeholders include: the American Physical Therapy Association (APTA); 2 APTA component organizations, the Academy of Physical Therapy Education (APTE) and the American Council on Academic Physical Therapy (ACAPT); the Commission on Accreditation of Physical Therapy Education (CAPTE); the American Board of Physical Therapy Specialties (ABPTS); the American Board of Physical Therapy Residencies and Fellowship (ABPTRFE); and the Federation of State Boards of Physical Therapy (FSBPT). The Educational Leadership Partnership (ELP) is a collaboration among the APTA, APTE, and ACAPT (Table 11-1).

LEADERSHIP

We learned that leadership is essential for physical therapist educational programs to achieve excellence. This is demonstrated both through strong central leadership and widespread distributive leadership. Distributed leadership means more than shared leadership or multiple individuals taking responsibility for leadership; it is the leadership practice through the collective interactions among leaders, their followers, and the situation that is critical.[6] In Chapter 8, we outline many actions that individuals and institutions can take to strengthen leadership and engage in distributive leadership practice. Here we address important steps that must be taken system-wide to ensure that physical therapist education has the leadership it needs to grow and excel.

First, we need to increase leadership skills across all faculty, academic, and clinical settings. As discussed in Chapter 8, distributed leadership is essential in today's complex work environments. The APTA Section on Health Policy and Administration has developed a strong, well-regarded program focused on clinical leadership, the Institute for Leadership in Physical Therapy (LAMP).[7] As mentioned before, the APTA also supports the Educational Leadership Institute (ELI), which focuses on developing small numbers of educators to take leadership positions.[8] These programs are just a starting point and currently not sufficient to meet the need for distributed leadership throughout physical therapist education.

TABLE 11-1

STAKEHOLDERS IN PHYSICAL THERAPIST EDUCATION

ENTITY	BRIEF DESCRIPTION
American Physical Therapy Association *www.apta.org*	The APTA is an individual membership professional organization representing more than 100,000 member physical therapists, physical therapist assistants, and students of physical therapy. The APTA seeks to improve the health and quality of life of individuals in society by advancing physical therapist practice, education, and research, and by increasing the awareness and understanding of physical therapy's role in the nation's health care system.
Academy of Physical Therapy Education *www.aptaeducation.org*	The APTE serves as a point of contact for those interested in patient and professional education, and a mechanism for networking and professional development.
American Council on Academic Physical Therapy *www.acapt.org*	The purpose of the ACAPT is to advance the enterprise of academic physical therapy by promoting the highest standards of excellence. For the purposes of the Council and its activities, academic physical therapy includes all aspects of physical therapist education, including clinical, and post-professional education. Member institutions are institutions of higher education located in the US with a CAPTE-accredited physical therapist education program.
Educational Leadership Partnership *www.apta.org/ELP*	The ELP includes representatives from the APTA, APTE, and ACAPT with the purpose of reducing unwarranted variation in practice by focusing on best practices in education.
Commission on Accreditation of Physical Therapy Education *www.capteonline.org*	The CAPTE is an accrediting agency that is nationally recognized by the US Department of Education and the Council for Higher Education Accreditation. The CAPTE grants specialized accreditation status to qualified entry-level education programs for physical therapists and physical therapist assistants
American Board of Physical Therapy Specialties *www.abpts.org*	The mission of the ABPTS is to advance the profession of physical therapy by establishing, maintaining, and promoting standards of excellence for clinical specialization, and by recognizing the advanced knowledge, skills, and experience by physical therapist practitioners through specialist credentialing.
American Board of Physical Therapy Residencies and Fellowship *www.abptrfe.org*	The ABPTRFE is the accreditation body for APTA for post-professional residency and fellowship programs in physical therapy.
Federation of State Boards of Physical Therapy *www.fsbpt.org*	The FSBPT is a member organization made up of representatives of the physical therapy licensing bodies in the state, with a goal to achieve a high level of public protection through a strong foundation of laws and regulatory standards in physical therapy, tools, and systems to assess competence, and public and professional awareness of resources for public protection.

- The APTA, with its components, including the Section on Health Policy and Administration, the ACAPT, the APTE, and the Private Practice Section, need to provide many more, widespread professional developmental activities to encourage physical therapists to participate in leadership in their clinical and educational settings.
- Educational programs must include development in distributed leadership as part of the preparation for practice. The CAPTE could augment this by making the requirement for this development in its standards of accreditation.
- While distributive leadership is essential, it is also essential that those designated as leaders of physical therapist educational programs have the knowledge and skills needed to ensure the necessary resources for their programs. Physical therapist education programs are located within a variety of administrative structures, some of which provide appropriate control over educational resources, but this is not uniformly the case. The organizations that set the standards for physical therapist education, both formally and informally, must address this issue.
- The ACAPT must develop resources for program directors to guide them in their efforts to garner resources, including publishing standards for equitable revenue sharing models in academia, advocacy, and leadership development, to place academic programs on sound financial standing within every academic institution.

This aspect of development for educational leaders has been neglected. Educational resources and opportunities should be made available that support leaders to have the knowledge to understand higher education financing, budget development, and resource acquisition, and the skills to negotiate for resources within the organization. In addition, leaders who have been successful in this area need to put aside concerns over competition and share strategies for success. Current leaders must consider the appropriateness of continuing to support educational programs in institutions that do not provide adequate resources for growth and development. Potential leaders must have the knowledge and skills to refuse to support the development of programs in institutions that do not demonstrate sound plans for equitable sharing of resources.

- **The CAPTE must strengthen the requirements for control of financial resources by professional programs.**

Table 11-2 shows the accreditation criteria related to financial management of physical therapist, medicine, and pharmacy educational programs. Medicine speaks directly to the need for diverse resources, without undue reliance on tuition. Pharmacy explicitly states that revenues should not be increased to support other educational programs. The CAPTE needs to review its criteria and the training it provides site visitors and commissioners about the importance of access to financial resources. For too long, physical therapists have allowed their can-do attitude to support acceptance of what amounts to subsistence-only funding for too many physical therapist education programs.

While we recognize that physical therapy programs can be a positive financial resource for academic institutions and that physical therapist education programs can excel in a variety of academic institutions and organizational structures within those institutions, there needs to be a just and equitable allocation of resources and control of those resources by the programs.

Partnership

The importance of vital partnerships in health care cannot be under-valued if excellence is the goal for our providers. These partnership opportunities for students, residents, and fellows in both the classroom and practice settings have become essential components of education for physical therapists.[9] Administrators are increasingly pursuing potential partners, identifying the types of educational or practice compacts that can be shared between each institution. The most significant transactions in this realm in physical therapist education address the need for clinical education (CE) opportunities. Academic programs have long relied upon clinical facilities to take their students for CE opportunities.

TABLE 11-2

ACCREDITATION CRITERIA RELATED TO FINANCIAL STATUS OF HEALTH PROFESSIONS EDUCATION PROGRAMS

PHYSICAL THERAPIST EDUCATION[1]

Standard 2: The program is engaged in effective, ongoing, formal, comprehensive processes for self-assessment and planning for the purpose of program improvement.

- 2B For each of the following, the program provides an analysis of relevant data and identifies needed program change(s) with timelines for implementation and reassessment. The assessment process is used to determine the extent to which:
  - ○ 2B2 program enrollment appropriately reflects available resources, program outcomes, and workforce needs.
  - ○ 2B4 program resources are meeting, and will continue to meet, current and projected program needs including, but not limited to, financial resources, staff, space, equipment, technology, materials, library and learning resources, and student services.

Standard 4: The program faculty are qualified for their roles and effective in carrying out their responsibilities.

Program Director

- 4H The program director provides effective leadership for the program including, but not limited to, responsibility for communication, program assessment and planning, fiscal management, and faculty evaluation.

Standard 8: The program resources are sufficient to meet the current and projected needs of the program.

- 8C Financial resources are adequate to achieve the program's stated mission, goals, and expected program outcomes, and to support the academic integrity and continuing viability of the program.

MEDICAL EDUCATION[2]

Standard 5: Educational Resources and Infrastructure—A medical school has sufficient personnel, financial resources, physical facilities, equipment, and clinical, instructional, informational, technological, and other resources readily available and accessible across all locations to meet its needs and to achieve its goals.

- 5.1 Adequacy of Financial Resources: The present and anticipated financial resources of a medical school are derived from diverse sources and are adequate to sustain a sound program of medical education and to accomplish other programmatic and institutional goals.
- 5.2 Dean's Authority/Resources: The dean of a medical school has sufficient resources and budgetary authority to fulfill his or her responsibility for the management and evaluation of the medical curriculum.
- 5.3 Pressures for Self-Financing: A medical school admits only as many qualified applicants as its total resources can accommodate and does not permit financial or other influences to compromise the school's educational mission.

(continued)

TABLE 11-2 (CONTINUED)

ACCREDITATION CRITERIA RELATED TO FINANCIAL STATUS OF HEALTH PROFESSIONS EDUCATION PROGRAMS

MEDICAL EDUCATION[3]

Finances

- ER-2 The present and anticipated financial resources of a medical school must be adequate to sustain a sound program of medical education and to accomplish other institutional goals.
  - The costs of conducting an accredited program leading to the MD degree should be supported from diverse sources, such as income from tuition, endowments, earnings by the faculty, support from the parent university, annual gifts, grants from organizations and individuals, and appropriations by government. Evidence for compliance with this standard will include documentation of adequate financial reserves to maintain the educational program in the event of unexpected revenue losses, and demonstration of effective fiscal management of the medical school budget.
- ER-3 Pressure for institutional self-financing must not compromise the educational mission of the medical school nor cause it to enroll more students than its total resources can accommodate.
  - Reliance on student tuition should not be so great that the quality of the program is compromised by the need to enroll or retain inappropriate numbers of students or students whose qualifications are substandard.

PHARMACIST EDUCATION[4]

Standard 23: Financial Resources—The college or school has current and anticipated financial resources to support the stability of the educational program and accomplish its mission, goals, and strategic plan.

Key Elements:

- 23.1 Enrollment support: The college or school ensures that student enrollment is commensurate with resources.
- 23.2 Budgetary input: The college or school provides input into the development and operation of a budget that is planned, executed, and managed in accordance with sound and accepted business practices.
- 23.3 Revenue allocation: Tuition and fees for pharmacy students are not increased to support other educational programs if it compromises the quality of the professional program.
- 23.4 Equitable allocation: The college or school ensures that funds are sufficient to maintain equitable facilities (commensurate with services and activities) across all program pathways.

1. Commission on Accreditation of Physical Therapy Education, Standards And Required Elements For Accreditation of Physical Therapist Education Programs http://www.capteonline.org/uploadedFiles/CAPTEorg/About_CAPTE/Resources/Accreditation_Handbook/CAPTE_PTStandardsEvidence.pdf Accessed January 7, 2018.

2. Liaison Committee on Medical Education, Functions and Structure of a Medical School. http://lcme.org/publications/ Accessed January 7, 2018.

3. International Association of Medical Colleges, LCME Accreditation Standards, http://www.iaomc.org/lcme.htm. Accessed January 7, 2018.

4. Accreditation Council for Pharmacy Education, Accreditation Standards and Key Elements for the Professional Program in Pharmacy Leading to the Doctor of Pharmacy Degree https://www.acpe-accredit.org/pdf/Standards2016FINAL.pdf. Accessed January 7, 2018.

While it is obvious that workplace learning is clearly crucial for the preparation of physical therapists, we now must consider wholly different approaches to developing vital partnerships. Two aspects of our call for reform address the importance of recreating and envisioning the needed partnerships.

- **The physical therapy profession must facilitate the creation of strong and equal academic practice partnerships that foster excellence.**

The growth in physical therapist educational programs, coupled with the growth in student numbers, impacts directors of CE and creates a culture of grasping for almost any CE sites for students. Larger academic health centers are increasingly choosing to provide CE only to students from the home university setting, leaving smaller physical therapist programs with more limited opportunities, particularly exposure to hospital-based student learning. It is likely that the pressures in academic settings will not encourage the creation of a culture of strong and equitable partnerships necessary to realize excellence. The ACAPT, in collaboration with the APTE and other relevant Sections of the APTA, and ABPTRFE, need to develop models that link CE, residency and fellowship education, and faculty practice, through equitable and responsible partnerships among the stakeholders in professional and post-professional education. Effective academic-practice partnerships are a non-negotiable component of excellence. These models need to allow for implementation across the variety of settings in which professional and post-professional education occurs. These models need to include the necessary infrastructures that can support partnerships between academic and clinical facilities that advance excellence in clinical learning and practice.

- **The APTA, ACAPT, and APTE working collaboratively, must invest considerable resources in or make a concerted effort to find funding for demonstration projects and research that illuminate the costs and benefits of clinical education from multiple perspectives.**

The ability to provide physical therapist students with the CE required for successful practice is threatened by real and perceived financial constraints in the health care system and a lack of data to support the value CE provides to clinical practices and patient outcomes. When an academic faculty member works to negotiate a partnership with a clinical setting, it can be difficult for the clinician to perceive the professional role and value of clinical teaching in the workplace. This attitude must be changed in the profession such that clinicians commit to educating young learners whenever possible. This is a difficult cultural change for the profession and the stakeholders should lead the charge by educating students and practitioners in the critical importance of these partnerships between academic and clinical organizations. Many potential clinicians have the options to choose whether to teach in the clinical setting, or for how long they may teach their students. Taking decisive action to demonstrate and increase the value of CE in the profession is a key call to action for the profession.

Changing the culture of valuing the opportunities for teaching and learning in the workplace is not the only component of enhancing our partnerships. Existing partnerships are not without challenge as weaknesses may be found in the clinical curricula, and there is cost sharing for the partners on both sides. Both the ACAPT and APTA have spent resources to identify possibilities for the future of CE. In 2014, the ACAPT hosted the Clinical Education Summit. The Summit was designed to bring together academic and clinical educators to assess the contemporary CE experience and anticipate future needs and directions. Education leaders were invited to provide background papers,[10] and the event was prefaced by interactive webinars. At the conclusion of the event, participants agreed on several topics, all based on the premise that "clinical education in physical therapy will have a common culture of teaching and learning based in strong partnerships with shared responsibility for preparing all students to enter and progress through their CE experiences prepared for practice."[11] Subsequently the ACAPT sponsored panels to explore 3 of those topics: updated and unified terminology; a description of knowledge, skills, and abilities that should be expected at entry into CE; and a fuller description of integrated CE. The ACAPT members adopted the recommendations from these panels in 2017.[12]

In a similar time frame, the APTA Board of Directors (BOD), in response to a motion from the APTA 2014 House of Delegates, created a Best Practice for Physical Therapist Clinical Education Task Force (BPCETF) and charged members to "identify best practice for physical therapist CE, from professional level through post-professional clinical training, and propose potential courses of action for a doctoring profession to move toward practice that best meets the evolving needs of society."[13] The BPCETF recommendations to the APTA BOD included: "That a framework for formal partnerships between academic programs and clinical sites that includes infrastructure and capacity building, and defines responsibility and accountability for each (eg, economic models, standardization, sustainable models), be developed." Following a period of public discussion the APTA BOD concluded, "that a long-term strategic plan for physical therapist professional and post-professional education, including staging of activities, be developed to create a work force prepared to meet the evolving needs of society. Engagement with relevant stakeholders will be critical to this effort."[13]

Should the profession fail to focus on the important role of partnerships, as identified in numerous types of medical and nursing health care partnerships,[4,5] we will be unable to support learning in the workplace setting that we believe is crucial. A variety of outcomes for partnering in physical therapist education would deliver a variety of excellent strategies, some that fit small community programs as well as academic medical centers.

PROFESSIONAL PREPARATION

A culture of excellence in professional education includes a value for innovation and risk taking among faculty and leaders who strive to address many limitations in the higher education environment, including a shortage of faculty. While inadequate numbers of faculty to meet the needs of physical therapist professional preparation programs in the United States is problematic, perhaps even more challenging is the inadequate number of highly qualified faculty who bring both the breadth and depth of expertise needed to ensure the potential for, and realization of, excellence in these programs. It is our belief that the faculty in professional preparation programs need to be not only adequate in numbers to meet program goals, curricular aims, desired graduate outcomes, and accreditation requirements, but the faculty also need to bring disciplinary/subject-matter expertise, a spirit of collaboration, and a desire to advance their own teaching and the learning of their students through the understanding and application of the learning sciences in the educational endeavor. The ability to achieve the goal of sufficient numbers and quality of faculty will be dependent on both external and internal factors. Critical internal factors are the characteristics and quality of academic leadership discussed earlier in this chapter and in Chapter 8. The following action item speaks to factors and activities that need to occur external to the program and at a systems level to address these concerns.

- **The CAPTE, supported by the APTA, APTE, and ACAPT, must place a hiatus on accrediting new programs and continued accreditation of programs must demand the depth and breadth of program director and faculty expertise needed to enact this culture of excellence.**

The shortage of qualified faculty and academic leadership is placing the academic enterprise at serious risk for mediocrity, if not failure. This risk requires that the CAPTE, with concurrence of the physical therapy community, pause accrediting new programs to establish criteria that ensure they have sufficient resources to succeed. Simultaneously, the CAPTE needs to move expeditiously to establish and apply rigorous standards for faculty, and for the program director, that emphasize the ability to lead and act collaboratively. Rigorously applied standards, while they may lead to more negative accreditation decisions, will set a bar that will better ensure every program has the required faculty and leadership resources to educate tomorrow's physical therapists.

There is a substantial and ever-growing body of theory, research, and literature from numerous disciplines on learning science.[14] Numerous questions are addressed and explored through theory and research in this area but at the heart of the matter are these crucial questions: How do people learn? How do people learn best? How can learning be supported, advanced, and optimized through teaching and experience? What features of learning environments and experiences constrain or are barriers to learning? This body of work on the learning sciences provides an exceptional resource for physical therapist educators to improve learning and teaching in a wide array of teaching/learning environments and across the continuum from professional preparation through post-professional education to ongoing professional development. Our study findings suggested that while there was some excellent teaching and learning occurring in the professional and post-professional educational settings we observed, there was a paucity of language for, and deep understanding of, learning theory and research; this gap was an impediment to the ability of teachers and learners to engage in rich dialogue about how to best promote learning in their settings and in the profession. All learners across the spectrum from professional to post-professional education and practice will be better served by faculty who enhance their knowledge and understanding of the learning sciences and translate that knowledge into skilled action in all learning environments. The time to infuse the learning sciences into the preparation of academic, clinical, residency, and fellowship faculty is now. The following 2 action items are linked to one another and draw focused attention to changes that are needed at a systems level to ensure that we use the best evidence possible as we prepare learners across their professional lives for present and future practice in the context of the constantly evolving and challenging health care environment.

- **Key stakeholders including the ACAPT, ABPTRFE, and APTE must work together to identify and create the needed resources to develop a coherent, sequential, and comprehensive approach to faculty development for all these educators.**

These faculty development programs should focus on (1) inculcating deep understandings of the profession's signature pedagogy, (2) designing effective teaching and learning strategies that are grounded in practice-based learning environments and focus on creating adaptive learners, (3) understanding how to optimize and advance learning in the robust workplace environment, and (4) preparing faculty to use the science of learning to enhance their teaching effectiveness in academic and clinical settings.

- **The APTA, ABPTRFE, ABPTS, APTE, and ACAPT should establish a systematic, widely accepted continuum for learners' competence, from preparedness for final clinical experiences, initial entry to practice, completion of residency education and ongoing professional practice to develop adaptive expertise.**

A foundational framework for professional performance standards is an essential structure for assessing competency over an entire learning continuum, as well as providing a framework for education research in the profession. While we observed the strong desire among faculty, students, and residents to achieve skilled practice and optimal outcomes for patients, the pursuit of excellence throughout a career in physical therapist practice can best be guided through developmental professional performance benchmarks. Learners must develop a lifelong commitment to continuous learning and the pursuit of excellence. The work being done in medicine and pharmacy that identifies entrustable professional activities (EPAs) grounded in professional practice expectations and defined competencies across multiple domains of competence is a framework that may be a model that could be used in physical therapy.[15-22] An important feature of the EPA framework in medicine is that it currently identifies expected milestones for professional performance across the learner continuum from undergraduate medical education and postgraduate medical education with further work anticipated for practicing professionals in various specialty areas.[15-19] The EPA framework, therefore, may be an example of one pathway toward establishing this continuum that physical therapy can follow. Furthermore, the development and ongoing refinement of the EPA framework has led to the creation of a systematic research agenda in medical education that has spawned numerous and robust investigations that are having a significant impact on teaching, learning, assessment, and practice in medicine.

PARTICIPATION IN SOCIETY

Among all our participating institutions, we discovered strong commitments towards preparing physical therapy professionals for clinical practice, teaching, and research. There was a great deal of learning that emphasized patient-centered care, the importance of professional comportment, the core values of the physical therapy profession,[23] and the Code of Ethics.[24] There were also instances of excellent community-centered clinical services aimed at addressing important health needs and of interprofessional, community-based learning opportunities for students. What we did not observe were widespread, systematic efforts to address the health needs of local communities and larger society at systemic levels. In Chapter 9, we offered recommendations that individual programs and clinics can pursue to truly prepare professionals who can act as responsible citizens and health professionals who meet their obligations to society. Here we emphasize the actions that are necessary among the major stakeholders in the profession if physical therapy is to meet its societal responsibilities.

- **The APTA, acting with the Health Policy and Administration Section, the Center on Health Services Training and Research, the FSBPT, and the Foundation for Physical Therapy must invest resources to further develop workforce models that accurately reflect the complex relationships in demand for and supply of physical therapists.**

If we are to design curricula that address societal needs, and if we are to graduate the right number of physical therapists who are willing and able to provide services where they are needed, then it is essential that the profession has a better understanding of the demand for physical therapy and the supply of physical therapists. Two examples of where the profession can devote resources on the understanding of the interplay between need and demand in physical therapy are (1) the mismatch that can occur between how the burden of disease and disability is experienced among different communities and populations; and (2) the effect of providing high-cost physical therapy that may not be effective as compared with cost effective primary care and preventive services. On the supply side, we need to understand the economic, social, cultural, and policy factors that influence (1) choices to become physical therapists, especially among people from disadvantaged backgrounds and from communities of color, and (2) where to practice, focusing on the needs of an aging population and underserved rural and urban communities.[25] The APTA, in cooperation with the FSBPT, ACAPT, federal and state agencies, and workforce researchers, needs to establish a robust data source that describes the current workforce (eg, inputs, deployment, outputs) and also identifies the workforce that is required to serve society now and into the future. These workforce demands go beyond simple numbers of physical therapists required for the population, but rather must begin to identify the size, quality, and utilization of a workforce that will be required to meet the profession's responsibilities to society. Understanding these relationships is essential as the US health system shifts to value-based payment and if the US health system commits to universal health coverage in which "…all people receive the quality, essential health services they need without financial hardship"[26(p6)] where there is an adequate number of practitioners with the appropriate skill mix who are distributed according to need and achieving the desired health outcomes.[25, 26]

- **The APTA, APTE, ACAPT, CAPTE, and the other relevant APTA Sections must work to ensure that there are student learning outcomes that are adopted by all physical therapist education programs that address population health, the needs of communities where health disparities exist, the social determinants of health, and needs of an aging population.**

The annual health care expenditures in the United States are expected to exceed $3 trillion and represents 17.9% of the US gross domestic product, yet our health outcomes fall far short when compared with other developed countries.[27,28] Also, despite the expenditures on health care, health care is a weak determinant of health, being far outweighed by the social and upstream factors, such as inadequate education, poverty, toxic environments, race and ethnicity, gender, disability, and stressful low-paying jobs. These social determinants of health are frequently rooted in structuralized inequalities that arise from economic factors, public policy, social forces, and ideologies.[29-32] These social determinants of health and their causes present a moral imperative for health professionals; there is a professional responsibility to work toward elimination of these social inequities and inequalities that affect health.[27-30]

Physical therapists, like many other health professions, have for far too long focused on meeting the needs of individual patients and professional education has not kept pace with the challenges in our interdependent world.[33] It is vital that we learn to meet the needs of populations, particularly more vulnerable communities.[34-36]

While educational programs and the profession need the will and commitment to address these challenges, the profession must ensure there are the necessary curricular resources to successfully meet those learning outcomes. The profession needs to develop a deeper understanding of population health and the role of public health that moves beyond individual health behaviors. How policies and practices that impact communities, such as economics, community development, transportation, food policy, and early childhood education, are best learned through program and learner engagement in communities in which we live. Learner engagement must be supported by preparing practitioners who exhibit systems-level thinking given that it is critical for successful practice, leadership, and the profession's ability to meet its vision. The profession and education programs need to identify the outcomes and resources needed to integrate community-based clinical learning experiences that are not only effective learning experiences for students, but that also make explicit their primary purpose of improving the health of the community being served. Thus, measuring the health outcomes at the individual and population level that result from these community-based learning experiences need to be an integral component of their design.

- **The stakeholders in Table 11-1 need to engage in an examination of the design, content, and standards for development of the National Physical Therapy Exam.**

In a profession characterized by an increasing scope of practice with direct access to services, there are concerns of curricular bloat as well as "curriculo-sclerosis," in which nothing can be changed. Given that overall licensure pass rates are a standard, essential outcome for physical therapist education programs, the stakeholders in Table 11-1 can engage in an analysis of the National Physical Therapy Exam from the values of our professional responsibility to society and the demand for high quality, accessible, and affordable health care.[37,38] There are also implications for accreditation in this call for action. We previously argued that accreditation needs to shift its focus to learning outcomes and lessen its focus on process. Given that such an effort is a major shift in accreditation, requiring time to achieve, there are immediate steps that can be taken. Accreditation criteria related to curricular content can be re-examined to ensure they are meeting society's needs.

- **The APTA and ACAPT must make an intentional, public, concrete effort to increase the diversity of students and faculty.**

In the face of an increasingly diverse society and overwhelming evidence of health disparities based on race, ethnicity, gender identity, sexual orientation, and disability, the profession must find the will to change from an overwhelmingly White profession to one that reflects the society we serve.

There is a major demographic shift facing the United States over the next decade with the number of high school graduates having peaked in 2010 to 2011 and significant declines in the number of high school graduates continuing in the Mideast and Midwest, the West remaining flat, and the South being the only region experiencing an increase.[39] During this same period, an increasing percentage of college-age students will be from Latino and Asian backgrounds, with the Black population staying about the same and the percentage of White students declining. Meanwhile, college attainment among Latino and Black students has remained significantly below that of Asian and White students. The US Census Bureau estimates that by 2060, the White population will no longer be a majority, and the Hispanic population will be just under 30% of the US population. Over this same period, the percent of Americans who are over 65 is expected to double, with the largest increase occurring from 2020 to 2030. In 2016, 85% of APTA members identified as White, 6.4% as Asian, 2.3% as Black, and 3% as Latino, far different ratios from the US population.[40] The applicant pool through the Physical Therapy Centralized Application Service presents similar ratios. Between 2008 and 2016, prospective students who identified as Black comprised 4.7% of the applicant pool and 2.6% of those admitted; Hispanics were 4.6% of the pool and 3.6% of those admitted and Whites were 67.2% of the applicant pool and 72.2% of those admitted.[41]

The abstract to the Institute of Medicine 2003 report *Unequal Treatment: Confronting Racial and Ethnic Disparities in Health Care*[42] opened this way:

> Racial and ethnic minorities tend to receive a lower quality of health care than non-minorities, even when access-related factors, such as patients' insurance status and income, are controlled. Consistent with the charge, the study committee focused part of its analysis on the clinical encounter itself, and found evidence that stereotyping, biases, and uncertainty on the part of health care providers can all contribute to unequal treatment...Minorities may experience a range of other barriers to accessing care, even when insured at the same level as Whites, including barriers of language, geography, and cultural familiarity. Further, financial and institutional arrangements of health systems, as well as the legal, regulatory, and policy environment in which they operate, may have disparate and negative effects on minorities' ability to attain quality care.

The Sullivan Commission[43] report included evidence of these disparities. Both reports concluded that the health professions need to make a concerted effort to recruit more diverse practitioners. Additionally, they made recommendations that the health care workforce be adequately prepared to address these disparities. Recent work on fostering cultural humility, and fostering the understanding of intersectionality and how it relates to people's identities as health care practitioners and as recipients of health care,[44] and specific training to address respect, cultural humility, and communication in health care[45] are learning approaches that show promise to address disparities in addition to recruiting a more diverse workforce.

In 2017, the APTA House of Delegates passed RC 11-17 to increase diversity and inclusion in the profession. The necessary work to increase diversity can build upon work done by ACAPT,[41] supported by the APTA policy on under-represented minority populations in physical therapy education.[46] The profession will benefit from consistent and current data on the members of the profession, including students. The profession needs to be more explicit and public about linking the demographic changes in the US population (eg, increasing number of older adults, a more diverse society, the critical social determinants of health and health disparities) to the profession's obligation in meeting these societal needs and to diversifying the profession.[47]

- **The APTA, ACAPT, and the APTE need to convene a panel of experts to develop curricular and learning guidelines and models that fully integrate the moral foundation of the profession into policy advocacy and population health practices and to identify the faculty development necessary to implement them.**

Learners across all levels need to understand and embrace the concept of joining a moral community. Individual involvement is certainly important, along with collective action and broader participation as a professional community that can facilitate change. Throughout professional and post-professional education, learners will be challenged with increasingly complex ethical and moral dilemmas that are of a complex and uncertain practice environment. While the skills of critical thinking and the ability to problem solve are important in professional education, society needs health professionals who believe and act from a deeper commitment to their professional role and obligation to society to make a difference as moral agents. Professional schools serve as important portals to professional life and potentially trustee institution as they have responsibility for what Sullivan calls "reliable formation in their students of integrity of professional purpose and identity."[48] In 2000, Purtilo[35] gave us a clarion call that the profession needs deeper digging and tilling of the soil that facilitates development of professionals who are not complicit but understand the concept of moral courage and what it means to be a moral agent as a health care professional. To be an effective trustee institution requires that students have developed throughout the academic and clinical curricula an understanding and concern for social justice and their social responsibility as professionals. As Gruen and colleagues wrote when addressing the importance of the collective voice of physician citizens, "although individual action is laudable, collective action is the hallmark of professionalism."[49(p97)]

EDUCATIONAL RESEARCH

We believe that education research is a fifth area for reform and is essential for continued and expanded, rigorous research in the 4 areas outlined in this chapter: leadership, partnership, professional preparation, and participation in society. Education research in physical therapy has long focused on basic educational structures, such as program development, curriculum models, and teaching strategies done in a program, classroom, or clinic site. This is not surprising because faculty with doctoral preparation in education find themselves quickly moving into educational administration; there is a paucity of funding for education research; this lack of funding makes it difficult to do large, multi-site investigations; and our education communities in the profession are challenged to move beyond the operational and tactical issues in educational programs.[50] Education research and educational researchers in physical therapy have not had the support nor the collective strength of a scholarly community, in contrast to our clinical research colleagues. Education research is critical to the future of physical therapist education in preparing graduates who can assume professional responsibility for improving the health of patients and communities we serve. Education researchers across disciplines share a similar challenge, the complexity of the learning environment where events, social interactions, problems, people, and processes are the raw material for study and are difficult, if not impossible to control.[50]

A task force appointed by the ACAPT published a perspective paper, "Education Research in Physical Therapy: Visions of the Possible."[50] The task force made recommendations in 4 areas (need for conceptual framing and vision for education research, development of a community of scholars, develop a data repository for education data, establish funding for education research). The ELP, which has representation from the APTA, ACAPT, and APTE, is using these 4 areas as a starting point for implementing targeted projects.

- **The APTA, ACAPT, and APTE need to continue to collaborate through the ELP in developing the necessary strategic vision and goals, infrastructure and funding for making education research a priority for the profession.**

The action items in this chapter were generated from review of our findings and recommendations, assessment of current initiatives in the profession, and a critical look at the influences of current external environments. As we have discussed in Parts II and III of this book, research grounded in the learning sciences is essential for exploring important questions in the teaching and learning environment. Our education researchers need to be able to go beyond drawing primarily from literature in physical therapy education to drawing on theory and research in the learning sciences found in a wide array of literature from disciplines such as education, sociology, psychology, and cognitive science. Education researchers in physical therapy need to use theoretically grounded knowledge as well as create new knowledge that can inform and advance education and practice.

- **The profession, through the work of education researchers, and the support of the APTA, ACAPT, and APTE, must develop strategies to engage and learn from and with the education research community across health professions.**
- **The physical therapy clinical research community has done well in implementing a clinical research agenda. The past efforts to either include education and professional development questions in the clinical research agenda or develop specific questions for education research has generated a list of questions but has not resulted in a robust agenda.[51-53] Our conceptual model, findings, and recommendations provide a working blueprint for the critical areas in need of research.**
- **Education researchers in physical therapy must identify the most urgent problems that should be explored and studied across sites through collaborative work.**

We believe we have an urgent need to develop and support education research, as it is a critical element in the profession's ability to ensure that these recommendations for reform can be implemented.

CONCLUSION

We believe that the educational enterprise will benefit from our proposed reforms across leadership, partnership, professional preparation, participation in society, supported by changes in education research. Adopting these changes will provide the physical therapy profession with a blueprint for stakeholders who have the obligation for this important work ahead. The success in making these changes is dependent on all stakeholders working collaboratively. Chesbro and Boisssonnault provide more details on potential mechanisms for this collaboration in Chapter 16 (Table 11-3).

TABLE 11-3
CALLS FOR REFORM

LEADERSHIP

The APTA, with its components, including the Section on Health Policy and Administration, the ACAPT, APTE, and the Private Practice Section, need to provide many more, widespread professional developmental activities to encourage physical therapists to participate in leadership in their clinical and educational settings.

Educational programs must include development in distributed leadership as part of the preparation for practice. The CAPTE could augment this by making the requirement for this development in its standards of accreditation.

While distributive leadership is essential, it is also essential that those designated as leaders of physical therapist educational programs have the knowledge and skills needed to ensure the necessary resources for their programs. Physical therapist education programs are located within a variety of administrative structures, some of which provide appropriate control over educational resources, but this is not uniformly the case. The organizations that set the standards for physical therapist education, both formally and informally, must address this issue.

The ACAPT must develop resources for program directors to guide them in their efforts to garner resources, including publishing standards for equitable revenue sharing models in academia, advocacy, and leadership development, to place academic programs on sound financial standing within every academic institution.

The CAPTE must strengthen the requirements for control of financial resources by professional programs.

PARTNERSHIP

The physical therapy profession must facilitate the creation of strong and equal academic practice partnerships that foster excellence.

The APTA, ACAPT, and APTE, working collaboratively, must invest considerable resources in, or make a concerted effort to find funding for, demonstration projects and research that illuminate the costs and benefits of CE from multiple perspectives.

PARTICIPATION PREPARATION

The CAPTE, supported by the APTA, APTE, and ACAPT, must place a hiatus on accrediting new programs, and continued accreditation of programs must demand the depth and breadth of program director and faculty expertise needed to enact this culture of excellence.

Key stakeholders, including the ACAPT, ABPTRFE, and APTE, must work together to identify and create the needed resources to develop a coherent, sequential, and comprehensive approach to faculty development for all these educators.

The APTA, ABPTRFE, American Board of Physical Therapy Specialties, APTE, and ACAPT should establish a systematic, widely accepted continuum for learners' competence, from preparedness for final clinical experiences, initial entry to practice, completion of residency education and ongoing professional practice to develop adaptive expertise.

(continued)

TABLE 11-3 (CONTINUED)

CALLS FOR REFORM

PARTICIPATION IN SOCIETY

The APTA, acting with the Health Policy and Administration Section, the Center on Health Services Training and Research, the FSBPT, and the Foundation for Physical Therapy must invest resources to further develop workforce models that accurately reflect the complex relationships in demand for, and supply of, physical therapists.

The APTA, APTE, ACAPT, CAPTE, and the other relevant APTA Sections must work to ensure that there are student learning outcomes that are adopted by all physical therapist education programs that address population health, the needs of communities where health disparities exist, the social determinants of health, and needs of an aging population.

The stakeholders in Table 11-1 need to engage in an examination of the design, content, and standards for development of the National Physical Therapy Exam.

The APTA and ACAPT must make an intentional, public, concrete effort to increase the diversity of students and faculty.

The APTA, ACAPT and APTE need to convene a panel of experts to develop curricular and learning guidelines and models that fully integrate the moral foundation of the profession into policy advocacy and population health practices, and to identify the faculty development necessary to implement them.

EDUCATIONAL RESEARCH

The APTA, ACAPT, and APTE need to continue to collaborate through the ELP in developing the necessary strategic vision and goals, infrastructure, and funding for making education research a priority for the profession.

The profession, through the work of education researchers and the support of the APTA, ACAPT, and APTE, must develop strategies to engage and learn from and with the education research community across health professions.

The physical therapy clinical research community has done well in implementing a clinical research agenda. The past efforts to either include education and professional development questions in the clinical research agenda or develop specific questions for education research has generated a list of questions but has not resulted in a robust agenda. Our conceptual model, findings, and recommendations provide a working blueprint for the critical areas in need of research.

Education researchers in physical therapy must identify the most urgent problems that should be explored and studied across sites through collaborative work.

REFERENCES

1. Sullivan W, Colby A, Wegner JW, Bond L, Shulman L. *Educating Lawyers: Preparation for the Profession of Law.* San Francisco, CA: Jossey-Bass; 2007

2. Foster C, Dahill L, Goleman L, Tolentino BW. *Educating Clergy: Teaching Practices and Pastoral Imagination.* San Francisco, CA: Jossey-Bass; 2006.

3. Sheppard S, Macatangay K, Colby A, Sullivan W. *Educating Engineers: Designing the Future of the Field.* San Francisco, CA: Jossey-Bass; 2009.

4. Benner P, Sutphen M, Leonard C, Day L. *Educating Nurses: A Call for Radical Transformation.* San Francisco, CA: Jossey-Bass 2010.

5. Cooke M, Irby D, O'Brien B. *Educating Physicians: A Call for Reform of Medical School and Residency.* San Francisco, CA: Jossey-Bass; 2010.

6. Spillane J. *Distributed Leadership.* San Francisco, CA: Jossey-Bass; 2006.

7. American Physical Therapy Association, Health Policy and Administration Section. LAMP Leadership Institute. http://www.aptahpa.org/page/LAMP. Accessed January 22, 2018.

8. American Physical Therapy Association. Education Leadership Institute (ELI) fellowship. http://www.apta.org/ELI/. Accessed January 22, 2018.

9. Jette D. 19th Annual Polly Cerasoli Lecture. Unflattening. *J Phys Ther Educ.* 2016;30:4-10.

10. Special issue on Clinical Education Summit. *J Phys Ther Educ.* 2014;28.

11. American Council of Academic Physical Therapy. Recommendations from the Summit. http://www.acapt.org/docs/default-source/pdfs/recommendations_from_the_summit_june_2015.pdf. Accessed August 31, 2018.

12. American Council of Academic Physical Therapy. Business meeting minutes (draft) October 13, 2017. http://www.acapt.org/docs/default-source/minutes/2017/acapt-business-meeting-minutes-2017--draft.pdf?sfvrsn=0. Accessed January 31, 2018.

13. American Physical Therapy Association. Best Practice in Clinical Education Task Force. http://www.apta.org/Educators/TaskForceReport/PTClinicalEducation/. Accessed August 31, 2018.

14. American Physical Therapy Association. American Council on Academic Physical Therapy. Report on Excellence in Physical Therapist Education Task Force. http://www.acapt.org/docs/default-source/default-document-library/excellenceinpteducationtf-final.pdf?sfvrsn=0./. Accessed January 22, 2018.

15. Alexander PA, Levine FJ, Tate WF, eds. *Education Research: A Century of Discovery. Vol. 40.* Washington DC: American Educational Research Association; 2016.

16. ten Cate O, Chen HC, Hoff RG, Peters H, Bok H, van der Schaaf M. Curriculum development for the workplace using Entrustable Professional Activities (EPAs). AMEE Guide No. 99. *Med Teach.* 2015;37(11):983-1002.

17. Englander R, Carraccio C. From theory to practice: making entrustable professional activities come to life in the context of milestones. *Acad Med.* 2014;89(10):1321-1323.

18. Carracio C, Englander R, Gilhooly J, et al. Building a framework of entrustable professional activities, supported by competencies and milestones, to bridge the education continuum. *Acad Med.* 2017;92:324-330.

19. Peters H, Holzhausen Y, Boscardin C, ten C. Twelve tips for the implementation of EPAs for assessment and entrustment decisions. *Med Teach.* 2017;39(8):802-807.

20. Association of American Medical Colleges. *Core Entrustable Activities for Entering Residency: Curriculum Developers Guide.* Washington, DC: American Association of Medical Colleges; 2014.

21. Pittenger AL, Chapman SA, Frail CK, et al. Entrustable professional activities for pharmacy practice. *Am J Pharm Educ.* 2016;80(4):1-4.

22. Chesbro S, Jensen GM, Boissonnault W. Entrustable professional activities as a framework for continued professional competence: is now the time? *Phys Ther.* 2018;98:3-7.

23. American Physical Therapy Association. Core Values. http://www.apta.org/CoreValuesSelfAssessment/Altruism/. Accessed January 22, 2018.

24. American Physical Therapy Association. Code of Ethics for the Physical Therapist. http://www.apta.org/Ethics/Core/. Accessed January 22, 2018.

25. National Academies of Sciences, Engineering, and Medicine. *Future financial economics of health professional education: Proceedings of a workshop.* Washington, DC: The National Academies Press; 2017.

26. Evans T, Araujo EC, Herbst CH, Pannenborg O. Addressing the challenges of health professional education: opportunities to accelerate progress towards universal health coverage. Doha, Qatar: World Innovation Summit for Health; 2016.

27. Lewis, Carole. 47th McMillan Lecture. Our future selves: unprecedented opportunities. *Phys Ther.* 2016:1493-1502.

28. Henry J. Kaiser Family Foundation. US Health Spending. https://www.kff.org/health-costs/. Accessed January 22, 2018.

29. The Commonwealth Fund. US Health Care from a Global Perspective. http://www.commonwealthfund.org/publications/issue-briefs/2015/oct/us-health-care-from-a-global-perspective. Accessed January 22, 2018.

30. Stone J. Saving and ignoring lives: physicians' obligations to address root social influences on health—Moral justifications and educational implications. *Cambridge Quarterly of Healthcare Ethics.* 2010;19:497-509.

31. Sharma M, Pinto A, Kumagai A. Teaching the social determinants of health: a path to equity or a road to nowhere? *Acad Med.* 2017;April. doi: 10.1097/ACM.0000000000001689.

32. National Academies of Sciences, Engineering, and Medicine. *A framework for educating health professionals to address the social determinants of health.* Washington, DC: The National Academies Press; 2016.

33. US Department of Health and Human Services. Social determinants of health. https://www.healthypeople.gov/2020/topics-objectives/topic/social-determinants-of-health. Accessed January 22, 2018.

34. Frenk J, Chen L, Bhutta ZA, Cohen J, et al. Health professionals for a new century: transforming education to strengthen health systems in an interdependent world. *Lancet.* 2010;376:1923-1958.

35. Purtilo RB. 32nd Mary McMillan Lecture. A time to harvest, a time to sow; ethics for a shifting landscape. *Phys Ther.* 2000;80:112-119.

36. Berwick D, Nolan T, Whittington J. The Triple Aim: care, health, and cost. *Health Affairs.* 2008;27(3):759-769.

37. Jensen GM, Nordstrom T, Mostrom EM, Hack LM, Gwyer J. A national study of excellence and innovation in physical therapist education: Part 1: design, methods, and results. *Phys Ther.* 2017;97:857-874.

38. Jensen GM, Hack L, Nordstrom T, Gwyer J, Mostrom E. National study of excellence and innovation in physical therapist education: Part 2: call for reform. *Phys Ther.* 2017;97:875-888.

39. Cox M, Blouin A, Cuff P, Paniagua M, Phillips S, Vlasses P. The role of accreditation in achieving the Quadruple Aim. National Academy of Medicine. https://nam.edu/the-role-of-accreditation-in-achieving-the-quadruple-aim/. Accessed January 22, 2018.

40. Selingo J. *2026: The Decade Ahead*. Washington, DC: The Chronicle of Higher Education; 2016.

41. American Council on Academic Physical Therapy. Diversity Task Force Report. http://www.acapt.org/docs/default-source/reports/diversity-task-force-final-report.pdf?sfvrsn=2. Accessed January 22, 2018.

42. Smedley B, Stith A, Nelson A, eds. Committee on Understanding and Eliminating Racial and Ethics Disparities in Health Care. Unequal Treatment: Confronting Racial and Ethnic Disparities in Health Care. National Academies Press; 2003.

43. Sullivan, LW. Missing Persons: Minorities in the Health Professions, A Report of the Sullivan Commission on Diversity in the Healthcare Workforce. http://health-equity.lib.umd.edu/40/. Published 2004. Accessed January 21, 2018.

44. Kumagai A, Lypson M. Beyond cultural competence: critical consciousness, social justice and multicultural education. *Acad Med*. 2009;84:782-787.

45. School of Nursing, University of California, San Francisco. Diversity in Action Committee. https://nursing.ucsf.edu/about/DIVA. Accessed January 31, 2018.

46. American Physical Therapy Association. Definition of Underrepresented Minority Populations in Physical Therapy Education. http://www.apta.org/uploadedFiles/APTAorg/About_Us/Policies/Education/DefinitionofUnderrepresentedMinorityPop.pdf#search=%22minorities%22. Accessed January 22, 2018.

47. Kirch D. Addressing the physician shortage: the peril of ignoring demography. *JAMA*. 2017;317:1947-1948.

48. Colby A, Sullivan W. Formation of professionalism and purpose: perspectives from the preparation for the professions program. *University of St. Thomas Law Journal*. 2008;5:404-426.

49. Gruen RL, Pearson SD, Brennan TA. Physician citizens—public roles and professional obligations. *JAMA*. 2004;291:94-98.

50. Jensen GM, Nordstrom T, Segal R, McCallum C, Graham C, Greenfield B. Education research in physical therapy: visions of the possible. *Phys Ther*. 2016;96:1874-1884.

51. Clinical Research Agenda for Physical Therapy. *Phys Ther*. 2000;80:499-513.

52. Goldstein M, Scalzitti D, Craik R, et al. The revised research agenda for physical therapy. *Phys Ther*. 2011;91:165-174.

53. American Physical Therapy Association. Education Division Strategic Plan. https://www.apta.org/uploadedFiles/APTAorg/About_Us/Policies/BOD/Plans/APTAEducationStrategicPlan.pdf. Published 2006. Accessed January 22, 2018.

IV

The Way Forward
Visions of What Could Be

An obvious question as one moves toward conclusion of any major study or volume such as this is: "Where do we go from here?" Our aim in Part IV, is to address this question drawing on reflections and insights from invited authors who were asked to join us in envisioning the future for physical therapist education. Our guests bring expert and unique perspectives, both national and international, on our work and this question. Importantly, they also provide emic and etic viewpoints, as we have invited authors from within and outside the profession of physical therapy.

In Chapter 12, Reeves, Fitzsimmons, and Kitto provide a review of the history and growth of interprofessional education efforts over the past few decades. In doing so, they highlight lessons learned from these efforts, nationally and internationally, that can help to improve education for successful collaboration among health professionals so that high quality, effective, and comprehensive health care is realized in everyday practice. They conclude by offering directions for future research and other activities that will help to expand and enhance interprofessional education and practice and shape health policy and health care delivery in the decades to come. In this realm, physical therapists have a great opportunity to become more visible and vocal participants in achieving this aim.

In Chapter 13, our colleague from Australia, Joy Higgs, argues convincingly for a visionary educational framework for physical therapist preparation that is grounded in practice-based education. She points out that we must bring education (and educators) and practice (and practitioners) together to achieve excellence and innovation in physical therapist education and to prepare clinicians for future-oriented practice. Higgs emphasizes that this will require the creation of curricular frameworks that are sustainable and coherent but also flexible and responsive to adaptations in practice and changes in higher education. The author submits that such curricula, in combination with the incorporation of practice-based pedagogies, will enable physical therapy programs and faculty to best realize the goal of preparing graduates for their future life and practice.

Drawing on their experience and expertise in medical education and research, Loftus and Huggett (Chapter 14) underline the importance of, and urgent need for, expanded scholarship and research in health professions education. Working from the model of Excellence in Physical Therapist Education put forth in this volume, the authors identify several intriguing research questions that arise from the elements in the model—especially those in the Praxis of Learning dimension where the learning sciences have much to offer. The questions they pose highlight the many possibilities and opportunities for educational research in physical therapy at both the instrumental/practical and conceptual/theoretical levels.

In Chapter 15, Purtilo and Benner bring their combined wisdom and philosophical perspectives to, as they say, "look through the telescope" and consider the role and importance of professional formation in the education of future physical therapists who will meet the needs and expectations of the profession and society. Together, the authors focus on the critical need for integration of the 3 apprenticeships in professional education (habits of head, hand, and heart) to meet these needs. Benner offers a vision of how the pedagogical demands of teaching a practice that truly integrates these apprenticeships might be met and how physical therapist educators can cultivate the thoughtfulness, clinical imagination, and ethical comportment that "is at the heart of becoming an excellent practitioner." Purtilo extends Benner's insights by exploring how physical therapist education can best position future therapists to be first adapters and professionals who individually and collaboratively become moral agents who possess professional humility in addition to the moral courage to act ethically in ambiguous situations. When these visions are met, we will be better equipped to address the needs of society.

The American Physical Therapy Association has a long history of developing priorities, initiatives, and resources for advancing the profession and physical therapist education. In Chapter 16, Chesbro and Boissonnault, 2 current leaders in the American Physical Therapy Association, provide an overview of this history and describe current activities by several components within the organization representing a variety of stakeholders to identify priorities and opportunities for enhancing physical therapist education in the future.

In the final chapter of this book, Chapter 17, we consider the wealth of perspectives and insights provided by our invited authors, and we draw on the understandings gained through our study. We envision a future for physical therapist education, research and practice, a way forward, that will ensure and improve not only the health of the profession but also the health of our society. We ask readers to imagine with us, what the physical therapist profession could contribute if we collectively re-imagine the profession, physical therapist curricula, and the educational enterprise. We propose these reimaginings, these visions, to invite robust and thoughtful engagement around the ideas presented here and with the hope that they will inspire action that will move us purposefully and positively forward in the 21st century.

12

Understanding and Embracing the Potential of Interprofessional Education

Scott Reeves, PhD, MSc; Amber Fitzsimmons, PT, MS, DPTSc; and Simon Kitto, PhD

The Triple Aim, proposed by Berwick et al[1], offers a vision of how the US health care system can work toward delivery of high-value health care. The Triple Aim posits that health care value can be linked to improvements in individual experiences of care, the health of populations, and reducing the per capita cost of health care.[1] Recently, the Triple Aim has evolved into the Quadruple Aim, to also include the improvement of the work life for the health care professional.[2] A recent review found evidence suggesting that interprofessional interventions, involving physicians, nurses, physiotherapists, social workers, pharmacists, and others, positively impact provider satisfaction and workplace quality.[3] Therefore, interprofessional education (IPE) and interprofessional collaboration (IPC) are important components for addressing the goals of the Quadruple Aim.[2,3]

The Physical Therapy and Society Summit, convened by the American Physical Therpay Association (APTA) in 2009, reframed the care paradigm from a traditional 1:1 physical therapist to patient relationship to one in which physical therapists are effective and thrive as part of a collaborative, interprofessional health care team with patients and families at its focus.[4] To support this move toward IPC when delivering physical therapy care, increasingly, physical therapy educators are looking toward the use of IPE.

IPE aims to provide students and practitioners with opportunities to learn together to develop the attributes and skills required to work in an effective collaborative manner. Interest in IPE has grown significantly in the past few decades. From a small number of IPE enthusiasts scattered across the world 30 to 40 years ago, the IPE movement has grown exponentially, and has now become a common and required feature in most health care curricula of higher education institutions across the globe.

In this chapter, we discuss IPE to begin to understand its key concepts, methods, and outcomes to show its potential for improving the quality of health professions education and helping address

Jensen GM, Mostrom E, Hack LM, Nordstrom T, Gwyer J.
Educating Physical Therapists (pp 175-187).
© 2019 Taylor & Francis Group.

problems with poor collaborative practice, which can seriously impede the delivery of high quality and safe patient care. The chapter is presented as follows. First, we outline the worldwide growth of IPE before describing different key learning and teaching approaches employed. Next, we discuss a series of lessons learned for successful implementation of IPE. Then, we provide an overview of the expansion of IPE research. Finally, we provide conclusions highlighting some directions for IPE in the future.

BACKGROUND

Spread of Interprofessional Education

IPE is defined as occasions "when 2 or more professions learn with, from, and about each other to improve collaboration and the quality of care."[5] Over the past 3 to 4 decades, globally, health policy makers have identified the key role of IPE in improving health care systems and outcomes.[6,7] However, in the past 20 years IPE has been at the forefront of much curricula, research, policy, and regulatory activity. The promotion of IPE is embedded in the complexity and multifaceted nature of patients' health needs and the health system, and research demonstrating that effective collaboration amongst different health care providers is essential for the provision of effective and comprehensive health care.

Ongoing difficulties with interprofessional communication and collaboration are well documented in the interprofessional and patient safety literature. For example, studies reporting failures of interprofessional collaboration were found to be at the center of several health settings across the globe, causing harm, injury, and death to patients.[8] In the United States, poor interprofessional communication was identified as a central cause of approximately 2/3 of all clinical errors.[9]

Health care professionals need education and training to provide them with the attitudes, knowledge, skills, and behaviors needed to work effectively together to deliver safe, high-quality patient care. Barr and colleagues[10] argue that the traditional uniprofessional approach to health professions education is insufficient to provide the competencies needed to be an effective collaborator. As a result, educational reforms advocating the introduction of IPE are being demanded. Education policies have identified that a key role for IPE is to ensure graduates can contribute as effective interprofessional team members, work together to better coordinate services and help deliver enhanced patient care.

Two major international reports have identified the need to reform health professions education systems toward providing learners with more opportunities to develop collaborative competence through the delivery of IPE.[7,11] The World Health Organization (WHO) stated that IPE is important for health care professions to develop the abilities needed to be ready to practice in a collaborative fashion.[7] This document also stressed the importance of IPE and collaborative practice in improving fragmented and struggling health systems throughout the world, arguing that interprofessional teamwork can provide better coordinated services, which provides better care to patients and their communities, which result in a strengthened health system and improved outcomes.[7]

Policy documents have provided an increased impetus for a range of health care education providers to begin to develop a range of IPE activities for both students and qualified practitioners to enhance their abilities to work in a more collaborative manner. For example, IPE centers and offices have been created at several universities across the globe, in countries such as Australia, Canada, Japan, Sweden, United Kingdom, and the United States. In these institutions, colleagues in different departments are working together to provide IPE opportunities for a range of different learners. Recognizing the outcomes associated with IPE and IPC, the Commission on Accreditation of Physical Therapy Education (CAPTE) recently mandated that by January 2018, all accredited physical therapy curricula must include both didactic and clinical IPE and learning activities that are directed toward the core competencies for IPC practice.[12] Additionally, Element 7D39 calls for participation in the health care environment to include participation in patient-centered, IPC practice:

TABLE 12-1
EXAMPLE RESOURCES FOR INTERPROFESSIONAL ORGANIZATIONS, CONSORTIA, JOURNALS, AND CONFERENCES

NATIONAL ORGANIZATIONS	American Interprofessional Health Collaborative: https://aihc-us.org
	Australasian Interprofessional Education Network: http://www.aippen.net
	Canadian Interprofessional Health Collaborative: http://www.cihc.ca
	Centre for Advancement of Interprofessional Education: http://caipe.org.uk
	National Center for Interprofessional Education and Practice: https://nexusipe.org
CONSORTIA AND ACADEMIES	American Council of Academic Physical Therapy: http://www.acapt.org/about/consortium/national-interprofessional-education-consortium-(nipec)
	Interprofessional Education Collaborative:[13,14] https://www.ipecollaborative.org
	National Academies of Practice: http://www.napractice.org/About-NAP/Mission-Vision-Values
SCHOLARLY JOURNALS	*Health and Interprofessional Practice*
	Journal of Interprofessional Care
	Journal of Interprofessional Practice and Education
	Journal of Research in Interprofessional Practice and Education
CONFERENCES	All Together Better Health (international)
	Collaborating Across Borders (United States and Canada)
	European Interprofessional Education Network (Europe)
	National Academies of Practice Conference (United States)
	National Center—Nexus Summit (United States)
	Nordic Interprofessional Network Conference (Nordic region)

- Element 6F: The didactic and clinical curriculum includes IPE.
- Element 6L3: Involvement in interprofessional practice.
- Element 7D39: Participate in patient-centered interprofessional collaborative practice.

Over the past 25 years, the interprofessional field has seen several important developments with the growth of national organizations, consortia/academies, journals, and conferences that have championed IPE and collaborative practice. These developments are presented in Table 12-1.

Collectively, these developments (the expansion of interprofessional organizations, consortia, journals, and conferences) demonstrate that the IPE field is both growing and maturing as an established domain in health professions education and critical in preparing graduates for collaborative practice.

KEY INTERPROFESSIONAL LEARNING AND TEACHING APPROACHES

Interactive Learning Methods

The definition of IPE outlined previously stresses the need for explicit interprofessional interaction between learners, as this interactivity can promote the development of the competencies required for effective collaboration. Educational strategies that enable interactivity are therefore a requirement of IPE. There are several different types of interactive learning methods used in IPE, including:[15]

- Exchange-based learning (eg, seminar-based discussions)
- Observation-based learning (eg, joint visits to patients/clients)
- Action-based learning (eg, problem-based learning)
- Simulation-based learning (eg, simulating clinical practice)
- Practice-based learning (eg, interprofessional clinical placements)
- e-learning (eg, online discussions)
- Blended learning (eg, combining exchange-based and e-learning)

The literature contains numerous examples of these learning activities within IPE initiatives. Brashers et al.[16] report the use of exchange-based learning in the form of interprofessional workshops in their IPE program, while Sanborn[17] reported introducing e-learning methods in the IPE programs for students. Combining different interactive learning methods in an IPE initiative can make the experience more stimulating, as well as contribute to a more profound level of learning.[18]

A key element of successful IPE is the use of interactive team-building activities. An ice-breaking session can help in facilitating interprofessional team cohesion. Such sessions may allow students to interactively and explicitly focus on any negative stereotyping or hostile professional assumptions they bring to their IPE. Team-building sessions can be particularly advantageous in unpacking and exploring issues of professionalism (eg, boundary protectionism) that are central to IPC.[19] They are also helpful in team-building, especially when a group of learners has not previously worked together. For established interprofessional teams, these sessions can also be useful in allowing them to deconstruct issues linked to hierarchy and power differentials that surround their daily practice.

Interprofessional Mix

Effective IPE requires a balance and presence of multiple professions. An equal mix of members from each profession involved in IPE means that a team is not skewed too heavily in favor of one profession, which can inhibit interaction, as the larger professional group can dominate. However, ensuring this balance of professions can be challenging. For students, finding mutually convenient space in different profession-specific timetables for IPE can be problematic. One strategy that may help navigate through timetabling difficulties is the introduction of extracurricular or elective learning, which can provide flexibility for IPE. For example, several academic institutions have offered an IPE Passport system, thereby allowing learners to select IPE activities of interest for inclusion, allowing them to choose activities based on their own schedules in their IPE experiences as required by their institution for graduation (find more at https://passport.health.ubc.ca).

For health care providers, team composition for IPE can be affected by the demands of clinical work, especially if sessions are held nearby the learners' clinical area (where individuals can be easily called back to the workplace). Also, if an IPE program occurs over several days or weeks, it can interfere with clinical work schedules. One way of overcoming this difficulty is to offer IPE to clinical teams offsite. This can be rewarding in terms of providing a more conducive learning environment for both formal and informal IPE activities. However, it is an expensive option, especially as one needs to secure clinical coverage for the team.

Effective Interprofessional Facilitation

Successful IPE facilitation requires skill, experience, and preparation to deal with the various responsibilities and demands involved. It is ideal to train facilitators from the diverse professional programs involved in IPE, and thus, the number of facilitators required can be large, particularly in a pre-qualification context, depending on the number of students. There are a range of attributes required for this type of work, including:[15]

- Experience of interprofessional work (to draw upon when facilitating)
- In-depth understanding of interactive learning methods
- Knowledge of group dynamics
- Confidence in working with interprofessional groups
- Ability to role-model and mirror collaborative learning
- Flexibility (to creatively use professional differences within groups)

Like other small-group education formats, facilitators need to focus on team formation and development; creating a supportive and safe learning environment; and enabling all participants to have the opportunity to participate equally. Another core skill of an interprofessional facilitator then becomes the ability to make explicit for participants learning moments that can surface the traditional power hierarchies amongst the professions and then move participants to common ground, which is most often an integrated plan for patient care. Specifically within a clinical environment, learning occurs in a complex setting with complex relationships.[20] In the midst of the clinical complexity, a substantial amount of informal and implicit education occurs.[21] This tacit workplace learning may make it difficult for students and clinical instructors (CI) to participate in, recognize, or value IPE opportunities, thus reinforcing the need to make the implicit and informal curriculum more explicit, formalized, and structured for the developing student and CI. Given the recent surge of interest in IPE as a means to develop a collaborative-ready health care workforce, current health profession practitioners (eg, physical therapists) are unlikely to have explicitly learned about common IPE principles and interprofessional core competencies in their own training.[14,22] Even if these are familiar, the art of facilitating discussions around these core competencies requires practice and a way of conversing/debriefing that is different than feedback to learners about their performance with more commonly discussed topics such as manual muscle testing, goniometry, mobilizations and/or other common tests and measures.

With the evolution of IPE, from the pre-clerkship years in classroom and simulation context to the intentional shift of IPE to the clinical practice settings, there is a need to develop interprofessional faculty preceptors. Shrader et al[23] describe interprofessional preceptoring as intentionally educating learners from multiple professions in authentic practice-based settings. This allows for both clinical teaching and patient care, combined with facilitated conversation around the benefits of IPC care. Interprofessional facilitation skill development has been described in the literature[23,24] (for a downloadable facilitation toolkit, see https://nexusipe.org/engaging/learning-system/preceptors-nexus-toolkit).

A Focus on Collaborative Competence

The call for an increased use of IPC has been underpinned by a growing body of literature on IPE competency frameworks.[14,25] These frameworks aim to provide a common lens through which professions can understand, describe, and implement IPC practices. IPC frameworks are designed to help guide the alignment of learning and teaching activities with assessment strategies so that the learners have attained competence in a set of knowledges, skills, beliefs, and/or attitudes. Barr[26] originally defined collaborative competences as "dimensions of competence which every profession needs to collaborate within its own ranks, with other professions, with non professionals, within organizations, between organizations, with patients and their carers, with volunteers and with community groups."[(p184)] Current challenges are now to incorporate the IPE competencies into existing curricula in a way that does not duplicate profession specific competencies[27] and ensures that the measurement of these competencies is robust.[28]

Assessment of Interprofessional Education

Formally assessing the changes in knowledge, skills and attitudes (ie, collaborative competence) following the delivery of an IPE program is critical.[29] Ideally, the assessment of learning should be an integral part of the IPE program. Assessment should be capable of not only differentiating between successful and less successful students, but also enabling program improvement. In general, informal formative assessment uses self-report surveys from students. However, increasingly, many IPE programs are moving toward summative assessment. This poses a challenge within phiiscal therapy clinical education (CE) environments. While the CAPTE standards continue to evolve to include minimum requirements of IPE and IPC, the commonly used APTA clinical performance instrument (http://www.apta.org/PTCPI) does not yet adequately capture the outlined standards, challenging CIs in providing focused formal summative assessment of IPE/IPC in the clinical environment. Conversely, the APTA credentialed CI program (http://www.apta.org/CCIP) is currently in its 5-year review, and there have been discussions about inclusion of explicit teaching around the IPE standards. Medical education literature has an increased focus on developing structured approaches to IPE assessment in the form of EPA and milestones, using formal observation-based assessment in the form of team-based or interprofessional objective, structured, clinical examinations.[29]

Learning Outcomes

Table 12-2 presents 6 key outcomes (Levels 1 to 4b) developed from the educational literature, which help explain the various learning outcomes which can be generated from an IPE program.[10] As presented in this table, IPE outcomes can cover changes to learners' reactions of their IPE program (Level 1), changes in attitudes/perceptions of different professional groups (Level 2), improvements to collaborative knowledge and skills (Level 2b), changes to an individual's behavior (Level 3), changes in organizational practice (Level 4a), and/or improvements to the delivery of care to patients (Level 4b).

This IPE typology has usefully been employed in systematic reviews of IPE to help classify the range of outcomes that can be generated from this type of education.[30]

A New Conceptual Model

Drawing upon the IPE literature, the Institute of Medicine recently developed a conceptual framework to help understand the different connecting components related to IPE learning and teaching approaches.[31]

As Figure 12-1 presents, IPE, both formal and informal, should ideally occur with increasing regularity along the learning continuum from foundational (prequalification) to graduate and then continuing professional development. This figure also shows several enabling or inferring factors that can affect the delivery of IPE, including professional and institutional cultures as well as workforce and financing policy. Collectively, these factors can impact the learning outcomes (see Table 12-2), health outcomes and system outcomes.

	TABLE 12-2
SIX KEY LEARNING OUTCOMES FOR INTERPROFESSIONAL EDUCATION PROGRAMS	
OUTCOME	DETAILS
Level 1: Reaction	Learners' views on the learning experience and its interprofessional nature
Level 2a: Modification of attitudes/perceptions	Changes in reciprocal attitudes or perceptions between participant groups/teams
Level 2b: Acquisition of knowledge/skills	Gains of knowledge and skills linked to IPC
Level 3: Behavioral change	Individuals' transfer of interprofessional learning to their practice setting and their changed professional practice
Level 4a: Change in organizational practice	Wider changes in the organization and delivery of care
Level 4b: Benefits to patients	Improvements in health or well-being of patients

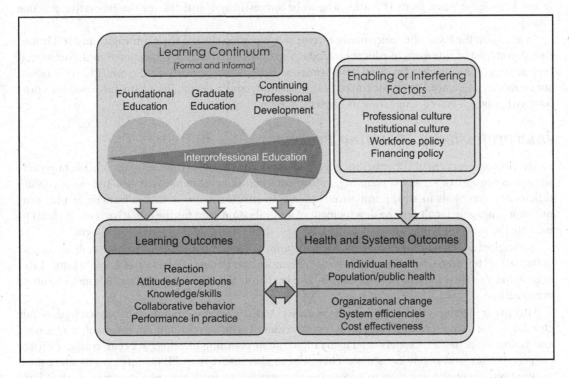

Figure 12-1. A conceptual framework representing various connecting components related to IPE learning and teaching approaches.[31]

SUCCESSFUL INTERPROFESSIONAL EDUCATION: LESSONS LEARNED

Senior Leadership and Organizational Support

It is both crucial and critical to have senior leadership with interest, knowledge, and experience to champion and forward IPE as a priority within an organization. Institutional policies and leadership commitment at all levels are also crucial given the resources required to develop and implement IPE.

The support required is often dependent on the stage of education. Planning and implementing prequalification (first professional degree education) IPE is challenging given the high number of organizational barriers, such as large numbers of students, professional accreditation requirements, and inflexible curricula and academic schedules that exist. This creates logistical difficulties over finding a suitable location for this type of education. In addition, differences in course timing for these student cohorts can create further problems around finding a suitable time to deliver IPE. Obtaining approval from each of the participating profession's regulatory bodies often adds additional complications, as well as agreeing on issues of accountability.

Although IPE for qualified professionals can be less problematic to plan because of the fewer organizational/logistical barriers, senior management support is still required to ensure professionals have sufficient time and resources to attend the IPE program. Furthermore, this type of support is critical if any knowledge gains from IPE are going to be successfully translated into collaborative practice changes.

In addition, the issue of finance needs careful consideration during the planning of any IPE initiative. As the cost of this form of education tends to span several different professional or departmental budgets,[32] agreement over financial arrangements can often be a main hurdle for IPE. As a result, senior faculty often need to be convinced of the feasibility and acceptability of any proposed interprofessional program before supporting its implementation.

Interprofessional Planning Processes

Developing a successful IPE program is a complex process. It will involve a range of different professions who engage in a variety of planning, implementation, and evaluation activities. Indeed, involving different professionals in an IPE initiative is crucial to ensure a sense of shared ownership and commitment. Engaging faculty in the development of an evaluation plan for the initiative is also crucial to increase the probability that the evaluation findings will be useful to program development.[32]

As developing IPE can take time and energy, planning team members need to have dedication and enthusiasm. However, when IPE programs are dependent on the input of a few key enthusiasts, it has been found that their long-term sustainability can be threatened when these individuals move to other organizations.

Effective leadership of all IPE programs is central to their success.[33] Importantly, such leaders can coordinate the activities and ensure progress is achieved with curriculum development, assessment and evaluation activities. Leaders need to arrange regular planning meetings to occur, consider different perspectives, and ensure consensus. They need to also ensure that IPE planning teams share their assumptions about the initiative to encourage all members to work toward a common goal. Where differences are identified, leaders need to ensure they are discussed and resolved.

Sustaining IPE is complex. It requires good communication among participants, enthusiasm and support for a range of curriculum development, assessment, and evaluation activities. It also needs a shared vision and understanding of the benefits of introducing IPE. One key challenge in sustaining and supporting IPE initiatives in the clinical environment relates to state practice act requirements. Currently in California, physical therapy students must be supervised by a licensed physical therapist when rendering physical therapy services. Therefore, other health care providers cannot legally provide supervision to a physical therapy student providing services, in lieu of a therapist, even for skills that are shared among providers, such as, common clinical monitoring skills, basic balance assessments, or other related health promotion and education activities. Technically, any health fair or other interprofessional clinical skill activity in which physical therapy students are participating requires direct physical therapist oversight. This requires multiple faculty/providers oversight for one team of interprofessional learners, even when overseeing the shared skills taught by these professions. To sustain quality IPE/IPC initiatives will require continued dialogue between the CAPTE, Federation of State Boards of Physical Therapy (FSBPT), and individual state-by-state practice licensing boards (for example in California, http://www.ptbc.ca.gov/laws/laws_pt_students.pdf).

Another challenge in sustaining IPE initiatives is providing recognition in the promotion and/or tenure process for IPE faculty champions. Many institutions see involvement of faculty/clinicians in IPE activities as service to the department and/or university and these efforts may not be as favorably rated compared to teaching, research, and/or clinical service activities. It has been found that successful IPE occurs in organizations that value and reward IPE efforts,[32] constantly evaluate and revise their learning, as well as remind all members, including promotion and tenure committee members, about the general goals of IPE, which is to improve interprofessional practice and patient care.[10,15]

Faculty Development

To ensure success with IPE, it is important that faculty development is offered for those involved in developing, delivering, and evaluating IPE. For most educators, teaching students how to learn about, from, and with each other is a new and challenging experience. Similarly, to students, staff, and faculty may also struggle with interprofessional and professional issues. Faculty development may reduce feelings of isolation, develop a more collaborative approach to facilitation, as well as provide opportunities for faculty to share knowledge, experiences, and ideas.[34]

There are a growing number of IPE faculty development activities. In general, they focus on offering a similar range of preparatory activities, such as understanding the roles and responsibilities of the different professions, exploring issues of professionalism, and planning learning strategies for interprofessional groups. There is also a need for IPE faculty development programs to enable individuals to promote change at the individual and organizational level, and thus should also target diverse stakeholders and address leadership and organizational change.[24]

To ensure that faculty maintain their knowledge of interprofessional facilitation, they need ongoing faculty development opportunities. Often, it is useful to consider team-teaching with more experienced colleagues to help develop the range of necessary skills, knowledge, and confidence that are vital for interprofessional facilitation. Regular opportunities for discussion and reflection can be a useful type of support for facilitators of IPE. Where formal training cannot be obtained, it is advisable to seek informal input from a colleague more experienced in this type of work. For IPE to be successfully embedded in curricula and training packages, the early experiences of staff must be positive. This will ensure continued involvement and a willingness to further develop the curriculum based on student feedback.

The challenge facing physical therapist education is the need to provide IPC practice experiences in contextually relevant clinical settings. Previous study findings suggest limited opportunities exist for students to participate in workplace communities that truly practice IPC and team-based care.[35] While results indicate that the most frequent and diverse interprofessional learning takes place in the inpatient setting,[35,36] we should recognize that most physical therapists practice in the outpatient setting. 2017 APTA membership demographic data indicates that approximately 59% of APTA members report practicing in an outpatient facility (private or hospital-based), while 18% report practicing in an inpatient facility (acute hospital, skilled nursing facility, or inpatient rehabilitation).[37] The combination of fewer inpatient clinical placement sites and a dominant outpatient workforce will continually force programs to rely heavily on outpatient settings for student CE placements. Outpatient settings will bear the burden of providing students with opportunities to achieve the mandated IPE and IPC competencies. In our current physical therapy CE paradigm, how will we provide collaboration and team-based experiences that offer students an opportunity to build their skills and to meet the required IPE competencies for graduation?

GROWING EVIDENCE FOR INTERPROFESSIONAL EDUCATION

During the past decade, several IPE systematic reviews have been conducted to examine and summarize the IPE evidence.[30] The reviews used different criteria for the studies to be included and thus, while there was overlap, each examined a different group of studies. To understand the overall nature of this evidence, these reviews were synthesized to provide an overall understanding of the evidence base.[38] We outline the main findings from this work to offer an indication of the current level of evidence for IPE.

Studies and Programs

In total, the synthesis located 6 systematic reviews of IPE that collectively reported on the effects of over 200 IPE studies spanning from 1974 to 2005. While the synthesis found that these 6 reviews reported on studies which differed in methodological quality and reported a range of different outcomes associated with IPE, all shared a similar definition of IPE.

The synthesis revealed that IPE was delivered in a variety of acute, primary, and community care settings and addressed a range of different health conditions (eg, asthma, arthritis) or acute conditions (eg, cardiac care). While different combinations of professional groups participated in the IPE programs, medicine and nursing were the consistent participants across learning groups. IPE was generally delivered as a voluntary learning experience to participants and few programs included any form of formal academic accreditation. The duration of programs varied, ranging from 1- to 2-hour sessions to programs delivered over a period of months; however, most IPE programs lasted between 1 and 5 days.

Most IPE programs were more commonly delivered to health care providers in their workplaces, although IPE was increasingly being delivered to students in a classroom or sometimes as a practice-based activity. While the synthesis revealed that IPE programs used a variety of interactive learning methods, seminar-based discussions, group problem-solving, and/or role-play activities were the most common employed. In general, most IPE programs employed formative assessments of learning, typically using assessment techniques in the form of individual written assignments and/or team presentations of participants' interprofessional experiences. Theoretically, the synthesis indicated that most IPE programs only drew implicitly upon theories of adult learning. Looking forward, IPE programs may consider the use of virtual simulation-based activities and/or telehealth options when creating opportunities for IPE.[39]

Interprofessional Education Impact and Quality

The synthesis used the different outcomes levels reported in the IPE typology (see Table 12-2) to understand the range of results reported in the reviews. Most studies report that IPE programs can result in positive learner reactions (Level 1), where the learner enjoyed their interprofessional experiences. IPE programs reported positive changes in learner perceptions/attitudes (Level 2a) in relation to changes in views of other professional groups, views of collaboration and/or views of the value attached to interprofessional work. In addition, the synthesis indicated that these types of programs reported positive changes in learner knowledge and skills of interprofessional collaboration (Level 2b), usually related to an enhanced understanding of roles and responsibilities of other professional groups, improved knowledge of the nature of IPC and/or the development of collaboration/communication skills.

It was found that few IPE programs reported outcomes related to changes in individual behavior (Level 3); of those programs that did provide this type of evidence, positive change in individual practitioners' interactions was usually cited. A small number of studies reported positive changes to organizational practices resulting from the delivery of IPE (Level 4a), as evidenced by changes to interprofessional referral practices/working patterns or improved documentation. A smaller amount of studies report changes to the delivery of care to patients/clients (Level 4b). These studies typically reported positive changes to clinical outcomes (eg, infection rates, clinical error rates), patient satisfaction scores, and/or length of patient stay.

In general, IPE programs for students reported outcomes in relation to changes to attitudes, beliefs, knowledge, and collaborative skills. While IPE programs for clinical staff report a similar range of learner-oriented changes, they also reported changes to organization practice and improvements in the delivery of patient care. However, these differences in outcomes may, in many ways, be inevitable, as developing collaborative attitudes, knowledge, and skills before students qualify is a timely outcome, while attempting to improve patient care is a more normal outcome for qualified practitioners.

The synthesis revealed that most studies provided little discussion of methodological limitations associated with their research. As a result, it was difficult to understand the nature of biases and the overall quality of a research study. Most IPE programs also paid little or no attention to sampling techniques in their work, or issues relating to study attrition. Across the studies, there was a propensity to report the short-term outcomes linked to IPE. As a result, there was little idea of the long-term impact of this type of education.

There was a widespread use of non-validated instruments to detect impact of IPE on learner and/or patient satisfaction. While the use of such tools can provide helpful data for local quality assurance issues, they limit the quality of the research as it is difficult to assess their validity or reliability. Measures to detect changes in individual behavior were particularly poor, often relying on simple self-reported descriptive accounts of this form of change. In addition, most IPE studies were undertaken in single site studies, in isolation from other studies, limiting the authenticity and generalizability of the research.

The synthesis also found that there was a common use of quasi-experimental research designs (eg, before-and-after studies; before-during-and-after studies) that can provide some indication of change associated with the delivery of IPE. Most studies did gather 2 or more forms of data (typically survey and interviews) and there is a growing use of longitudinal studies to begin establishing the long-term impact of IPE on organizations and patient care. Importantly, the synthesis indicated that the evidence for the effects of IPE rests upon a variety of different program elements (eg, duration, balance of professional participation), different methods (eg, quantitative, qualitative studies) of variable quality, as well as a range of outcomes (eg, reports of learner satisfaction to changes in the delivery of care).

An Update

In 2017, this work was updated and found 8 additional IPE reviews.[40] Despite a growth of the international IPE evidence contained in this newer review, the key results in relation to use of learning activities, methods of evaluation and outcomes reported in the initial work remained unchanged. As a result, the evidence for the effects of IPE continues to rest upon a variety of different interprofessional programs (eg, in terms of learning activities, duration, and professional mix) and study methods (eg, experimental studies, mixed methods, qualitative designs) of variable quality. Nevertheless, this updated review revealed that IPE can nurture collaborative knowledge, skills, and attitudes. It also found more limited, but growing, evidence that IPE can help enhance collaborative practice and improve patient care. Mindful of these and other limitations to the IPE evidence base, Reeves and colleagues recently published guidance for improving the quality of IPE studies to support evaluation teams, in their future work, to generate more rigorous interprofessional scholarship.[40]

CONCLUSION

As presented in this chapter, IPE has achieved many successes over the past 40 years. As a result, IPE is now recognized globally as an important form of education that help improve IPC and the delivery of high-quality and safe patient care. Ongoing organizational engagement, support, and commitment remain critical for the continuing success of IPE. Physical therapy education efforts should prioritize and support faculty development activities, specifically CE instructors. We should continue to:

- Develop academic and workplace cultures that explicitly endorse IPE. Education and professional development should focus on the Interdisciplinary Professional Education Collaborative competencies[14] to identify and capitalize on IPE teachable moments, most urgently in the CE and workplace settings.

- Leadership from professional associations, universities, and clinical organizations will also be key to encourage and support students and practitioners fully engaging in IPE programs.

- Future investment in IPE must be based on rigorous evidence. It is encouraging that the evidence base for IPE is growing. Indeed, IPE reviews have shown that this type of education can have positive outcomes. With the expanding number of IPE studies, it is hopeful that the evidence of this field will, over time, also become increasingly more rigorous and show evidence of impact and sustainability.

REFERENCES

1. Berwick D, Nolan T, Whittington, J. The Triple Aim: care, health, and cost. *Health Aff.* 2008;27:759-769.
2. Bodenheimer T, Sinsky C. From triple aim to quadruple aim: care of the patient requires care of the provider. *Ann Fam Med.* 2014;12(6):573-576.
3. Brandt B, Lutfiyya M, King J. A scoping review of interprofessional collaborative practice and education using the lens of the triple aim. *J Interprof Care.* 2014;28(5):393-399.
4. Kigrin C, Rodgers M, Wolf S. The Physical Therapy and Society Summit (PASS) meeting: observations and opportunities. *Phys Ther.* 2010;90:1555-1567.
5. Centre for the Advancement of Interprofessional Education. Interprofessional education: a definition. Fareham, UK: CAIPE; 2002.
6. World Health Organization. *Continuing Education of Health Personnel.* Copenhagen, Denmark: WHO; 1976.
7. World Health Organization. *Framework for Action on Interprofessional Education and Collaborative Practice.* Geneva, Switzerland: WHO; 2010.
8. Wachter R. *The Digital Doctor: Hope, Hype, and Harm at the Dawn of Medicine's Computer Age.* New York, NY: McGraw-Hill; 2015.
9. Dow A, Reeves S. How health professional training will and should change. In: Hoff T, Sutcliffe K, Young G, eds. *The Health Care Professional Workforce: Understanding Human Capital in a Changing Industry.* Oxford, UK: Oxford University Press; 2017:147-176.
10. Barr H, Koppel I, Reeves S, Hammick M, Freeth D. *Effective Interprofessional Education: Assumption, Argument and Evidence.* Oxford, UK: Blackwell; 2005.
11. Frenk J, Chen L, Bhutta ZA, et al. Health professionals for a new century: transforming education to strengthen health systems in an interdependent world. *Lancet.* 2010;376:1923-1958.
12. Commission on Accreditation in Physical Therapy Education. http://www.capteonline.org/AccreditationHandbook/ Updated January 5, 2018. Accessed September 4, 2018.
13. Interprofessional Education Collaborative. *Core Competencies for Interprofessional Collaborative Practice: Report of an Expert Panel.* Washington, DC; 2011.
14. Interprofessional Education Collaborative. *Core Competencies for Interprofessional Collaborative Practice: 2016 Update.* Washington, DC: 2016.

15. Reeves S, Kitto S. Collaborating interprofessionally for team-based care. In: Turco M, Davis D, Rayburn W, eds. *Continuing Professional Development in Medicine and Health Care: Better Education, Better Patient Outcomes.* Philadelphia, PA: Wolters Kluwer; 2017:121-134.

16. Brashers V, Erickson J, Blackhall L, Owen J, Thomas S, Conaway M. Measuring the impact of clinically relevant interprofessional education on undergraduate medical and nursing student competencies: a longitudinal mixed methods approach. *J Interprof Care.* 2016;30(4):448-457.

17. Sanborn H. Developing asynchronous online interprofessional education, *J Interprof Care.* 2016;30(5):668-670.

18. Wise H, Frost J, Resnik C, Davis B, Iglarsh A. Interprofessional education: an exploration in physical therapist education. *J Phys Ther Ed.* 2015;29(2):72-80.

19. Baker L, Egan-Lee E, Martimianakis M, Reeves S. Relationships of power: implications for interprofessional education and practice. *J Interprof Care.* 2011;25:98-104.

20. Wenger E. *Communities of Practice: Learning, Meaning and Identity.* Cambridge, UK: Cambridge University Press; 1998.

21. Nisbit G, Lincoln M, Stewart D. Informal interprofessional learning: an untapped opportunity for learning and change within the workplace. *J Interprof Care.* 2013;27(6):469-475.

22. Kogan J, Holmboe E. Preparing residents for practice in new systems of care by preparing their teachers. *Acad Med.* 2014;80(11):1436-1437.

23. Schrader S, Zaudke J, Jernigan S. An interprofessional objective structured experience (iOSTE): an interprofessional preceptor professional development activity. *J Interprof Care.* 2018;32(1):98-100.

24. Hall L, Zierler B. Interprofessional education and practice guide no. 1: developing faculty to effectively facilitate interprofessional education. *J Interprof Care.* 2015;29(1):3-7.

25. Canadian Interprofessional Health Collaborative. A National Interprofessional Competency Framework. https://www.cihc.ca/files/CIHC_IPCompetencies_Feb1210.pdf. Published 2010. Accessed September 4, 2018.

26. Barr H. Competent to collaborate: toward a competency-based model for interprofessional education. *J Interprof Care.* 1998;12(2):181-187.

27. Thistlethwaite J, Forman D, Matthews L, Rogers G, Steketee C, Yassine T. Competencies and frameworks in interprofessional education: a comparative analysis. *Acad Med.* 2014;89(6):869-875.

28. Reeves S. The rise and rise of interprofessional competence. *J Interprof Care.* 2012;26:253-255.

29. Simmons B, Wagner S, Reeves S. Assessment of interprofessional education: key issues, ideas, challenges and opportunities. In: Wimmers P, Mentkowski M, eds. *Assessing Competence in Professional Performance Across Disciplines and Professions.* New York, NY: Springer; 2016:237-252.

30. Reeves S, Fletcher S, Barr et al. A BEME systematic review of the effects of interprofessional education: BEME guide no. 39. *Med Teach.* 2016;38(7):656-68.

31. National Academies of Science, Engineering, and Medicine. *Measuring the Impact of Interprofessional Education on Collaborative Practice and Patient Outcomes.* Washington, DC: The National Academies Press; 2016.

32. Reeves S. *Developing and Delivering Practice-Based Interprofessional Education.* Munich, Germany: VDM Publications; 2008.

33. Brewer M, Flavell HL, T Franziska, Smith M. A scoping review to understand "leadership" in interprofessional education and practice, *J Interprof Care.* 2016;30(4):408-415.

34. Schrader S, Hodgkins R, Laverentz D, et al. Interprofessional education and practice guide no. 7: development, implementation, and evaluation of a large-scale required interprofessional education foundational programme. *J Interprof Care.* 2016;30(5):615-619.

35. Fitzsimmons A, Topp K, O'Brien BC. Investigation into physical therapist students' perceptions of interprofessional education experiences during an 8-week clinical clerkship: a qualitative study. *J Phys Educ.* 2017;31(2):44-53.

36. Robson M, Kitchen S. Exploring physiotherapy students' experiences of interprofessional collaboration in the clinical setting: a critical incident study. *J Interprof Care.* 2007;21(1):95-109.

37. American Physical Therapy Association. 2017. Physical therapy workforce and membership data. Published September, 2014.

38. Reeves S, Goldman J, Sawatzky-Girling B, Burton A. A synthesis of systematic reviews of interprofessional education. *J Allied Health.* 2010;39:(S)198-203.

39. Taylor MS, Tucker J, Donehower C, et al. Impact of virtual simulation on the interprofessional communication skills of physical therapy students: a pilot study. *J Phys Educ.* 2017;31(3):83-90.

40. Reeves S, Palaganas J, Zierler B. An updated synthesis of review evidence of interprofessional education. *J Allied Health.* 2017;46:56-61.

13

Practice-Based Education
Realizing Excellent Education for Future-Oriented Practice

Joy Higgs, AM, BSc, MHPEd, PhD, NSW, PFHEA

In this chapter, I argue that the pursuit of excellence and innovation in professional education, and education of health professionals where the quality of people's lives is a direct result of education and learning, requires deep consideration of each of the fundamental purposes that educators are aiming to achieve, along with a visionary educational framework. The visionary educational framework I am advocating is practice-based education. My foundation premises are as follows:

- *Higher education* is for the public as well as private good. Individuals, groups, and society gain from the glorious endeavor of higher education. The public benefit is not just a backdrop or historical artifact of traditional professional education; it is also a reasonable current expectation of the investment from the public purse into the nation's education.
- *Professional education* (eg, physical therapy education) is a key means for shaping society. Societies provide and expect high quality human services, in this case health care, and it is important to recognize that the nature and character of education shapes the quality and commitments of the graduates who provide these services.
- *Professional socialization* is a core dimension of professional education. It would be expected that individuals are encultured into a world of professionalism where their individual life and learning for practice gains through their education become capabilities and commitments that serve the interests and needs of the public.
- *Excellence and innovation* are challenging concepts. On the one hand, excellence is a matter of judgement and is inarguably situationally determined. Educational standards and frameworks require the possibility of adaptation and contextual relevance. As for innovation, we tend to, all too readily, relate innovation to the use of advanced educational and communication technologies. We need to remember that sometimes professional education that has people (the end users) seeking better health may well need to translate innovation as human strategies, systems, and processes that most benefit people. Innovation in such education could

Jensen GM, Mostrom E, Hack LM, Nordstrom T, Gwyer J.
Educating Physical Therapists (pp 189-199).
© 2019 Taylor & Francis Group.

involve including in curricula multiple languages, multicultural ways of dealing with patients or clients, and recognizing the advanced health information literacy of these clients by valuing their knowledge and input in clinical decision making. Innovation, like excellence, is primarily a way of seeking better practices that can be justified through argument and theory, not just quantitative evidence, and it needs to be directed toward good health care and education.

- *Professionalism,* like each of the previous key terms, is an evolving concept. The white-coat, clinically distant concepts of professionalism from the past are not unquestionably transferable to today's professionalism. But neither should the personal benefits for students who are paying high fees give rise to future generations of graduates who place self-gain and self-interest above the needs, wishes and benefits of their patients and clients. Similarly, the escalating costs of health care, particularly in high-cost and high-technology areas of health care, often become an excuse for deciding that the single bottom line of economic determinants of health care is the primary thing that matters. Perhaps the most excellent, innovative, human-centered, and person-beneficial health care encompasses strategies that are less expensive and more strongly based on triple bottom line parameters (ie, social, environmental/ecological, financial), to redefine quality, sustainability, access, and affordability of health care more broadly.

- *Innovation* and other terms like quality care also draw to our attention to the question of which time, era, and/or populations we are educating our graduates. In developed countries, we typically educate graduates to be global citizens able to work across cultures and with their own career trajectories involving working in areas beyond the country of their birth or education. Yet, this poses some interesting challenges to the scope and busyness of curricula. We are clearly educating people who can enter their national practice worlds at the time of graduation and be highly contributing practitioners. In physical therapy, this graduate work would typically not involve high levels of direct supervision or intensive internship training in the early post-graduation years. We could call these *work-ready graduates.* We also must be educating graduates for the next phase of practice, not just through the ability to be lifelong learners, but also with the vision and capability to contribute to future practice themselves. Curricula need to balance learning for near and far practice.

BRINGING EDUCATION AND PRACTICE TOGETHER

Education is not just a means of preparing for professional practice. Both education and professional practice are, in fact, complex practices with their many inherent situational, multivariate, and multi-stakeholder dimensions of practice. In this section, I am exploring the importance of bringing higher education practices and professional practices together.

In Chapter 3, the conceptual model developed by the study research team poses several important aspirations and possibilities for high quality courses that aim to produce well educated health professional graduates. First, we see that the model consists of 3 major dimensions:

1. *Leadership and partnership*: These are key dimensions in the practice of education and professional practice.

2. *Organizational imperatives*: The importance of viewing practice as a contextualized phenomenon is evident in both practice arenas, and in both education and professional practice, choice and responsibility go together with making sound defensible decisions associated with consequential practice and leadership. The situatedness of learning is built around organizational structures and resources, as well as their values and aspirations. We see this in the following questions: What type of educational institution do we want to be? What do we stand for? What do we want our graduates to remember us for? What type of role models will we be for them?

3. *Advancing learning/learning sciences*: In education, we face the dual responsibilities of advancing the learning capabilities and attainments of our students and of building the excellence of our

educational sciences and teaching capabilities. In professional practice, practitioners and practice managers similarly face the responsibilities of advancing the practice capabilities of individuals and groups as well as advancing practice itself. Ideally our students should see their educators role-modeling high quality performance and building quality into future educational practice. Seeing these strategies in action and preferably participating through shared educational leadership, students will graduate with a commitment and ability to carry both responsibilities into their professional practice of physical therapy.

Second, through this model we are challenged to pursue and reshape cultures of educational excellence that manifest and aspire to excellent practices in relation to shared beliefs and values, leadership and vision, drive for excellence with high expectations and mutually respectful partnerships. These challenges can be met by making the links between professional practice and education strong, overt and participatory. In practice-based education such goals are eminently attainable.

Third, the educational excellence in this model sets the Praxis of Learning as a hero. Practice-based education is a highly suitable and achievable whole-of-curriculum model for linking the Praxis of Learning and the Praxis of Practice.

Finally, this model presents a Nexus where patient- and learner-centeredness are critically interdependent. We should celebrate the explicit attention the model gives this Nexus. We might also question why this Nexus is not the cornerstone of all health sciences curricula. We can conclude from the following discussion:

- Learning in an environment where the process and responsibility of learning is transparent and shared between learners, teachers, and educational managers is highly desirable because it:
  - Models through teaching and learning the very dispositions and abilities (eg, shared responsibility and professionalism) that we want graduates to embody in post-graduation practice
  - Recognizes the importance of the learner's journey in becoming a better learner and practitioner as well as the teacher's journey of becoming a better facilitator of learning and a better learner about education
  - Deliberately supports and challenges learners, novice practitioners, educators, and experienced practitioners, all of whom are involved in education of the next generation of practitioners, to realize what good practice means for them and to build practice identities and practice models that allow them to manifest their values and professional practice goals in the way they interpret and shape their practice
  - Emphasizes the ephemerals as well as the fundamental realities of the human worlds of practice (including education, practice, and health care), particularly the inherent culture, needs and deep praxis pursuit in their deliberately owned practice, that comprise these worlds
- Health sciences curricula should be coherent. They are messages of clarity, purposeful frameworks of shared purpose, and organized living structures and systems of operations. Avoiding schedules of heavy and discipline-driven content and courses that are merely technology-driven, market-packaged commodities is vital.
- Professional education is about visioning what the practice of this profession entails and is becoming. Curricula that do not realize (understand and accomplish) such a vision fail our students.

Practice, Praxis, and Practice-Based Education

Higher education discourse places a high priority on preparation of graduates for work and practice. This involves socialization into the relevant occupational culture, gaining work-readiness capabilities, developing agency for future practice and employability, understanding one's role, and creating a chosen pathway and approach for pursuing practice. In pursuing these goals, we can recognize the value of conceptualizing professional practice as comprising knowing, doing, being and becoming.[1] These simple words take us to the depth of practice and practice ownership. It is about being, embodying and becoming a practitioner and owning, valuing, and morally enacting the type of practice that practitioners espouse and wish to provide to their clients. It is also a journey of growth in knowledge and capability, including the capacity to work in unknown and unpredictable circumstances, and expansion in self-determined practice and career management capabilities, rather than doing a job in an externally controlled, legislated, and legitimated environment. In being and becoming the practitioner, the person and the professional combine the following key dimensions of advanced professional practice:[2-4]

- *Practice epistemology*: The way knowledge is determined and created within that practice world; taking an epistemological stance in one's practice
- *Practice ontology*: What really exists in practice, what is real; adopting a worldview of practice
- *Epistemic fluency*: Encompassing flexibility and adeptness in relation to different ways of knowing for and about the world[5]
- *Employability*: Translated as the degree to which a person is employable or prepared for/capable of employment, in general, or in relation to a job, and the ability and agency of a person to act positively in the maintenance and pursuit of his or her desired employment options, situation, and directions[6]
- *Authenticity*: The capacity to be true to self, capable in practice, and authentic in professionalism
- *Practice wisdom*: Realized as an embodied state of being that imbues and guides insightful and quality practice; it comprises self-knowledge, action capacity, deep understanding of practice, and an appreciation of others
- *Professional judgement*: The capacity of practitioners to make highly skilled judgements that are optimal for the given circumstances of the client and the context; such judgements are grounded in the unique knowledge base, frame of reference, self-knowledge, metacognitive ability, wisdom, and reasoning capacity of the practitioner in the task of solving complex practice problems such as: demanding, moral and ethical issues; questions of value, belief and assumptions; and the intricacies of health issues as they impact people's lives

Figure 13-1 provides a diagrammatic synthesis of these terms and ideas.

Creating Purposeful Curricula

In professional practice situations, there are times when patient management protocols have great merit. Following routine surgery, for instance, where different patients' conditions demonstrate low variability, the benefits of particular surgical approaches are well known, and the risks of complications are low, and the use of post-surgical treatment regimens, where all staff know their roles, the collaboration and efficiency of treatment protocols can be great. However, as soon as we start to add variables, such as differences in venue location and resourcing, staff stability, experience and expertise, and patient comorbidities, age differences, and cultural backgrounds, the uncritical use of standardized, non-flexible care becomes problematic.

In education, the situation is the same. Standardized curricula fail to recognize the variable needs of students, the range of abilities and experience of staff, the logistics of the organization, the availability and nature of workplace learning opportunities, and the many other variations that can occur across different learning and teaching situations. Further, at national and regional levels there can be many stakeholder-driven expectations set in terms of national higher education qualifications frameworks and higher education institution accreditation requirements as well as professional accreditation standards. Even in consideration of one discipline, physical therapy, and utilizing knowledge of signature pedagogies[8,9] the idea of a curriculum that meets all such requirements is nonsensical.

The term *curriculum* refers to the sum of the experiences students engage in and acquire because of learning at university and the factors that create these experiences. This includes explicit, implicit and hidden aspects of the learning program, and experiences that occur incidentally (alongside) the formal curriculum. The curriculum is intentional teaching, content and assessment, as well as unintentional messages to learners created through role-modelling by

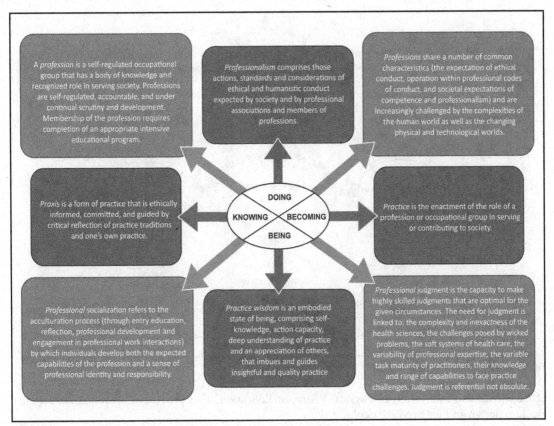

A *profession* is a self-regulated occupational group that has a body of knowledge and recognized role in serving society. Professions are self-regulated, accountable, and under continual scrutiny and development. Membership of the profession requires completion of an appropriate intensive educational program.

Professionalism comprises those actions, standards and considerations of ethical and humanistic conduct expected by society and by professional associations and members of professions.

Professions share a number of common characteristics (the expectation of ethical conduct, operation within professional codes of conduct, and societal expectations of competence and professionalism) and are increasingly challenged by the complexities of the human world as well as the changing physical and technological worlds.

Praxis is a form of practice that is ethically informed, committed, and guided by critical reflection of practice traditions and one's own practice.

DOING

KNOWING × BECOMING

BEING

Practice is the enactment of the role of a profession or occupational group in serving or contributing to society.

Professional socialization refers to the acculturation process (through entry education, reflection, professional development and engagement in professional work interactions) by which individuals develop both the expected capabilities of the profession and a sense of professional identity and responsibility.

Practice wisdom is an embodied state of being, comprising self-knowledge, action capacity, deep understanding of practice and an appreciation of others, that imbues and guides insightful and quality practice

Professional judgment is the capacity to make highly skilled judgments that are optimal for the given circumstances. The need for judgment is linked to: the complexity and inexactness of the health sciences, the challenges posed by wicked problems, the soft systems of health care, the variability of professional expertise, the variable task maturity of practitioners, their knowledge and range of capabilities to face practice challenges. Judgment is referential not absolute.

Figure 13-1. Exploring the professional practice and education context.[1,3,4,7]

teachers and fieldwork educators, through assessment schedules, learning climate, infrastructure (resourcing, facilities, staffing, administrative and support systems), university communities and additional experiences (eg, sporting, social) that are part of university life.[10(p4)]

Taking this notion of a curriculum, course managers and curriculum designers are faced with the task of coming up with a curriculum frame of reference within which a living, evolving, and engaging curriculum can be built. Figure 13-2 presents a framework for planning curricula based on the interpretation of practice as doing, knowing, being and becoming.[1] This framework is based on the following principles.

Knowing

Practice

The designers need to know deeply and to appreciate the practice that underpins their curriculum and the practice arena they are preparing their students to enter. What is it like to be a member of that profession and to become the type of practitioner the novice aspires to be? What do professional practitioners in this field need to know and be able to do, and what capabilities do they need to help them achieve these goals? What does it mean to be a member of a profession in this community of practice and in the broader health care arena? What is required of practitioners in this field? What is their role in cocreating their practice and of imagining future practice?

Education and Curricula

From the educational perspective, similar questions are asked of program managers, designers, and educators. They need to be knowledgeable, fluent, capable, and purposeful. Do they understand and subscribe to the curriculum framework? One such framework is the conceptual model from the study

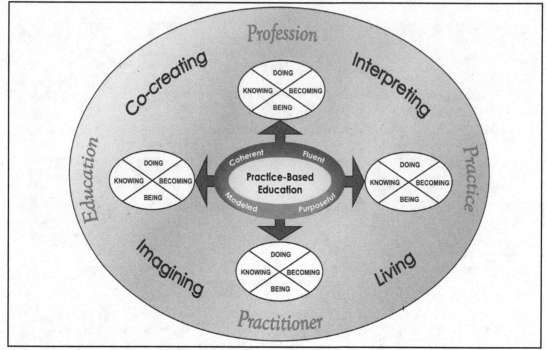

Figure 13-2. Creating purposeful curricula.

of Excellence and Innovation in Physical Therapist Education. This provides the foundation for curriculum design and for lived curricula.

Doing

Doing, as in designing, managing, and implementing curricula, involves modelling and fluently integrating coherent and purposeful educational programs that draw all the players together (ie, students, educators, workplace learning educator-practitioners, members of the profession, other stakeholders, clients). Education and professional practice go hand in hand in practice-based education.

Many pedagogies can be used in practice-based education; they do not need to be occurring in practice, they need to be about practice and for practice learning. The term *pedagogies* can be used to refer to learning and teaching approaches, including modes of interpersonal engagement as well as the teaching and learning strategies utilized in their educational programs. Pedagogies have purpose, such as socialization and preparation for professional practice, as well as actions. Pedagogies may be shared (eg within a discipline) or personal/personally owned by an individual educator or learner.

Signature Pedagogies

Characteristic forms of learning and teaching linked to professions (see Chapter 6). Signature pedagogies incorporate surface dimensions that consist of concrete, operational acts of learning and teaching, a deep structure or set of assumptions about optimal strategies for imparting the relevant professional or disciplinary knowledge and know-how, and an implicit moral dimension comprising the profession's beliefs, values, attitudes, and dispositions. Signature pedagogies for physical therapy such as presented in Chapter 6 (the human body as teacher, early authentic clinical experiences, and shared language on the role of movement) are entirely commensurate with the principles and practice of practice-based education.

Transcending Pedagogies

Rise above/are not limited to course modes, goals, cohorts, spaces, and pathways. They enhance the flexibility, sustainability, and accessibility of learning and enrich learning experiences and outcomes. This means that such pedagogies are not limited to a course or module mode of engagement (eg, on campus, in the workplace, online learning). Taking a transcending pedagogies approach means that educators and students are not limited to traditional teaching and learning strategies or roles; they can also share leadership and decision making in curricula, they can use pedagogy mixtures that transcend the old idea of blended learning (adding some online learning to on campus learning), they can pursue liberating strategies and challenge role, place, ideas, and purpose stereotypes, and they can question the time and place of the students' transition to graduate roles and responsibilities. Becoming a professional starts at enrollment, not at graduation. This approach blurs the boundary between education for life and work. Higher education is a path to citizenship, not just the pursuit of a professional practice occupation.

Being and Becoming

Being a curriculum designer of a purposeful curriculum requires having a vision and living it, plus helping students participating in this curriculum to share the course vision and live within it to become who and what they are able and wish to be: people with agency and a career pathway ahead of them; people who can contribute to society; people who, through their occupation (eg, physical therapy), can make the lives of others better.

PRACTICE-BASED EDUCATION CURRICULA

Practice-based education[11] as a concept and practice provides a deep way of knowing and practicing education. The term refers to university education that is grounded in the preparation of graduates for practice. This mode of education provides an approach to education that prepares students for entry to professions, disciplines, or occupations.

The key pedagogical foundations of practice-based education are:
- Situated or contextualized learning
- Learning in multiple communities of practice (including workplace, academic, multidisciplinary communities)
- Socialization into professional, industry, occupational worlds, roles, identities, and career paths
- Engagement, through teaching-learning relationships and industry partnerships, in practice-based learning and teaching activities
- Development of capabilities and behaviors that will enable graduates to contribute to local communities and society as responsible citizens and professionals who display ethical conduct and duty of care

An Australian Learning and Teaching Fellowship[10] produced a model of practice-based education. Eight key social practice dimensions were identified as underpinning the pedagogy of practice-based education (Table 13-1). Eight key practice-based education pedagogies were also identified (Table 13-2). Figure 13-3 demonstrates how practice-based education emerges from these practices and pedagogies. This figure depicts key pedagogy dimensions and practices. It illustrates relationships among these aspects of practice-based education and reflects the key words that epitomize practice-based education.

Following this fellowship research, a second study was conducted through the Education for Practice Institute at Charles Sturt University to develop standards for the implementation of practice-based education. These standards include standards related to expected learning outcomes for professional education courses conducted through higher education institutions; standards for learning and teaching; and standards for infrastructure needed to support practice-based education. These standards are valuable for curriculum managers and educators implementing practice-based education. The standards have recently been published.[13]

TABLE 13-1

PRACTICE-BASED EDUCATION PEDAGOGIES—EIGHT KEY SOCIAL PRACTICE DIMENSIONS[12]

1. Pedagogical frame	Pedagogy refers to a form of social practice that seeks to shape the educational development of learners. Practice-based education is a pedagogy that prepares students for a practice/occupation.
2. Practice and higher goals	Practice-based education aims to realize the goals of developing students' occupationally relevant social, technical, and professional capabilities, forming their occupational identities, and supporting their development as positively contributing global citizens.
3. Education in context	Practice-based education inevitably occurs within contexts shaped by the interests and practices of students, teachers, practitioner role models, university and workplace settings and society. Both planned processes (eg, curricula, resources, pedagogies) and unplanned factors (eg, changes in workplace access, student numbers) need to reviewed and enhanced to address these goals.
4. Understanding the practice	The students' prospective practice needs to be appraised and evaluated on an ongoing basis to provide a relevant frame of reference to situate students' curriculum and pedagogical experiences.
5. Socialization	Through pedagogical practices students are socialized into the practices of their occupation/profession and into the multiple communities and circumstances of practice that their working worlds comprise.
6. Engaging in relationships	Practice and pedagogy are essentially about relationships. These are realized through partnerships between learners and academics, workplace learning educators and practitioners, among learners (eg, peer learning), across universities and industry/practice-worlds, among university and practice-based educators, and with universities and regulatory authorities, professional groups, society etc.
7. Authenticity and relevance	Authenticity and relevance are themes that are embedded in the goals, venues, activities, student assessment, and program evaluation of practice-based education programs. That is, the curriculum and the key pedagogical perspective are focussed on relevance to graduates' future practice. The education approach, including educators' role-modelled behaviors, should reflect and be grounded in the expectations, norms, knowledge, and practices of the profession.
8. Reflecting standards, values, and ethics	A dimension that needs to permeate all aspects of curricula and pedagogies is the concept and practice of standards; standards as reflective of practice expectations and professionalism and professional codes of conduct or industry standards that are part of practice/professional socialization, standards as accepted pedagogies across the discipline and standards of higher education, good educational practice.

TABLE 13-2

PRACTICE-BASED EDUCATION PEDAGOGIES—EIGHT KEY PRACTICES[12]

Practice	Description
1. Supervised workplace learning	This pedagogy involves students learning through engaging in practice in real workplace placements with formal or informal supervision by workplace educators and/or more experienced practitioners. Examples include nursing practicums and pre-service teachers' professional experience. The educators or practitioners act as mentors and role models.
2. Independent workplace learning and experience	In some courses, there is no tradition of, or capacity for, supervision of workplace learning. In such cases students may participate in unsupervised work experience or may organize their own independent learning programs/projects. Some curricula encourage and recognize for course credit students' paid work as a means of gaining work experience and learning.
3. Simulated workplaces	Universities can establish actual or simulated workplaces where students provide services to clients. Examples of actual workplaces include health services clinics (eg, podiatry, physiotherapy), farms, and veterinary clinics. Universities can also simulate workplaces (eg, radio stations, restaurants) that provide community and on campus services and enable experiences that simulate real practice/work.
4. Simulated practice-based learning	Practice can be simulated by creating practice environments (eg, a simulated police training village), e-learning programs and tools to simulate practice tasks (eg, online learning of professional decision making), problem-based learning (by focussing on cases and problem solving to promote practice-based learning), practical classes (eg, learning resuscitation on mannequins), role plays in tutorials, peer learning projects for clients (eg, advertisements), moot courts, and avatar programs to learn about client services.
5. Distance and flexible practice-based learning	Much practice-based education is conducted through distance, distributed and flexible pedagogies, recognising students' need or preference for learning at times, places and paces of their choosing. This trend is particularly common for graduate entry, international/interstate, regional/isolated and mature age students. An example is students participating in distance practical experiences during their night time study via technological communication systems (eg, multi-site videoconferencing) to real locations operating in other countries/hemispheres.
6. Peer learning	Peer learning facilitates exploration of emerging occupational identities, capabilities, and knowledge with other students and with a diminished authority of teachers. Such learning can occur in person, at a distance and via flexible and e-learning (eg, peer projects, Skype, chatrooms, intranet sites). Peer assessment is a useful means of developing/critiquing shared perspectives.
7. Independent learning	Professional practitioners and workers in many occupations must rely on their own judgements, critique, standards, and self-development. Practice-based learning can include encouragement of self-directed learning, self-appraisal, reflection, and self-development.
8. Blended learning	No single pedagogy is sufficient to meet all the needs of all the students in relation to all the learning tasks and goals of the curriculum. Blended learning addresses this challenge and bridges traditional and innovative pedagogies, on and off campus learning, individual and group learning, real, theoretical, and simulated learning situations.

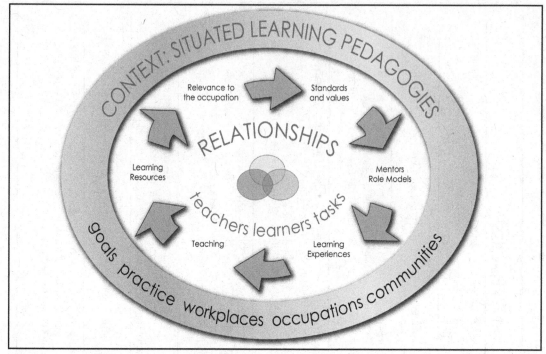

Figure 13-3. Implementing practice-based education.[12]

CONCLUSION

When we think about professional education we need a vision of higher education that deals with the education of a university graduate entering the workforce with graduate attributes. We also need a vision of education that prepares graduates to be professionals in their chosen professional disciplines with generic professional attributes and profession-specific capabilities. Practice-based education provides a powerful framework and strategy for achieving these goals and preparing graduates for their future life and practice.

REFERENCES

1. Higgs J. Doing, knowing, being and becoming in professional practice. Presented at: Master of Teaching Post Internship Conference; September 1999. Sydney, Australia.
2. Higgs, J, Richardson B, Abrandt Dahlgren M, eds. *Developing Practice Knowledge for Health Professionals*. Oxford, UK: Butterworth-Heinemann; 2004.
3. Higgs J. Practice wisdom and wise practice: dancing between the core and the margins of practice discourse and lived practice. In: Higgs J, Trede F, eds. *Professional Practice Discourse Marginalia*. Rotterdam, Netherlands: Sense; 2016:65-72.
4. Higgs, J. Re-interpreting clinical reasoning: A model of encultured decision making practice capabilities. 4th ed. In: J. Higgs, G. Jensen, S. Loftus, & N. Christensen (Eds.). *Clinical reasoning in the health professions*. Edinburgh, Scotland: Elsevier; 2019:13-31.
5. Markauskaite L, Goodyear, P. *Epistemic Fluency and Professional Education: Innovation, Knowledgeable Action and Actionable Knowledge*. Dordrecht, Netherlands: Springer; 2017.
6. Higgs J. Employability, The Education, Practice and Employability Network. www.epen.edu.au/definition. Published 2016. Accessed December 5, 2017.
7. Higgs J, McAllister L, Whiteford G. The practice and praxis of professional decision making. In: Green B, ed. *Understanding and Researching Professional Practice*. Rotterdam, Netherlands: Sense; 2009:101-120.
8. Chick NL, Haynie A, Gurung RAR, eds. *Exploring Signature Pedagogies: Approaches to Teaching Disciplinary Habits of Mind*. Sterling, VA: Stylus Publishing; 2012.

9. Shulman LS. Signature pedagogies in the professions. *Daedalus.* 2006;134(3):52-59.

10. Higgs J. *Professional and Practice-Based Education at Charles Sturt University (Occasional Paper 1).* Sydney, Australia: The Education for Practice Institute, Charles Sturt University; 2011.

11. Higgs J. *Practice-Based Education: Enhancing Practice and Pedagogy* (Final Report for ALTC Teaching Fellowship). Australian Learning and Teaching Council. Sydney, Australia; 2011.

12. Higgs J. *Practice-Based Education: A Framework for Professional Education.* Sydney, Australia: Australian Learning and Teaching Council; 2011.

13. Higgs J. Practice-based education: setting quality standards, In: Patton N, Higgs J, Smith M, eds. *Developing Practice Capability: Transforming Workplace Learning.* Rotterdam, Netherlands: Sense-Brill; 2018; 81-93.

Directions for Education Research in Health Professions
Opportunities for Physical Therapy

Stephen Loftus, PhD and Kathryn Huggett, PhD

The need for research and scholarship into the education of health professionals has always been important. This need has not always been recognized. For example, there are reports going back as far as 1863 that the curriculum for the education of doctors was overloaded with content.[1] If we had engaged in serious research and scholarship much earlier, then we might have been able to provide an education that was more effective and less burdensome a long time ago. Now that nearly all health professions require a rigorous university education to accredit new practitioners there is an urgent need to engage in scholarship and research to ensure that new graduates really are given the best preparation for the workplace.

We want to take as our point of departure the model devised by the National Study of Excellence and Innovation in Physical Therapist Education.[2] The model has played a prominent role in much of the rest of this book. We support this model but want to emphasize that, like any model, it cannot provide final and definitive answers to all the issues confronting the physical therapy profession. Such a model provides provisional answers. In this chapter, we take a critical look at some of the components of the model to explore some possible future directions. We begin with a look at the need for creating adaptive learners. This can be seen as a need for criticality.

THE PURSUIT OF CRITICALITY (ADAPTIVE LEARNING)

There is a need for all health professionals to become critical thinkers. Being critical means being willing and able to ask hard questions and make judgments about both the good and the bad

Jensen GM, Mostrom E, Hack LM, Nordstrom T, Gwyer J.
Educating Physical Therapists (pp 201-209).
© 2019 Taylor & Francis Group.

and to be aware of why something is good or bad. It also means being willing to change our minds as we find answers to critical questions. Asking the hard questions also means raising awareness of what issues there may be and how they may be approached. There is an old story about a cohort of eager new health care students sitting in their first lecture on the first day of their program, listening to their dean. The dean gives them some bad news. It seems that there are 2 major problems with the curriculum. The first problem is that the teachers now realize that half of what the students will be taught in the curriculum is wrong. The second problem is that nobody knows which half is wrong!

The story is apocryphal, but it has an important message. In the world of health care there are major reversals in what we know and what we practice occurring on a regular basis.[3] These reversals are in addition to a steady stream of innovations demanding implementation. This puts pressures on practitioners. In response to a recommended reversal or innovation, should they change their practice immediately or should they wait until more evidence is available to substantiate the change? How do we prepare practitioners so that they are able to make such decisions? There are, therefore, real demands on all health professions to educate newcomers so that they are ready, both for the practice of today and ready to cope with the practice of tomorrow, even though we cannot be certain what the practice of tomorrow will look like. What we can be certain of is that the practice of tomorrow will be different. It will be characterized by more complexity and more uncertainty. Indeed, it has been claimed that we now live in an age of supercomplexity.[4] *Supercomplexity* is defined as a state of affairs where the fundamental frameworks by which we understand what it means to know, to act, and to be are challenged. In other words, the professional habits of head, hand, and heart are going to be challenged and the underlying value systems and assumptions are themselves open to question. Important educational research questions for the future are:

- How can we teach criticality in the professions?
- How can we know if we have been effective in developing adaptive learners?
- What counts as effectiveness in the teaching of criticality in physical therapy education?

Critical thinking alone will not be enough. We need to go beyond developing critical thinking and move toward developing students' powers of critical action and critical being.[5] We have often construed critical thinking too narrowly as a set of intellectual games. Critical thinking is more than finding faults in statistical tests and sample sizes in research reports. But, if we really develop critical capacities in our students then there are serious implications. Barnett argues, "We cannot leave our students sensing that there is a givenness to the knowledge structures that they are encountering or that those structures are socially neutral."[5(p5)] Our students need to graduate with a sense that those knowledge structures are contestable and contested, and always will be. They need to be able to join in the conversations around those contests. For example, much of the knowledge in the health professions is dominated by the assumptions underlying the biomedical sciences. One common and contestable assumption is that only the scientific view of an issue is valid. It can be argued that this view has led to the widespread and simplistic misunderstanding that a health professional does nothing more than apply scientific knowledge in practice.[6]

A purely scientific view excludes insights from other disciplines, such as the humanities and social sciences. These other disciplines can, and do, provide useful insights into how health professionals work and how they learn to do that work.[7,8] A future challenge for health professional education and its research is to be more interdisciplinary and explore ways of integrating insights from these other disciplines so that new practitioners can begin their careers with a more balanced and varied set of views of what their practice entails. Questions that arise are:

- What does it mean to be an interdisciplinary professional practitioner?
- How do we provide an interdisciplinary professional education?

This should not be confused with interprofessional education (IPE), where the emphasis is more on learning with, through and about other health professions, rather than using other academic disciplines. IPE itself is set to grow and can be a fruitful direction for future scholarship and research. Encouraging more criticality in professional education has other implications for educational research and scholarship. Students will question much of what we teach them, and that is a good thing. This means teachers will often need to move away from didactic teaching alone to more collaborative inquiry with their students to foster these critical and adaptive attitudes.

- What curriculum structures and pedagogies foster criticality?
- How can we know if these structures and pedagogies have been successful in fostering criticality?
- How do these curriculum structures and pedagogies foster excellence in education and practice?

THE PURSUIT OF EXCELLENCE

The National Study model places great emphasis on excellence. This is an understandable and admirable position to take. However, even the notion of excellence can be critiqued. Readings[9] argued that excellence in the university has become a vapid concept as it can be interpreted in any way whatsoever. Readings begins with the notion that excellence, as it is currently understood, has been imported from the discourse of managerialism. There is too much emphasis on productivity and efficiency, as if education was nothing more than a specialized form of industrial production. What is lacking, according to Readings, is a critical reappraisal of what excellence can mean in an educational setting. While the position of Readings may be extreme, the notion of excellence is not straightforward. For example, what it means to be an excellent researcher or teacher is not straightforward and is fiercely debated.

Unpacking what excellence means in physical therapy education can be seen as an attempt to engage with the supercomplexity mentioned earlier. The theoretical frameworks and underpinning values that we use to understand what constitutes excellence are contestable and open to question. We need deep conversations that articulate what goes into professional and educational excellence and these conversations should be a part of future educational research and scholarship. Having a better articulation of excellence can, in turn, help us critique what is seen as the signature pedagogy of the profession.

SIGNATURE PEDAGOGY

Another element of the Praxis of Learning in the conceptual model is signature pedagogy.[2] Signature pedagogies, as defined by Shulman, are the "types of teaching that organize the fundamental ways in which future practitioners are educated for their new professions."[10(p52)] The signature pedagogy of physical therapist education has been described as the "focus on the human body as teacher."[2(p867)] Specifically, teachers help learners focus on what they see, feel, and hear when working with patients. The theory of embodiment can help here (see later). Shulman proposed 3 dimensions of a signature pedagogy, surface structure, deep structure, and implicit structure. Each dimension of the signature pedagogy of physical therapist education offers a rich source of ideas for educators who wish to enlarge the evidence base for physical therapist education and explore emerging phenomena. Shulman also encouraged educators to identify what is missing from the signature pedagogy and to understand how absences of approaches or characteristics in the teaching of the profession also define the pedagogy.

Surface Structure

The first dimension, surface structure, is composed of "concrete, operational acts of teaching and learning."[10(p54)] These everyday activities for both the teacher and learner may seem time-honored and routine, but all warrant the systematic investigation offered by a well-designed research study. All aspects of teaching and learning, including preparing and facilitating learning sessions, assessment of learning, simulation, and supervised clinical practice offer questions for research. For example, there is a persistent need for research to investigate the implementation and efficacy of new instructional methods. Although faculty frequently present and publish descriptive reports of new or innovative approaches, there remains relatively less literature outlining the comparative effectiveness of instructional methods. This is particularly evident with respect to active learning approaches. Although there is substantial and compelling evidence across the health science literature that active learning is more effective than passive lectures, there is still a dearth of literature explaining which active learning approaches work best, under what conditions, for which learners, and at what point along the continuum of physical therapist education. For example, both team-based learning (TBL) and problem-based learning have received substantial scholarly attention in the health sciences literature.[11] Both are considered effective active learning approaches. How should an instructor decide which method is optimal? Often the determination is made for purely resource-related reasons (ie, absent a sufficient roster of small group facilitators) the lead instructor may design a TBL exercise because the benefits of small group work can be realized in a large-group setting, requiring only a single faculty member. Research examining the comparative instructional requirements and learning outcomes is still needed to guide instructors and curriculum deans. There is a similar need for published evidence to guide the design and implementation of distance or e-learning.

Fortunately, there are 2 important sources of scholarship to guide education researchers who wish to better understand the surface structure of a signature pedagogy: adult learning theory and learning sciences. First, decades of scholarly work across multiple social science fields, including psychology, sociology, and anthropology, have contributed and examined theories of adult learning.[12] These theories describe core assumptions about adult learners and what motivates and sustains learning. Educators can apply learning theory to shape learning environments and instructional approaches. Learning theory may also be used as a framework to develop research questions and ground scholarly inquiry about teaching, learning, and assessment.

A second, and closely related, source of scholarship is the growing interdisciplinary field of cognitive and learning sciences. Research in the learning sciences draws from disciplines such as cognitive psychology, philosophy, artificial intelligence, cognitive anthropology, and linguistics.[13] Discoveries in the learning sciences offer fascinating new insights into how people learn, including the factors that contribute to knowledge acquisition, retention, and transfer. Learning sciences research in the health professions has established a foundation for understanding cognitive processes such as retrieval practice, spaced learning, and clinical reasoning.[14-16] This work, coupled with the conceptual frameworks offered by adult learning theory, offers education researchers both a foundation and scaffolding to explore new questions about the most recognizable features of the signature pedagogy.

Deep Structure

The second dimension of a signature pedagogy, deep structure, is defined by Shulman as the "set of assumptions about how best to impart a certain body of knowledge and know-how."[10(p55)] These assumptions provide myriad opportunities for researchers who wish to test assumptions and pose hypotheses about the core competencies (ie, the knowledge and skills required for each stage of preparation and transition to professional practice). This includes the competencies required for entry to professional and post-professional programs, progression from unsupervised to supervised clinical practice, graduation and licensure, and continuing professional practice.

Each element of a competency offers its own line of scholarly inquiry. Research about the knowledge required for preparation and practice must begin by examining the content of the curriculum. This may include posing questions about the sources and accuracy of scientific and practice-based knowledge. Education researchers must also consider the appropriateness of curricular content as well as the breadth and depth. Finally, understanding the deep structure requires careful consideration of the progression of learning objectives and their relationship to the overall goal of the program, and the assessment plan.

Another facet of the deep structure of a signature pedagogy is the role and authority of the teacher. This is a much-overlooked area in the literature. Education in the health professions has a long tradition of engaging peer and near-peer instructors (eg, senior learners, residents, fellows), but the benefits and limitations of this model have not been studied as systematically as other curricular features. The question of the role of the teacher also has implications for active learning approaches, where learners work in teams of peers with occasional facilitation by the faculty instructor (eg, TBL) or groups of peers with a tutor who may not be a content expert (eg, problem-based learning). Similar questions arise in distance learning programs where learners engage with teachers asynchronously and in IPE where instruction may be offered by teachers from an entirely different profession.

Understanding the deep structure of a signature pedagogy requires scrutiny of the core essence of the profession and expectations for preparation. It is not unlike an exercise in critical reflection, albeit at a meta-profession level. As such, it can be uncomfortable and challenging at times. A research agenda that pursues systematic investigation of these questions, however, offers the potential to introduce the evidence to affirm or upend old assumptions.

Implicit Structure

The third and final dimension of a signature pedagogy, implicit structure, is defined by Shulman as "a moral dimension that comprises a set of beliefs about professional attitudes, values and dispositions."[10(p55)] Shulman refers to this as the hidden curriculum of the pedagogy. This dimension offers a very different set of research questions to advance education in the profession. Instead of examining visible and tangible elements of the curriculum, teaching encounter, or learning environment, the researcher must often employ methods to uncover and explicate complex and sometimes sensitive topics. Examples include bias (explicit and implicit) in the learning environment or faculty messages that are incongruent with professional norms and standards. Both examples can be particularly challenging when the learning occurs at sites outside of the academic health center setting. Education in the health professions relies heavily upon community preceptors at affiliated sites. An important area for research is the influence of the culture at these sites. For example, do learners receive different messages about interprofessional practice or evidence-informed care depending upon the site or preceptor? Do these messages reinforce or contradict the formal curriculum?

Yet another area of implicit structure for study is program characteristics and requirements. Research in this area might ask whether these characteristics and requirements are aligned with stated program goals. For example, programs that seek diversity in their student population may find their degree program design favors students who do not have work or family responsibilities. Similarly, a program may rely on the lecture modality, despite research indicating active learning approaches can significantly improve learning for some subgroups of learners, especially women[17] and under-represented minority students.[18] Some of these questions may be addressed at the local level as part of routine program evaluation. These findings, in turn, may generate questions and hypotheses to be explored as part of larger, systematic studies of multiple programs or institutions.

PROFESSIONAL FORMATION

Professional formation is another element of the Praxis of Learning dimension of the conceptual framework for physical therapist education.[2] The authors define professional formation as "an intentional focus on the development of professional identity and commitment to the profession."[2(p868)] This element extends earlier understandings of teaching and learning professionalism in the health professions. For example, Cruess et al. commented that in medical education "15 years ago it seemed appropriate to stress the active teaching of professionalism as an important component of the medical curriculum."[19(p1446)] They noted further that learning objectives for professionalism curricula focused upon the knowledge base of professionalism, the values of the medical profession, and the "demonstration of behaviors expected of a professional."[19(p1446)] They argued that this focus is too limited and should be expanded to address professional identity formation. Other reports and commentaries, including the Carnegie Foundation report, have advocated for this shift in emphasis to professional identity development or formation.[20-23] The shared understanding is that professionalism is not a fixed body of knowledge to be taught and learned. Rather, teachers must assist learners as they develop and integrate their professional expertise, moral sensibility, and personal values. Professional formation training is believed to help learners integrate, rather than sacrifice, their personal and professional values. Professional formation also prepares learners to navigate situations where the hidden curriculum challenges their beliefs and values. This, in turn, makes learners less vulnerable to unprofessional behavior.[21]

Rabow et al[21] offered a summary of essential elements for the future of professional formation. Their list, derived from the literature and divided into 3 categories, offers a ready-made research agenda for those who wish to investigate professional formation as an element of the Praxis of Learning model.

The first category, *learners*, includes topics such as mindfulness, positive role-modeling and mentoring, reflection, and evaluation and feedback about values and choices. The second category, *faculty*, includes faculty development, support for teaching, training in feedback and mentoring, and serving as a positive role model, and evaluation and feedback about teaching performance. The final category, *institutions and the profession*, includes valuing moral character at 4 critical milestones in health professions education: admission, licensure, hiring, and promotion. In addition, the list for institutions and the profession includes 3 specific strategies to promote professional formation, appreciative inquiry, inclusive participation, and mission-based budgeting.

Fortunately, education researchers across the health professions have already started to investigate many of these recommended elements. This means there are opportunities to test hypotheses, clarify existing findings, and replicate studies within physical therapist education or across multiple sites for education and practice. For example, the mini multiple interview format has been adopted in many health professions education admissions processes.[24] This admissions strategy, designed to minimize bias in the admissions process, offers great potential to enhance selection and professional formation. The first generation of research findings are encouraging, but many questions remain about the optimal conditions for the mini multiple interview, details of cases and interviewer training, and potential outcomes for the applicant and entering cohort. Investigation of these questions and other elements of professional formation will ultimately improve practice, ensure quality, and reinforce the integrity of the educational experience. It is also clear that much professional formation will need to take place in practice settings.

PRACTICE-BASED EDUCATION

In recent years there has been a growing recognition of the importance of Practice-Based Education (PBE). It is not enough to emphasize theory and expect students to be able to readily apply this in practice. Much health professional education needs to take place in settings where they can start doing the work they will be expected to do as fully qualified practitioners. This is not to deny the usefulness of pedagogies such as simulations which are rightfully growing in importance. Simulations provide opportunities for students to try things out in a safe environment where nobody gets hurt. As simulations become more varied and sophisticated they provide an important direction for future research and scholarship in themselves. However, the day must come when students must confront real world practice with all its uncertainties and uniqueness. In PBE, students can discover for themselves the "primacy of practice"[25] and that:

Practice sets the tasks and serves as the supreme judge of theory, as its truth criterion. It dictates how to construct the concepts.[26(p1)]

In other words, students need good practice experience to integrate theory with practice in meaningful ways that help them start to develop their own expertise and practice wisdom.

PRACTICE-BASED EDUCATION, EXPERTISE, AND PRACTICE WISDOM

Expertise goes well beyond the competency of a beginning practitioner. Our education needs to prepare practitioners who are not only competent but are willing and able to build on their basic competency and develop professional expertise throughout their working lives. They need to develop what has been called *practice wisdom*. This is the capacity to exercise clinical judgment and cope with complexity and uncertainty. It comes as a surprise to many students in the health professions to find that clinical practice is characterized by complexity and uncertainty. Many begin by believing that because our scientific knowledge is growing then complexity and uncertainty must be diminishing. If anything, the opposite is true. We have a growing, and aging, population with more and more chronic problems. Very often the combination of problems will be unique to a patient, preventing simplistic application of theory and technical procedures, and requiring thoughtful clinical judgment to bring about the best possible outcome for that patient. Our education needs to prepare practitioners for such a world and we need to research the best ways of doing this. Some discourses that can inform such education and its research include, but are not limited to, the following.

The signature pedagogy of physical therapy, as noted earlier, is the body. This includes the body of the patient and the body of the practitioner. We not only have bodies, but we are bodies. We are body-subjects acting and living in the world. There is a growing literature on embodiment that focuses on the body as subject.[27] There is much scope to build on this literature with educational scholarship and research that takes the body-subject as a starting point. For example, the clinical encounter normally takes place with patient and practitioner engaging with each other in a physical and bodily manner. It is not a simple meeting of minds. What does this bodily engagement bring to the clinical encounter and what are the educational implications for someone trying to behave bodily like other physical therapists?

Our education prepares people to join a community of practice called a profession.[27] There is a need for our students to interact with other and more experienced practitioners who can guide them into full membership of the profession. The community of practice provides fellow travelers who can share 'war stories' about patients and practice events that are not in any textbook and that everyone, new and old, can learn from. The more experienced members not only help the newcomers develop their practice but also help them develop a sense of professional identity. Research questions for the future include:

- How does the community of practice cope with new practitioners and the new knowledge they can bring?
- What can experienced practitioners do to improve the assimilation of newcomers into the community and help them develop expertise?

Improving expertise can be conceptualized in terms of phronesis and praxis that come from the discourse of Neo-Aristotelianism.

Aristotle's notions of episteme, techne, and phronesis are generating growing interest in professional education.[28] Episteme is conventional textbook knowledge and techne is technical know-how. Phronesis has been defined as the disposition to act wisely. It is the ability to think through a new, uncertain, and complex situation. It is often said that we cannot teach phronesis, but we can provide people with the opportunity to learn it. Phronesis needs to be learned in practice settings where novel and challenging situations arise. Newcomers to the profession will need mentors to guide them through the thinking and judgment required so that the appropriate lessons are learned. Phronesis is closely related to praxis. *Praxis* has been defined as morally informed and morally committed action.[29] In other words, there is a strong commitment to doing what is best for the patient and modifying practice protocols depending on what is needed in each case. Blindly following protocols and working through procedures in just the way you were trained is not enough. The procedures need to be seen against the background of the patient and what is best for him or her. Therefore, carefully managed PBE is a key aspect of becoming a professional. Research questions based on these insights include:

- What are the characteristics of the best PBE?
- How do we provide the best PBE and evaluate it?
- Where in the curriculum does PBE occur?
- How much PBE is needed?

These questions are particularly relevant today. There is a looming shortage of physical therapists in many countries that have a growing population of older people. Some countries, to meet the growing demand for physical therapy, may be tempted to provide short training programs that can only produce technicians. Another viewpoint is that we need longer and more nuanced educational programs that can help people develop into professional practitioners. The debate on this issue is complex. There are different views about what constitutes a physical therapist, who is also a professional, that come down to underlying and conflicting values. These values need further articulation and critical discussion. These values will inform the design of any studies that aim to provide data that can resolve the debate one way or another.

CONCLUSION

Physical therapy, like other health professions, is in a process of change. There are many questions surrounding this change and most have implications for education. This is an exciting time to be involved in the education of any health profession as there are so many possibilities for scholarship and research. These range from the more instrumental questions of how we can improve what we already do to the more conceptual questions of what values and assumptions are needed to underpin physical therapy and its education and what theories can best help us to engage in such inquiry. In this chapter we have attempted to open a few of the directions such inquiry could take based on the National Study model. These range from the issue of excellence to questioning how we can better understand the signature pedagogy of physical therapy and its ramifications.

ACKNOWLEDGEMENTS

Dr. Stephen Loftus would like to thank Dr. Deb Doherty and Dr. Kris Thompson of Oakland University for their helpful insights into physical therapy education.

REFERENCES

1. General Medical Council. Tomorrow's Doctors. Education Committee of the UK General Medical Council. 1993.
2. Jensen GM, Nordstrom T, Mostrom E, Hack LM, Gwyer J. National study of excellence and innovation in physical therapist education: Part 1–design, method, and results. *Phys Ther*. 2017;97(9):857-74. doi:10.1093/ptj/pzx061.
3. Sukel K. Misguided medicine. *New Sci*. 2016;231(3088):34-38. doi.org/10.1016/S0262-4079(16)31564-0.
4. Barnett R. Supercomplexity and the university. *Soc Epistemol*. 1998;12(1):43-50. doi: 10.1080/02691729808578859.
5. Barnett R. *Higher Education: A Critical Business*. Buckingham, UK: Open University Press; 1997.
6. Loftus S. Thinking like a scientist and thinking like a doctor. *Med Sci Educ*. 2018;28(1):251-254. doi: 10.1007/s40670-017-0498-x.
7. Frank, AW. *The Renewal of Generosity: Illness, Medicine and How to Live*. Chicago, IL: University of Chicago Press; 2004.
8. Mattingly C, Fleming MH. *Clinical Reasoning: Forms of Inquiry in a Therapeutic Practice*. Philadelphia, PA: FA Davis; 1994.
9. Readings B. *The University in Ruins*. Cambridge, MA: Harvard University Press; 1996.
10. Shulman LS. Signature pedagogies in the professions. *Daedalus*. 2005;134(3):52-60. doi:10.1162/0011526054622015.
11. Huggett, KN, Jeffries, WB, eds. *An Introduction to Medical Teaching*. 2nd ed. Dordrecht, Netherlands: Springer; 2014.

12. Taylor DC, Hamdy H. Adult learning theories: implications for learning and teaching in medical education: AMEE Guide No. 83. *Med Teach.* 2013;35(11):e1561-1572. doi:10.3109/0142159X.2013.828153.

13. Patel VL, Yoskowitz NA, Arocha JF, Shortliffe EH. Cognitive and learning sciences in biomedical and health instructional design: A review with lessons for biomedical informatics education. *J of Biomed Inform.* 2009;1;42(1):176-97. doi:10.1016/j.jbi.2008.12.002.

14. Karpicke JD, Blunt JR. Retrieval practice produces more learning than elaborative studying with concept mapping. *Science.* 2011;331(6018):772-775. doi:10.1126/science.1199327.

15. Ariel R, Karpicke JD. Improving self-regulated learning with a retrieval practice intervention. *J Exp Psychol Appl.* 2018;24(1):43-56. doi:10.1037/xap0000133.

16. Woods NN, Mylopoulos M. How to improve the teaching of clinical reasoning: from processing to preparation. *Med Educ.* 2015;49(10):952-953. doi:10.1111/medu.12823.

17. Lorenzo M, Crouch CH, Mazur E. Reducing the gender gap in the physics classroom. *Am J Phys.* 2006;74(2): 118–122. doi:10.1119/1.2162549.

18. Eddy SL, Hogan KA. Getting under the hood: how and for whom does increasing course structure work? *CBE Life Sci Educ.* 2014;13(3):453-468. doi:10.1187/cbe.14-03-0050.

19. Cruess RL, Cruess SR, Boudreau JD, Snell L, Steinert Y. Reframing medical education to support professional identity formation. *Acad Med.* 2014;89(11):1446-1451. doi: 10.1097/ACM.0000000000000427.

20. Cooke M, Irby DM, O'Brien BC. *Educating Physicians: A Call for Reform of Medical School and Residency.* San Francisco, CA: Jossey-Bass; 2010.

21. Rabow MW, Remen RN, Parmelee DX, Inui TS. Professional formation: extending medicine's lineage of service into the next century. *Acad Med.* 2010;85(2):310-317. doi:10.1097/ACM.0b013e3181c887f7.

22. Jarvis-Selinger S, Pratt DD, Regehr G. Competency is not enough: integrating identity formation into the medical education discourse. *Acad Med.* 2012;87(9):1185-1190. doi:10.1097/ACM.0b013e3182604968.

23. Goldie J. The formation of professional identity in medical students: considerations for educators. *Med Teach.* 2012;34(9):e641-e648. doi:10.3109/0142159X.2012.687476.

24. Rees EL, Hawarden AW, Dent G, Hays R, Bates J, Hassell AB. Evidence regarding the utility of multiple mini-interview (MMI) for selection to undergraduate health programs: A BEME systematic review: BEME Guide No. 37. *Med Teach.* 2016;38(5):443-455. doi:10.3109/0142159X.2016.1158799.

25. Higgs J, Fish D, Goulter I, et al. eds. *Education for Future Practice.* Rotterdam, Netherlands: Sense; 2010

26. Vygotsky LS. *The Historical Meaning of the Crisis in Psychology: A Methodological Investigation.* (trans. R. van der Veer). New York, NY: Plenum; 1927/1987.

27. Loftus S. *Exploring Communities of Practice: Landscapes Boundaries and Identities.* In: Higgs J, Fish D, Goulter I, Loftus S, Reid J, Trede F, eds. *Education for Future Practice.* Rotterdam, Netherlands: Sense; 2010:41-50.

28. Kinsella EA, Pitman A, eds. *Phronesis as Professional Knowledge: Practical Wisdom in the Professions.* Rotterdam, Netherlands: Sense; 2012.

29. Kemmis, S, Smith, TJ. Personal praxis: learning through experience. In: Kemmis S, Smith TJ, eds. *Enabling Praxis: Challenges for Education.* Rotterdam, Netherlands: Sense; 2008:17-35.

Educating for Professional Responsibility
Integration Across Habits of Head, Hand, and Heart

Patricia Benner, RN, PhD, FAAN and Ruth Purtilo, PT, PhD, FAPTA

We were given the opportunity to look through the telescope into the yet unrealized future to speculate about some key aspects of professional formation and the integration of the 3 apprenticeships (ie, head, hand, and heart) that will continue to ensure physical therapy has a relevant role in health care. We turn then to some existing and emerging themes that we propose will help yield a physical therapy workforce that meets its own and society's high standards of excellence.

Fortunately, a gaze into the physical therapy cosmos reveals many constellations that help to orient us and the reader regarding visions of what could be. Upon reviewing chapters authored by outstanding educational and clinical leaders in physical therapy and other disciplines, we are encouraged by the impressive progress in pedagogy and other key components of physical therapy education that are laid out on these pages. We join readers in welcoming the promise that future physical therapists can remain relevant in their society, and there is no greater indicator of excellence than remaining relevant for the right reasons. This result will be realized in large part due to changes by educators who are willing to adapt their approaches in accordance with key suggestions and guidelines offered in this volume, while at the same time building on current strengths and caveats also highlighted in these pages.

All practice disciplines have the challenge of preparing students to practice in the present while adapting and enlarging their practice for the inevitable future changes. Physical therapists must constantly integrate their knowledge and skills as they interact with patients. Like other professions, physical therapy has long placed strong emphasis on both knowledge and clinical skills. In this chapter, the authors address the critical integration that must occur across all 3 apprenticeships (habits of head, hand, and heart). As noted in earlier chapters, the challenge and goal are to help students become adaptive learners as well as moral agents who understand their professional responsibilities. This chapter highlights the important pedagogical demands in preparing professionals for good practice, present and future, aligned with societal needs.

Jensen GM, Mostrom E, Hack LM, Nordstrom T, Gwyer J.
Educating Physical Therapists (pp 211-221).
© 2019 Taylor & Francis Group.

EXPLORING LEARNING FOR PRACTICE

In a practice discipline, the student will have to revise and extend learning not only in theory and principle, but also embody these changes in actual ways of practicing physical therapy. As a practice discipline, physical therapy has many domain-specific pedagogies[1] related to enhancing patient mobility and movement. The signature pedagogy is human body as teacher in learning and relearning movement. One of the key findings of the Excellence and Innovation in Physical Therapist Education Study was that the learning sciences are essential in order to advance pedagogical development in physical therapy.[2,3] In particular, learning sciences provide guidance in discovering, articulating, and further developing domain-specific pedagogies in physical therapy practice.[1] For example, domain-specific pedagogies will attend to learning about the use of one's own body in demonstrating movement, and learning to be observant in assessing the clients' need for particular corrections in posture and movement and specific therapeutic strategies for particular clients.

In the Carnegie studies of 5 professions (clergy, engineering, law, medicine, and nursing[4-8]) the goal was to examine the pedagogical requirements to effectively educate practice professionals for the present and future. This study of physical therapy adds to the cumulative knowledge of the Carnegie studies, while adding new insights on what is required for teaching and learning in a professional practice. Physical therapy is unique in its pedagogies and mission. Diagnosing and describing patterns of clients' existing movement patterns, and the need for change, create unique teaching and learning challenges. Physical therapy, like all practice disciplines, must link and translate theory of movement and assessment of problems in movement into a therapeutic action plan. The pedagogical challenges include teaching physical therapist students to become aware of their own bodily movement, as well as the styles of movement in their clients.

This study highlights pedagogies related to situated cognition. Robbins and Aydede[9] note in a short primer on situated cognition that it includes a cluster of interrelated concepts: (1) the embodied mind, (2) the embedded mind, and (3) the extended mind. Embodied mind refers to the role of the body in cognition. They state:

> Without the cooperation of the body [integrated, functioning whole body] there can be no sensory inputs from the environment and no motor outputs from the agent—hence, no sensing or acting. And without sensing and acting to ground it, thought is empty.[(p3,4)]

Many embodied actions are caught through automatic mimicking through mirror neurons rather than taught explicitly. Without mirror neurons, the interactive demonstrations between physical therapist and client would be impossible. The embedded mind refers to the ways that the person is embedded in the social and physical environment. Physical therapists attend to "the complex interplay of processes spanning mind, body, and world."[10(p7)] Gallagher[11] states:

> It is not that I simulate the action of the other; it is rather that the other's actions elicit the resonant responses in my system. In this affectivity we find ourselves pulled into a situation that is already intersubjective...the theory of the body is already a theory of perception and already a theory of intersubjectivity.[(p45)]

The embodiment and embedded aspects of a situated cognition view of the brain already goes past an inner representational view of the brain further as noted by Robbins and Aydede[9] and van Gelder.[12] The Cartesian tradition is mistaken in supposing that the mind is an inner entity of any kind, whether mind-stuff, brain states or whatever. Ontologically, it is much more than a matter of what we do within environmental and social possibilities and bounds. Twentieth century anti-Cartesianism thus draws much of mind out, and in particularly out of the skull.[12]

The Cartesian view of the representational inner mind and the older computational models of the brain in old fashioned artificial intelligence are inadequately demonstrated in the contextual embeddedness of the practice of physical therapy. In practices related to the embodied, embedded, and extended mind, physical therapists have much to offer learning sciences and much to learn from examining practice-based studies related to use of situated cognition in practice.

The practice of physical therapy is unique in the health care practices in that it deals with micro and macro physiological levels of functioning, while addressing the integrated and whole patterns of movement of clients. Consequently, articulating the knowledge embedded in this robust and effective practice is essential through improving practice by using the latest scientific discoveries, and theory development from cutting edge effective practice. As detailed in Chapter 9 on learning, much of the knowledge embedded in the practice of physical therapists is tacit, and not well described and articulated. Thus, the burden of transmission of much of physical therapy knowledge rests on articulating the knowledge already embedded in physical therapy practice.

All 6 of the Carnegie studies of practice disciplines[2,3,4-8] (clergy, engineering, law, medicine, nursing, and now physical therapy) were based upon 3 universal apprenticeships, referred to in earlier chapters as education for the head, hand, and heart. The premise is that these apprenticeships must be integrated. Compartmentalizing the apprenticeships prevents effective integration and performance as a physical therapist. A quick review of the apprenticeships reveals their interrelatedness:

- *The Knowledge, Science, Theory, and Technology of the Profession*
- *Practice:* Knowing how to engage in actual practice including practice know-how and clinical reasoning. Practitioners require situated cognition and knowledge use and a grasp of the particular in relation to the general to be good practitioners.
- *Ethical Comportment and Formation:* Learning to embody and enact good practice in specific situations. An apprenticeship to the ethical standards, social roles, and responsibilities of the profession, through which the novice is introduced to the meaning of an integrated practice of all dimensions of the profession, grounded in the profession's fundamental purposes.[13]

The third apprenticeship is the most integrative because, without adequate knowledge of the first 2 apprenticeships (knowledge and skilled know-how, head, and hands), one cannot act ethically in practice. Substandard practice, by its nature, is unethical.

The word *apprenticeship* is used metaphorically in the Carnegie studies not to mean on-the-job training, but to indicate that students require situated guidance by expert practitioners (ie, practice-based learning) in order to develop the skilled know-how and situated cognition required in practice. For example, learning to assess range of motion for a patient requires initial guidance by an expert teacher. It is impossible to learn the skilled practices related to assessing and enhancing clients' movement without being shown how movement works in clients and seeing how that movement is embodied by physical therapist's practice. Productive thinking is required both in acquiring scientific, theoretical knowledge ("knowing that and about") and equally in the situated thinking and using of knowledge in practice situations ("knowing how and when"). Situated cognition is more than mere application of well-established techniques that are standardized and replicable with little or no interpretation. In practice disciplines situated cognition, perception, and skilled know-how require an expert teacher who embodies the practice.

Dreyfus[14,15] points out that "tele-presence," such as a video camera placed on the forehead of the clinician, cannot teach the student observer how to position themselves to see what they need to see to examine a patient or perform surgery or other procedures. The skill of seeing and perceptual acuity are forms of skilled know-how developed by situated practice over time. Practitioners learn to position themselves to see the most salient details in the clinical situation relevant to their planned intervention.

Teaching a practice requires integrating the 3 apprenticeships in practice and in teaching and learning. Learning a complex practice such as physical therapy requires the following teaching and learning strategies and more.

Experiential Teaching and Learning

Experience is more than passage of time. To count as experience, learners must have their thinking turned around or nuances added to their understanding by the demands, challenges, novelty, or situated possibilities in the clinical situation.[16] Interpretation and reflection on practice enhances and solidifies experiential learning. For example, a first-person account of learning something new or where the student was upended[17] allows an opportunity to engage in inquiry and reflect on the experiential learning. This aspect of learning a practice has been referred to as *practice-based learning* and *consciousness raising.*

Situated Cognition and Thinking-In-Action

Clinical situations are by their nature dynamic and unfolding. Bourdieu[18] notes that the logic of practice requires that situated thinking begin by recognizing the nature of the whole situation and proceeding to the most salient or pressing aspects of the clinical situation. Novice students lack the experiential background to grasp the nature of the whole situation and require initial interpretive guidance to understand or have a perspective view on the whole situation. This understanding of the whole departs from simplification pedagogical strategies used with novices. Simplification, such as breaking the situation down into more manageable elements is essential for the novice. But breaking the situation down into elements provides only a temporary bootstrapping for initial learning that must progress to an ability to recognize the nature of the whole clinical situation that establishes perspectives and a way to proceed in client situations.

Sequential Teaching and Learning

Curricular content must be sequenced so that the student is prepared for new learning by prior learning. On the surface this is an obvious requirement for any curriculum, however, within a practice discipline, much thinking goes into sequencing learning for students. For example, meeting clients and learning to build a therapeutic relationship is necessary before the student is ready to design a plan for therapy.

Since all practice-based learning is situated in an ongoing, unfolding clinical situation, students require situated coaching to develop multiple perspectives on a situation, and to ensure that the student can identify key aspects that must be addressed in the situation. The student must learn to recognize changes in the client over time, as well as changes in their own interpretation and understanding of the client's needs. Teachers can proceed by first getting the student's perspective on the nature of the situation, and then work with increasing perspectives and correcting misconceptions in the situation. Situated coaching enables students to develop a sense of salience in unstructured, uncertain clinical situations. By sense of salience, we mean coming to experience the situation as meaningful, where some things stand out as important, while others are considered unimportant or irrelevant in the situation. This is a universal demand in all practice disciplines because, without understanding the most salient aspects in a clinical situation, the practitioner, like any novice, is apt to consider too many possible clinical concerns rather than just attending those that must be addressed in the situation. This is a common dilemma for all practice disciplines, in that if physical therapists (clergy, engineers, lawyers, nurses, or physicians) try to list all the possible variables, concerns, and perspectives in a situation, they confront the limits of formalism in any complex practice. Many more variables are identified than can be addressed. The list of variables can be neverending in a complex practice situation, thus, the problem of the older attempts to build programs that would enable robots to act intelligently in a practice situation through building the situation up element by element failed.[15] The clinician must develop perspectives, and a sense of salience about what is most and least important to address in a situation. This is achieved, in part, by the ability to recognize the nature of demands, challenges, and possibilities inherent in clinical situations.

Reflection on Cases and Clinical Imagination

Learning to be a clinician requires learning generalizations from aggregate population data. However, to learn how to practice, one must encounter, and learn from, preferably authentic cases with real assessments and changes in the client's condition across time. Clinical practitioners learn to use evidence-based practice clinical situations that entail individual variations and adjustments to guidelines based upon the patient's condition. Fabricating teaching cases seldom captures what practitioners are most likely to see in clinical cases across time. Consequently, fabricated cases do not provide realistic clinical physiological changes or laboratory changes for a patient across time. All clinicians must engage in inquiry and thoughtful practice about the relationship of the case to the generalizations gleaned from aggregate studies (evidence-based practice).[13]

Developing clinical imagination is at the heart of becoming an excellent practitioner. Clinical imagination is essential in working with all clients. Both thinking-in-action and reflection on experiential learning can help the student to enrich clinical imagination situations. Good, situated coaching provided by faculty in practice-based learning can enhance the student's clinical imagination.

Development of Ethical Comportment

Everyday ethical comportment requires the skillful embodiment of the moral standards of practice. Skillful embodiment includes not just beliefs and decisions but also evidence of *dispositions and actions*. Humility, respect, openness, curiosity, honesty, attentiveness, and so on must be embodied in actual relationships in clinical practice. Consciousness raising about the clinician's quality of engagement and relational attunement requires thinking-in-action, situated cognition, and reflection on how well the client is responding to the physical therapists' interventions and progressing with therapeutic goals of movement.

Dialogue with students about their experiential learning with clients can uncover effective novel or well-established strategies, negative biases, blind spots, silences, and so on. Reflecting on specific clinical situations can make these hidden issues visible to the student. For example, the ways the student was taught in their family about anger and anger expression will often need to be explored with the student before habitual social responses to angry patients can change to openness and curiosity rather than avoidance or judgment of the patient for being angry.

We are encouraged by the impressive progress in pedagogy and other key aspects of physical therapy education laid out in this book. Educators' further development of pedagogies of practice-based learning will assist both faculty and students in articulating knowledge embedded in physical therapy. Articulating knowledge embedded in practice requires observation and reflection on tacit aspects of practice, including blind spots, silences, and puzzles. Physical therapy experts must at least participate in this articulation because it requires a deep understanding of the practice to make the taken-for-granted areas of practice knowledge accessible and public.

Much has been learned about body movement and the nature of embodied skilled know-how by physical therapists and clients. Physical therapists have practice capacities and knowledge embedded in their practice that is not yet visible and public. Both the science and practice of physical therapy rely on enhancing the understanding of movement and changes across time in physical capacities because of physical therapy. As noted in Chapter 9 on learning:

> The best way to learn about improving movement is through direct experience with the human body—learning the skills of guided touch, how to apply theories of movement in practice, how to listen sensitively for information about what the patient is experiencing and how they need to move to fulfill social roles.[p127,128]

Learning how movement works, and changes in health as well as in different injuries and diseases, promises to advance physical therapy knowledge and practice. In addition to further articulating and developing the knowledge embedded in physical therapy practice, physical therapists will need to stretch their skills of shaping social and health care policy. The following 2 aims can further the impact of physical therapy on population health and improved health care policies:

1. Physical therapists and their professional associations increase active participation in shaping health care–related structures. Although not a new educational goal, the challenge for educators lies in the likelihood that substantive changes during the students' tenure will take place at a much greater pace than, and in ways that, even current mentors themselves have experienced.[19]

2. The formation of students' professional identity and clinical imagination prepares clinicians for effective decision making shaped by their participation in a triad of educator/mentor, patient, and student-clinician encounters that are woven into the DNA of their curriculum. In Chapter 9, this teaching-learning arrangement is described as a *triadic dialogue and dance*, preparing future professionals to truly honor each party in an encounter, everyone having their unique knowledge, skills, experience, and vested interest in the outcome incorporated into the decision.

These 2 aims for maximizing physical therapists' impact on the health of the society depend on a united effort at enlarging the knowledge base for physical therapy with a united commitment to engage in shaping and addressing health care inequities and improving health care policies for better health promotion and health care outcomes. The voice and perspectives that come from the practice of physical therapy are unique in health care and population health and have much to offer in the areas of illness and disability prevention, promotion of health and rehabilitating persons with injuries and disabilities.

It follows that in this educational framework, the mentor's major function is to help students become prepared to envision themselves as shapers of their professional structures and practices and readiness to fully integrate the complementary contributions each party makes in a situation. They will also envision how this overall preparedness will translate into their profession's success as a relevant contributor to society's health related needs.

Regarding the mentor's role, it is noteworthy that the terms *integration* and *integrity* come from the same root prefix, meaning "fit for purpose" as described later in this chapter. Therefore, the content of what is being integrated is the variable determining the value of integration. In short, ensuring that students are becoming fit for purpose means that mentors must prepare students for full participation in a professional life aligned with the tenets of their individual and professional integrity. This research uncovers weak areas in the current conceptual and methodological structures of physical therapy education that need to be expanded.

PROFESSIONAL FORMATION FOR THE FUTURE

Preparing Students for Rapid Change

A lag in therapy education strategies that will prepare students for rapid change may be due in part to current leadership, including faculty and practitioners who are just catching up with the fact that apparently subtle societal changes have the power to dramatically affect physical therapy practice and are doing so at an accelerating rate. In a quickly moving situation, customary assumptions and practices can destabilize what formerly appeared to be fit for purpose and, worse, may obscure a vision for welcomed improvement rather than supporting desired outcomes. Changing social patterns and the health of a population will radically change how physical therapy is practiced. In his book *The Tipping Point: How Little Things Can Make a Big Difference*, Malcolm Gladwell[20] popularized this fact of life that many entrepreneurs recognize but educators in the professions find easy to overlook. The tipping point is "the moment of critical mass, the threshold, the boiling point."[20(p4)] The processes of reaching this point are brought about by sometimes apparently small sociological changes that are operative in everyday life. Physical therapy excellence into the future requires that students be prepared to become professional entrepreneurs in areas where participation for needed change depends on their preparedness and capacities to be adaptive and active learners over time. Physical therapists will need to be first adapters in key situations. This challenge is a tall order but not impossible. Physical therapists are known for their skill in making improvements through adaptations at more immediate levels of practice, such as setting shared but fluid treatment goals with patients and clients and adapting processes and tools for improved patient function. Expanding this focus on innovativeness in working with individual clients needs to be expanded to maintaining excellence and planned change in the overall system. Translating new insights learned directly from practice that challenge current practices or theories requires strategies for making this private practice knowledge public and translatable into the discourse and decisions about physical therapy research agendas.

For the integration of this challenge facing physical therapy educators with that of preparing students for full participation in everyday decision making, we explore other aspects of the student's professional formation.

Preparing Students to Be Fit for Purpose

What adaptations are called for so that education and practice will be aligned to fit the student's current and future role? What can the physical therapy educational process offer that will produce physical therapists who are fit for purpose in the several roles they may be asked to assume over the long haul of their careers? Being fit for purpose includes inevitable new purposes, and needed innovations in practice, research, and health care policy. The following are some broad tenets related to professional formation in physical therapy education that we believe are essential for all physical therapist students.

Moral Agency, Autonomy, and Deep Respect for Another

In recent years, much attention has been devoted to professionals as moral agents. An agent is someone who is willing and freely able to act for him- or herself and for others. It follows that the person is presumed to be able to take responsibility legally and ethically for his or her own actions and will be held accountable accordingly.[21] It is easy to see that this notion is related to a prevalent theme in the physical therapy professional literature in recent years. Becoming recognized as a full profession entails the ability of its members to engage in and be judged by fitting and astute decision making within their appropriate scope of practice. A moral agent is a person who takes an active role in changing substandard and unjust situations on the behalf of clients and a better practice environment for good practice.[22,23] In other words, a professional is also bound by ethical standards of right behavior and is held accountable for those standards in everyday ethical comportment.

An emphasis in educational curricula on what and how to prepare a student for the demands and privileges of being a professional includes demonstrating courageous moral agency in practice. The goal is to prepare the student for ensuring that their skilled know-how and excellence in relational and motivational skills with clients is supported by the institutional and organizational environments of practice. Collaborative interdisciplinary teamwork is essential and replaces an insular professional autonomy, formerly defined as independence. Autonomy has come to be better represented by moral agency, considered relational and contextual instead of a manifestation of independence from influence from others. Autonomous decision making of the individual therapist is now being replaced by interprofessional approaches calling for an understanding of shared moral agency. Professional responsibility has evolved into a more communal one that must be integrated with other professionals acting from their own stance of shared professional responsibility.[23,24]

Classroom and practice-based education in physical therapy must integrate moral agency, moral courage, and a more collaborative vision of professional practice. Students must be prepared to practice in more complex interprofessional contexts. The goal is for students to learn how to achieve optimum patient outcomes with shared moral agency at the core, but this is a work in progress.

Moral agency is a relational concept insofar as the agent takes responsible action in relationship and attunement to the professional, therapeutic goals of other practitioners. From this relational perspective, the moral agents must develop the emotional capacity and will to recognize the effects of their actions on other parties in an encounter.[24] This relational basis of moral agency can be introduced to help future professionals gain a better understanding of why claims made by all parties in a relationship must be considered in a decision.

However, cognitive understanding does not necessarily lead to action that honors the spirit and goals of shared collaborative moral agency. Moral agency requires more than a sense of an objective trans-action based upon efficiency.[25] Respect and respectfulness of all health care team members requires that each team member remain open, curious, active listeners to fellow team members.[26] Teaching and learning interdisciplinary collaboration requires situated teaching and learning. Teachers cannot assume that students will recognize when their practices fall short of effective collaboration.

Respect and Respectfulness

Facilitating the student's development of self-respect and respect for others counteracts the short-comings of professional autonomy in the past when it was understood as independence. Respect is an inherently relational concept, known to others through the agent's respectful treatment of others and their own respect for what they have to offer the health care team as physical therapists. Respect, from the Latin root *respicere,* means that the agent's attitude toward another is to hold him or her in high regard.[26] Respect for others does not call for the agent to abdicate his or her own professional authority and responsibility in working with other professionals. Staying open and curious will enable the physical therapist to discover the strengths and gaps in knowledge or skill of other parties in an encounter.

Respectfulness, at the superficial level of everyday politeness, is essential for communication but must go beyond mere protocols and etiquette. A more profound level of respect involves at least 3 additional components: A recognition that the other holds something which warrants one's attention in this encounter; further exploration and acknowledgement of the knowledge and skills of other team members and how these may be used effectively in the current situation; respect includes acknowledgement that other team members have worthwhile contributions to make.[27] In short, profound respect involves being disposed to give a person your attention, openness, and the conscious intent to explore the talents and knowledge of this person for the best care of the client. A stance of respect toward others requires an excellence of character and skill that honor all members as legitimate participants, each with valuable contributions to make.

Our conclusion is that preparing students to go into practice having wedded professional responsibility to a disposition of respect more fully equips them to foster their and others' effective team functioning. Moral courage must be coupled with professional humility to sustain the openness, respect, and curiosity in relationships with other team members.

Moral Courage

Historically speaking, moral courage is a relative newcomer compared to the traditional lists of traits essential to the health professionals' character formation, though the idea of courage goes back to the very roots of western society as one of the cardinal virtues (ie, character traits that help societies to survive and thrive). A *New England Journal of Medicine* article titled "Perspective: Health Care Professionals and the Law" by a respected physician-lawyer-ethicist analyzes an encounter between a policeman and nurse, the latter who refused to go along with police demands that she cooperate in a manner she believed to breach her professional obligation.[28] The author concludes that moral courage is the most reliable resource to maintain professional integrity, as an individual, and the integrity of professional practice.[28]

A good general explanation of moral courage defines it as readiness for voluntary purposeful action in the face of realistic reticence related to risks. Action is undertaken to uphold high ethical standards in the face of not knowing what the actual outcome of one's action might be. Moral courage almost always occurs in the context of ambiguity. Depending on the nature of the unacceptable situation, moral courage may prompt the agent to speak out, step up or stand firm for what is right.[29]

No professional escapes the need to exercise courage in complex practice environments with competing demands. Professionals are taught to be careful and circumspect in their practice relationships, but this must be balanced with a professional responsibility to be a client's advocate. Knowing that one is equipped with courage—the ancients called it fortitude—helps the professional to take actions that protect the well-being of clients and the work environment for effective practice.

Physical therapists must work within their organizational contexts to develop ethical and legal institutional changes. Moral courage is required to take corrective action in existing situations and to alter substandard practice environments and policies. Organizational structures and processes must be aligned with best professional practices. Some threats and dangers to clients make considered interventions worth the risk involved. Exercising one's agency courageously to shape a better practice environment comes with ambiguity. It is impossible to fully predict the outcomes of any planned change, and courageous change agents must be prepared to change and adapt the aspects of the change that are not working well. Preparing students in professional humility can complement their courage to ensure attentiveness, curiosity, and openness in the situation. Great qualitative distinctions exist between arrogance and moral courage. The professional's moral courage occurs in risky and high-stakes situations, and, consequently, the professional must have humility to stay open and be willing to change when needed.[23]

Professional Humility

Professional humility is a capacity that does not seek to achieve success alone as an autonomous agent. Health care teams perform better when they collaborate and hold all members accountable for results.[30] With deep respect for the contributions of these other parties, the credit and responsibility fall to each and all. Humility prepares an agent to embrace reasonable limits and honestly explore the issues in a clinical situation. Humility creates openness to better understand the situation. Far from rendering the actor paralyzed or vulnerable, humility tempers and corrects foolhardy assumptions or courses of action and explores what members of the interdisciplinary team can effectively contribute. Humility can prevent rash snap judgments, and foster attentiveness and respectful listening.

Almost all professional education is based on a goal of mastery. Mastery entails knowing, and knowing creates self-confidence for successfully performing the functions of the professional role. Mastery is believed to minimize risk; however, minimizing risk, as a rigidly held stance, may prevent moral courage in risky situations. Within a mastery framework, many physical therapy educators recognize the limits to mastery in ambiguous and novel situations and emphasize operating within the profession's scope of practice and the importance of acknowledging mistakes.

Professional humility allows the practitioner to see both opportunity and risk and explore openly the nature of the clinical situation. Humility can enhance professional discernment and judgment. At the center of the discernment is to fully consider one's limitations and to stay open and curious to participate effectively in creating perspectives and a narrative understanding of the situation. Physical therapy excellence into the future requires that students are prepared to become professional entrepreneurs when innovation and the courage to be first adapters in key situations are required.

CONCLUSION

Physical therapy is a rapidly developing practice discipline with opportunities to further develop theories and a dynamic science of movement. The pedagogies for such a complex practice require experiential learning, situated cognition and coaching, and more. Clinical practices must come to terms with the relationship between the particular and the general. Physical therapy, like medicine, is a science using profession.[31]

While science is essential to progress and correction within the discipline, the clinician must learn how to navigate the situated challenges and demands of clients with varied and unique histories, while confronting knowledge gaps in practice situations. Not everything encountered in practice will be covered by science. Clinicians require curiosity, inquiry skills, situated thinking in action to relate science, theory, and practice. More attention and investigation are needed to identify and describe effective and ineffective relational and communication skills for therapeutic effectiveness with clients for effective interdisciplinary collaboration. Descriptive and interpretive studies of relational qualities of highly effective physical therapists could open a new discourse about effective skills of involvement and motivation in the practice of physical therapy. Such investigation cannot focus on finding "rules" for relationship quality, but rather uncover the dynamics of what is experienced as needed for motivating, encouraging, and supportive by diverse clients.

With a clinically focused doctorate, physical therapy is poised to engage in studies highly relevant to the theory and practice of physical therapy. There is still much to learn about the theory and science of movement as well as domain-specific learning science. These studies will require innovativeness, courage, humility, curiosity, and a commitment to strengthen the practice of physical therapy and to increase the discipline's reach into health care improvement and policy.

REFERENCES

1. Shulman L. *The Wisdom of Practice, Essays on Teaching, Learning , and Learning to Teach*, San Francisco, CA: Jossey-Bass; 2004.
2. Jensen GM, Hack L, Nordstrom T, Gwyer J, Mostrom E. National study of excellence and innovation in physical therapist education: part 2: call for reform. *Phys Ther.* 2017;97:875-888.
3. Jensen GM, Nordstrom T, Mostrom EM, Hack LM, Gwyer J. A national study of excellence and innovation in physical therapist education: part 1–design, methods, and results. *Phys Ther.* 2017;97:857-874.
4. Foster C, Dahill L, Goleman L, Tolentino BW. *Educating Clergy: Teaching Practices and Pastoral Imagination*. San Francisco, CA: Jossey-Bass; 2006.
5. Sullivan W, Colby A, Wegner JW, Bond L, Shulman LS. *Educating Lawyers: Preparation for the Profession of Law*. San Francisco, CA: Jossey Bass; 2007.
6. Sheppard S, Macatangay K, Colby A, Sullivan W. *Educating Engineers: Designing the Future of the Field*. San Francisco, CA: Jossey-Bass; 2009.
7. Benner P, Sutphen M, Leonard C, Day L. *Educating Nurses: A Call for Radical Transformation*. San Francisco, CA: Jossey-Bass; 2010.
8. Cooke M, Irby D, O'Brien B. *Educating Physicians: A Call for Reform of Medical School and Residency*. San Francisco, CA: Jossey-Bass; 2010.
9. Robbins A, Aydede M, eds. *The Cambridge Handbook of Situated Cognition*. Cambridge, UK: Cambridge University Press; 2009.
10. Hutchins E. *Cognition in the Wild*. Cambridge, MA: MIT Press; 1995.
11. Gallagher S. Philosophical antecedents of situated cognition. In: Robbins A, Aydede M, eds. *The Cambridge Handbook of Situated Cognition*. Cambridge, UK: Cambridge University Press; 2009:35-51.
12. van Gelder T. What might cognition be if not computation? *J Philos*. 1995;1:345-381.
13. Benner P, Hooper-Kyrakidis P, Stannard D. *Clinical Wisdom and Interventions in Acute and Critical Care: A Thinking-in-Action Approach*. 2nd ed. New York, NY: Springer; 2009.
14. Dreyfus HL. *On the Internet (Thinking in Action)*. 2nd ed. New York, NY: Routledge Publishing; 2009.
15. Dreyfus H. *What Computers Still Can't Do, A Critique of Artificial Reasoning*. Cambridge, MA: MIT Press; 1992.
16. Gadamer HG. *Truth and Method*. London, UK: Sheed and Ward Publishing; 1975.
17. Kerdeman D. Pulled up short: challenging self-understanding as a focus of teaching and learning. In: Dunne J, Hogan P, eds. *Education and Practice: Upholding the Integrity of Teaching and Learning*. London, UK: Blackwell Publishing; 2004:144-158.
18. Bourdieu P. *The Logic of Practice*. Palo Alto, CA: Stanford University Press; 1990.
19. Sullivan W. *Work and Integrity: The Crisis and Promise of Professionalism in America*. 2nd ed. San Francisco, CA: Jossey-Bass; 2005.
20. Gladwell M. *The Tipping Point: How Little Things Can Make A Big Difference*. Boston, MA: Little Brown & Co; 2000.
21. Garner BA, ed. *Black's Law Dictionary*. 7th ed. Saint Paul, MN: West Group; 1999.
22. Purtilo R. 31st Mary McMillan Lecture: a time to harvest, time to sow: ethics for a shifting landscape. *Phys Ther.* 2000;80(11):1112-1119.
23. Purtilo R. Moral courage: unsung resource for health professional as friend and healer. In: Thomasma D, Kissel J, eds. *The Health Professional as Friend and Healer*. Washington, DC: Georgetown University Press; 2000:106-112.
24. Doherty R, Purtilo R. *Ethical Dimensions in the Health Professions*. 6th ed. St. Louis, MO: Elsevier Publishing; 2016:56-57.
25. Hardingham LB. Integrity and moral residue: nurses as participants in a moral community. *Nurs Philos*. 2016;5(2):127-134.

26. Purtilo R. New respect for respect in ethics education. In: Purtilo R, Jensen GM, Royeen C, eds. *Educating for Moral Action: A Sourcebook in Health and Rehabilitation Ethics*. Philadelphia, PA: FA Davis Company; 2005:1-10.

27. Haddad A, Doherty R, Purtilo R. Respect in the professional role. In: Haddad A, Doherty R, Purtilo R. *Health Professional and Patient Interaction*. 9th ed. St. Louis, MO: Elsevier; 2019:3-4.

28. Derse A. Perspective: health care professionals and the law. *New Engl J Med*. 2017;37:2515-2517.

29. Purtilo R. Moral courage in times of change, visions for the future. *J Phys Ther Educ*. 2000:14(3):4-7.

30. McGee S, Silverman RD. Treatment agreements, informed consent and the role of state medical boards in opioid prescribing. *Pain Med*. 2015;16(1):25-29.

31. Hunter KM. *Doctors' Stories: The Narrative Structure of Medical Knowledge*. Princeton, NJ: Princeton University Press; 1991.

Opportunities and Priorities for Physical Therapist Education
Perspectives From the Profession

Steven B. Chesbro, PT, DPT, EdD and
William G. Boissonnault, PT, DPT, DHSc, FAAOMPT, FAPTA

HISTORICAL OVERVIEW OF THE PROFESSION'S ROLE IN PHYSICAL THERAPIST EDUCATION

Meeting the needs of society through quality physical therapist practice has always had a significant influence on determining the requisite educational needs of the profession.[1,2] Historically, the profession of physical therapy has had many stakeholders in physical therapist education, including the American Physical Therapy Association (APTA), and 2 of its components—the Academy of Physical Therapy Education (APTE) and the American Council of Academic Physical Therapy (ACAPT). The APTA has had a significant role since the 1920s, most notably by establishing overall educational expectations and aspirations for the profession.[3-5] More recently, the APTE and ACAPT have been established to also assume leadership roles within the profession.

American Physical Therapy Association

In 1942, the APTA created an Office of Education to ensure adequate infrastructure and support to achieve the profession's goals. Much of the APTA work related to education has evolved through policies and positions adopted by its Board of Directors (BOD), and House of Delegates (HOD). These 2 bodies collectively form the vision and strategic agenda for the APTA, which has included topics such as accreditation, credentials/degrees, educational expectations, practice expectations, residency and fellowship education, and many others. The policies and positions adopted by the BOD and HOD have recognized the essential links among education, practice, and

Jensen GM, Mostrom E, Hack LM, Nordstrom T, Gwyer J.
Educating Physical Therapists (pp 223-235).
© 2019 Taylor & Francis Group.

research, as outlined in the APTA's 2 guiding visions crafted since 2000 for the profession's development: *Vision 2020*[6] (2000-2013) and *Transforming Society by Optimizing Movement to Improve the Human Experience*[7] (2013).

A recent example of a significant outcome associated with physical therapist education was *Vision 2020*'s aspiration of becoming a doctoring profession. The tenet of "the Doctor of Physical Therapy as the clinical doctoral degree reflects the growth in the body of knowledge that a professional physical therapist must master, along with expected clinical responsibilities to provide best practice to the consumer,"[6] and gave academic programs the national support needed to institute degree change. The elements of the 2013 vision to transform society similarly identified priorities expected to influence the future of physical therapist education. Although early in its implementation, significant work has already occurred, including: (1) establishment of the definition and description of the movement system, (2) development of the Frontiers in Research, Science, and Technology Council, (3) development and implementation of the Physical Therapy Outcomes Registry, (4) a renewed focus on embracing the concepts of diversity, equity, and inclusion within the profession, and (5) participation in the Education Leadership Partnership (ELP), a collaboration of the APTA, ACAPT, and APTE.

The APTA recognizes that creating a culture of educational excellence through collaboration and partnership is required for the profession to evolve and continue to meet society's needs. The ACAPT and APTE, both components of the APTA, are key organizational leaders committed to excellence in education. While sharing common visions for excellence in physical therapist education, these 3 organizations represent different constituencies within the profession. Where the APTA is responsible to the entire association membership and represents the profession at-large, the ACAPT is responsible to its institutional members, comprised of accredited physical therapist education programs (in 2017, 217 of 242 institutional members), and the APTE is responsible to its members, individuals representing education across a spectrum of academic and clinical interests (in 2017, approximately 3100 members).

Academy of Physical Therapy Education of the American Physical Therapy Association

In 1942, the profession adopted its first specialty component, the Schools Section, known until 2018 as the Education Section and now known as APTE,[4(p7,8)] making it the "oldest continuous special interest group in APTA" (written communication, Gini Blodgett, February 2018). The APTE's purpose is "to provide a means by which members having a common interest to meet the needs of all persons concerned with the progress, growth, and development of education in physical therapy, and to this end may meet, confer, and promote these interests."[8] The APTE serves as the home to several special interest groups representing academic administrators and faculty, clinical educators, physical therapist assistant educators, residency and fellowship educators, and those focusing on the scholarship of education. Much of the scholarship related to physical therapist education is disseminated through the APTE's publication, the *Journal of Physical Therapy Education*, and through peer-reviewed presentations and posters at the APTA annual Combined Sections Meeting, and the annual Education Leadership Conference it cohosts with the ACAPT. The APTE also sponsors faculty development workshops for new and early-career professionals.

American Council for Academic Physical Therapy

The ACAPT was officially recognized in 2013 by the HOD as an APTA component "to take a leadership role in setting direction for physical therapist academic and clinical education."[9] Significant outcomes of the ACAPT efforts to date include the establishment of admissions traffic rules and shared prerequisite course expectations among programs, creating benchmarks beyond minimal accreditation standards, and engaging institutions in efforts to support consortia with special areas of interest, including clinical educators, clinical reasoning, curricula, and assessment; doctor of Physical Therapy terminal internship; early assurance programs, education and pedagogy; humanities, ethics, and professionalism; interprofessional education; and research-intensive programs.[10] Additionally, the ACAPT's 2014 Clinical Education Summit and the subsequent 3 panel reports (common terminology, integrated clinical education[CE], and student readiness),[11] were instrumental in realizing key recommendations identified by stakeholders to improve CE.

Education Leadership Partnership

Because of 2 House actions,[12,13] RC 12-13: Promoting Excellence in Physical Therapist Professional Education, and RC 13-14: Best Practice for Physical Therapist Clinical Education, the APTA board appointed 2 task forces charged to produce reports with recommendations. The Excellence in Physical Therapist Education Task Force (EETF) was charged to "provide information regarding current and emerging issues impacting the ability of physical therapist education to produce practitioners to meet the needs of the current and evolving health care system" with a report to the BOD in November 2015.[14] The EETF report outlined 6 recommendations (Table 16-1), all of which were approved by the board. Importantly, the EETF recommendations included "That a steering committee be established to oversee implementation of the recommendations of the EETF" with the assurance that "leaders from ACAPT, the Commission on Accreditation in Physical Therapy Education (CAPTE), the Education Section of the APTA, the APTA BOD, the APTA education staff, and representatives from the clinical community" would be included in addressing the identified priorities.[15]

The Education Steering Committee was later renamed the ELP after a series of year-long discussions among the presidents of the 3 organizations. Believing that working collaboratively would facilitate realization of the priorities identified by the EETF, the partners formalized their participation through a Memorandum of Understanding in 2016. Other non-voting participants in the partnership include representation from the CAPTE, members from the clinical community, and stakeholder groups. In 2016, the ELP adopted the purpose statement of "reducing unwarranted variation in practice by focusing on best practices in education"[15] to guide its work.

In 2017, the Best Practices for Physical Therapist Clinical Education Task Force (CETF) was charged to "consider strategies and identify best practice for physical therapist CE, from professional level through post-professional clinical training, and propose potential courses of action for a doctoring profession to move toward practice that best meets the evolving needs of society."[16] The task force submitted its report to the Board, outlining 6 recommendations (see Table 16-1). The recommendations included 3 topics clearly aligned with previous recommendations of the EETF: Availability and use of data, education research, and structure/standardization of educational processes. New areas of focus were included specific to academic-clinical partnerships and a model of physical therapist education that included professional education, a structured clinical internship, staged licensure, mandatory residency, and board certification. While the Board did not approve the recommendation on a model of physical therapist education, they did ask the ELP to further investigate future options.

The ELP agreed to incorporate the APTA board-approved recommendations into its work and subsequently has created multiple categorical sub groups (Figure 16-1). The concepts of "excellence in physical therapist education" and "best practices in physical therapist clinical education" were merged, recognizing that education occurs in many environments, and that compartmentalizing education into didactic and clinical components would detract from an overarching goal of improving student and graduate outcomes to meet the needs of society.

TABLE 16-1

RECOMMENDATIONS FROM THE EETF AND CETF
ADOPTED BY THE EDUCATION LEADERSHIP PARTNERSHIP

EXCELLENCE IN PHYSICAL THERAPIST EDUCATION TASK FORCE	BEST PRACTICES FOR PHYSICAL THERAPIST CLINICAL EDUCATION TASK FORCE
That essential, rigorous, and progressively higher levels of outcome competencies for physical therapist graduates that are responsive and adaptive to current and future practice be identified and adopted.	That a structured physical therapist CE curriculum that includes, but is not limited to, the following elements be developed and implemented: Amount of full-time CE required; define role and structure of CE experiences; define essential CE settings, experiences, and exposures; define role of simulation and technology in CE; define essential competencies and create tools to measure them; and enhance existing residency and certification processes.
That essential resources to initiate and sustain physical therapist education programs that include, but are not limited to, faculty, clinical sites, finances, and facilities, be determined.	That a framework for formal partnerships between academic programs and clinical sites be developed that includes infrastructure and capacity building, and defines responsibility and accountability for each (eg, economic models, standardization, sustainable models). Infrastructure and capacity must be developed across all stages of CE, to include: Models of clinical supervision; mandatory CI training; effective communication among stakeholders; student readiness at all levels of CE; and a comprehensive evaluation plan for CE.
That a comprehensive and progressive data management system for physical therapist education that is accessible to stakeholders and includes the following be established: Curriculum management system; standardized performance-based outcomes; integrating existing data sets; and identify new data needs.	That CE be incorporated into the recommendations approved by the BOD that were forwarded to the ELP regarding education data management systems, and include but not be limited to the following elements: Creation of a unique identifier; development of a national clinical matching program; integration of student performance data with outcome registries; interoperability of data management systems; and accessibility to data by researchers and others.
That the adoption of a system of standardized performance-based assessments that measure student outcomes and establish benchmarks be developed and promoted.	That the physical therapy profession's prioritized education research agenda include a line of inquiry specific to clinical education
That a prioritized educational research agenda be developed with identified mechanisms for research funding and support.	That a long-term strategic plan for physical therapist professional and post-professional education, including staging of activities, be developed to create a workforce prepared to meet the evolving needs of society. Engagement with relevant stakeholders will be critical to this effort.
That needs for faculty development in content expertise and best practices in education are identified with coordinated mechanisms developed to address faculty needs across programs and professions.	

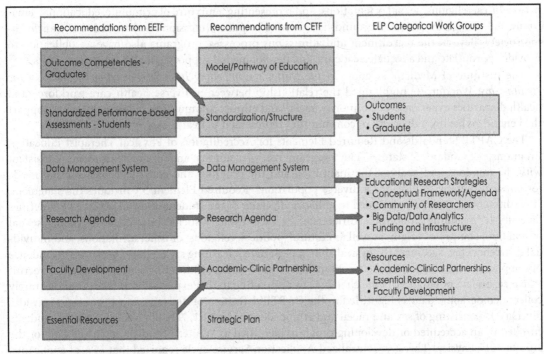

Figure 16-1. Recommendations of the EETF and CETF adopted as priorities of the ELP.

CURRENT AND FUTURE OPPORTUNITIES TO DRIVE EXCELLENCE IN EDUCATION

Recommendations from the EETF, CETF, and Clinical Education Summit, combined with work from previous task forces and work groups, have provided guidance for the profession and its pursuit of excellence in physical therapist education. Three specific priorities have been selected to describe in detail. One opportunity is related to improving diversity, equity, and inclusion in education, an ongoing priority of the profession. The others include advancing education research efforts, including the development of a continuum of professional performance expectations, and sufficient numbers and readiness of faculty to support excellence in physical therapist education.

Commitment to Diversity, Equity, and Inclusion

To meet the needs of an evolving society, it is imperative that the profession remain fully committed to advancing diversity (individual and group-social differences), equity (being fair and impartial), and inclusion (active, intentional, ongoing engagement with diversity). The profession has engaged in various efforts to address this over the years, including the APTA *Blueprint for Teaching Cultural Competence*,[18] which outlined 8 primary and 6 secondary dimensions of diversity. In addition, the APTA BOD and HOD have adopted more than 20 policies and positions related to diversity, equity, and inclusion. The HOD positions on *Increasing Professional Diversity* (RC 11-17),[17] and *Defining of Underrepresented Minority in Physical Therapy* (RC 14-14),[13] the ACAPT report on diversity,[19] and the recently created the APTA staff work group on diversity, equity, and inclusion are recent efforts by the APTA. Despite these efforts, the profession has not yet made the impact it desires.

Increasing diversity, equity, and inclusion across the profession begins with student recruitment, and admissions practices and policies associated with our academic programs, who serve as gatekeepers for the profession. Recruiting students of varying ages, abilities, races, ethnicities, gender identities, nationalities, religions, sexual orientations, and representing a mixture of economic, educational, environmental, and geographic backgrounds is needed to help the profession reach its vision of transforming society. Beyond the recruitment and admissions processes, programs also have an obligation to provide appropriate and adequate academic and developmental supports for all admitted students.[20,21]

The Institute of Medicine's report *In the Nation's Compelling Interest: Ensuring Diversity in the Health-Care Workforce*[22] highlighted the relationship between a diverse health care workforce and health disparities experienced by minority, racial, and ethnic, communities. Similar resources support the benefits of having a diversity of communities represented in health care.[23-25]

The CAPTE Standards and Required Elements for Accreditation of Physical Therapist Education Programs,[26] Standard 5 states, "The program recruits, admits and graduate students consistent with the missions and goals of the institution and the program and consistent with societal needs for physical therapy services for a diverse population." Required Element 5A includes the statement, "Recruitment practices are designed to enhance diversity of the student body." The CAPTE[26] defines diversity as "including group/social differences, eg, race ethnicity, socioeconomic status, gender, sexual orientation, country of origin, as well as cultural, political, religious, or other affiliations, and individual differences (eg, age, mental/physical ability, personality, learning styles, life experiences)." Evidence of compliance with this required element includes a description of "the efforts of the program to recruit a diverse student population." One challenge to responding to this expectation is that programs rarely collect demographic data as identified in the CAPTE definition of diversity. Most programs consider diversity as consisting of sex and racial and ethnic identity. In 2017, 76% of physical therapist students enrolled in an accredited or developing program identified as White.[27] Student applicant data for the 2016 to 2017 Physical Therapy Centralized Application Service cycle reported that 65% of applicants, and 70% of accepted students identified as White (not of Hispanic origin). These percentages have remained relatively unchanged since the 2011 to 2012 application cycle (+/- 2%).[28]

Professional academic programs have historically relied on grade point average (GPA) and Graduate Record Examination (GRE) scores in their admissions processes, and many use fear of "the risk to accreditation status" to support their limited admissions review practices. Other programs identify the *U.S. News & World Report* program ranking criteria in their rationale for not changing admissions review processes. For a variety of reasons described in higher education and health professions education literature, these narrow admissions criteria significantly limit diversity, equity, and inclusion.[22-25,29-31] Reliance on GPA and GRE to determine applicant readiness may make meeting the CAPTE standard and required element related to diversity difficult to achieve.

Many medical and dental education programs have moved from dependence on GPA and standardized test scores for determining applicant admissions to what is known as a holistic review process.[29-30] A holistic review process includes consideration of non-cognitive variables.[31] The Association of American Medical Colleges (AAMC)[29] defines holistic review as "a flexible, individualized way of assessing an applicant's capabilities by which balanced consideration is given to experiences, attributes, and academic metrics and, when considered in combination, how the individual might contribute value as a medical student and physician." The AAMC identifies 4 core principles in a *holistic review process:*

1. Selection criteria are broad-based, clearly linked to school mission and goals, and promote diversity as an essential element to achieving institutional excellence.

2. A balance of experiences, attributes, and academic metrics is (1) used to assess applicants with the intent of creating a richly diverse interview and selection pool and student body; (2) applied equitably across the entire candidate pool; and (3) grounded in data that provide evidence supporting the use of selection criteria beyond grades and test scores.

3. Admissions staff and committee members consider how each applicant may contribute to the medical school learning environment and practice of medicine, weighing and balancing the range of criteria needed in a class to achieve the outcomes desired by the school.

4. Race and ethnicity may be considered as factors when making admission-related decisions only when such consideration is narrowly tailored to achieve mission-related educational interests and

goals associated with student diversity, and when considered as part of a broader mix of factors, which may include personal attributes, experiential factors, and demographics, or other considerations (under federal law and where permitted by state law).

The American Dental Education Association created workshops for admissions personnel and faculty in these 4 areas to support the dental profession's adoption of holistic review in admissions processes, like AAMC.[30] Their experiences could be used by physical therapist education programs to explore the concepts, practices, and benefits of a holistic admissions review framework and how this may compliment current admissions efforts.

Another strategy to consider for increasing diversity is the creation of a student recruitment pipeline strategy that spans the educational experiences of school children through college-age students. Introducing school-age children to physical therapy as a career opportunity is vital to developing a diverse pipeline of students who prepare themselves academically and experientially to meet education program application requirements. This effort can include developing education materials to support elementary, middle, and high school curricula that introduce and describe the role of physical therapists in society. This should be coordinated on a national level to be maximally effective.

To change the culture in physical therapist education related to diversity, equity, and inclusion, faculty and students should engage in critical reflection to identify prejudices and biases, and participate in activities that enhance understanding of oppression, privilege, and power. These processes, coupled with the study of individual and population health issues, will allow members of the profession to better appreciate societal needs and the challenges associated with health disparities, and to view health equity through a social justice lens. In some cases, programs may need to seek assistance or guidance from outside individuals or organizations to help faculty and students navigate through the complex process of personal reflection, self-awareness, and social action.

Advancing Education Research

A learning science approach to improving educational processes should be at the core of the profession's research efforts. According to Jensen and colleagues[32] in their National Study of Excellence and Innovation in Physical Therapist Education, this educational research approach should be used to "guide the profession on what constitutes excellence" in physical therapist education.(p858) The need for access to and centralization of data and prioritized education research were adopted by the ELP and merged into a single priority. The profession has long recognized the critical importance of education research that drives the evidence-based decisions leading to best-practices in physical therapist education. As noted in the CETF report, "these calls have frequently been unanswered due to the dearth of research funding and infrastructure, and/or to the lack of researchers with the requisite skill set. The need to promote interest in education research, and to invest in the development of educational researchers has been identified as a critical starting point for efforts."[16]

The ELP initial approach to addressing the EETF recommendations on education research and data was to develop a subgroup that focuses on multiple aspects of education research. In January 2017, this subgroup focused on the 4 areas identified by Jensen and colleagues[33] for building education research capacity: (1) conceptual framing of educational research, (2) community of education researchers, (3) big data and data analytics, and (4) funding and infrastructure. Four work groups were assigned to focus on these interrelated and strategically aligned areas to advance the education research efforts of the profession.

Conceptual Framework to Support Education Research

The group determined there was a need in professional and post-professional education to bridge the gap between academic teaching, faculty preparation, and clinical practice, and the future needs of the education and health care systems. Developing a foundational structure of education research and identifying student performance-based outcomes to support improved educational practices would be a way to begin this process. The profession's education research agenda should build on what is known at the individual, group, organizational, environmental, and societal levels, with information coming from within and outside of the physical therapy profession. The development of a robust, longitudinal set of learner performance-based outcomes that span the continuum of professional education through post-professional levels, like those in academic medicine, was also identified as being an essential element of this initiative.

Investigating competency-based physical therapist education, including the use of milestones, competencies, and entrustable professional activities (EPAs) across the education continuum was identified as a priority. The AAMC initiated implementation of 13 undergraduate medical education EPAs (accompanied by education research pilot studies) at 10 institutions in 2014,[34] and at the graduate medical education level in 4 pediatric residency programs beginning in 2013.[35] In 2016, the American Association of Colleges of Osteopathic Medicine[36] and the American Association of Colleges of Pharmacy[37] were both considering opportunities to implement EPAs. Now may be the time to consider the creation of a set of physical therapy-specific competency-based assessments to guide professional and post-professional development, including self- and peer-assessment processes for practicing physical therapists. Chesbro, Jensen, and Boissonnault[38] recently questioned, "Will the development of EPAs provide the [physical therapist] profession with opportunities to promote education research as an essential strategy to advance education and practice?"[(p5)] They believe that "as a doctoring profession, physical therapists are more entrusted with the health and well-being of society," and suggest, "now is the time for the profession to establish an assessment framework that includes an EPA model... harnessed through collaboration among many stakeholder groups."[(p6)] As key stakeholders in physical therapist education, the ACAPT, the American Board of Physical Therapy Residency and Fellowship Education, the American Board of Physical Therapy Specialties, the CAPTE, and the Federation of State Boards of Physical Therapy would be ideal collaborators for such an effort, with the ELP being the ideal facilitator for this initiative.

Additionally, the ELP subgroup determined there is value in establishing a roadmap for a prioritized education research agenda. The profession has previously established education research agendas and priorities,[39] yet the impact of truly changing the trajectory of physical therapist education has been limited. Central components of this future agenda should include an emphasis on academic-practice partnerships to support education outcomes; imbedding education research projects within all the initiatives; and then developing a communication strategy, emphasizing the value proposition for this work and how an individual stakeholder can get involved.

Data to Support Research

The work group on Big Data and Data Analytics works under the assumption that the patterns, trends, and associations revealed by large data sets can help make processes more efficient and effective, resulting in enhanced outcomes of physical therapist education. Our physical therapist education programs generate large volumes of data that could be analyzed to drive innovation in academic and CE, practice, and the workforce. The work group identified data priorities for the profession, including (1) the need for a comprehensive data needs assessment, (2) a creation of a unique student/practitioner identifier for physical therapist education to connect datasets, facilitating research for education and workforce purposes, and eliminating duplicate records, (3) a creation of a centralized and searchable education research repository to facilitate access to past journal articles, session abstracts, and poster abstracts, and (4) the exploration and development of a centralized institutional data repository for physical therapist education.

This work group has identified the need to construct a data catalog that identifies existing data resources, accessibility of data, and interoperability among identified data sources. The APTA has identified funding for this project and anticipates hiring a consulting firm to complete this project in 2018. Once developed, the data catalog should provide a starting point for meeting the research needs of physical therapist education.

The creation of a unique identifier that would allow for tracking an individual's progress and outcome (eg, academic, clinical, continued competence, from program applicant to seasoned clinician) has been developed in medicine. The AAMC created such an identifier for academic medicine in 2008. Currently, their database collects data from multiple sources (eg, medical school application data, student academic progress data, licensure board data, continuing medical education information). Researchers can submit requests to access data stored in this confidential, protected repository, which has proven to be of significant value to medical education researchers.

Community of Education Researchers

The EETF noted that, although the volume of published basic science and clinical research in physical therapy has increased through growth in the numbers of funded physical therapist researchers, the profession still lacks a robust and vibrant community of education researchers. While there appears to be a strong interest in educational research among some physical therapy faculty, as evidenced by growth in related consortia and special interest groups, the actual number of interested and/or trained faculty members is not known. Many physical therapist educators have expressed interest in mentorship and continued learning opportunities in educational research. This interest includes the concepts of literacy in educational research, education research methods, writing for dissemination, and grantsmanship.

One component of this initiative is providing support to faculty who have little or no background in education research. By preparing faculty to be good consumers of education research literature, the profession ensures that dissemination of research findings can be fully appreciated and accurately applied in context. The profession should also support the development of researchers who want to focus their scholarly agendas on education research. This will require mentorship across the research spectrum, including theoretical foundations, research design and methods, writing for presentation/publication, and grant writing, as well as collaborative opportunities that advance their line of study. Whether through an apprenticeship or a mentorship model, creating opportunities for networking among mentors and mentees at various stages of research development will be required.

To facilitate programming that supports education research literacy, the ELP began licensing and sponsoring the AAMC Medical Education Research Certificate (MERC)[40] courses in 2017. Currently, 12 courses related to data analysis, collection, research methods, and statistics are currently available. Completion of 6 courses is required to earn a MERC; however, individual courses can be taken without intention to pursue the certificate. In addition, the ELP workgroup's efforts have led to the development of the Education Research Network. This multi-site network of mentors was established to organize the profession's education research mentor resources, and to facilitate connections with prospective mentees.

Research Funding and Infrastructure

The funding and infrastructure workgroup determined that the profession's education communities are facing significant challenges, including few grant writers prepared to pursue education research funding opportunities, and limited access to research funding. To increase our profession's education research capacity, this workgroup proposed a grant writing workshop titled Grants and Mentorship in Educational Research (GAMER) that is based on the successful Training in Grantsmanship for Rehabilitation Research (TIGRR) workshops. The goal of GAMER is to support the development of education researchers by providing mentorship and skill-building opportunities specific to grant seeking.

There continues to be a need to prioritize the use of available education research dollars and align research grants with education research priorities. This includes working with the Foundation for Physical Therapy to ensure that education research is clearly identified, when appropriate, to existing funding opportunities. Current grant opportunities within the Foundation with an education focus include the Bella May Scholarship Fund and the Mildred L. Wood Endowment Fund. Additionally, research support is available through 2 levels of Promotion of Doctoral Studies scholarship awards. New monies should be raised to support high-priority grants, scholarships, and fellowship opportunities. Thus, the education community will need to seek other funding opportunities to support its education research efforts.

Faculty Sufficiency and Readiness

The numbers of core, associated, and clinical faculty needed to meet the needs of the profession have grown with the increasing numbers of physical therapist, physical therapist assistant, and residency and fellowship education programs. This growth challenges the profession's ability to ensure that qualified faculty are available.[41] Faculty needs of the profession should be viewed on 2 levels: (1) sufficient number of qualified faculty and (2) readiness of individuals to succeed in a faculty role. Beyond numbers and readiness, there must be a strong relationship between professional and post-professional programs, and CE facilities. Academic and clinical faculty should be valued equally and should work in a coordinated and collaborative manner to ensure that the needs of the learner are met.

Sufficient Number of Qualified Faculty

Faculty qualifications vary among clinical, professional, and post-professional education programs. Unlike other professions, such as medicine, dentistry, and pharmacy, the physical therapy profession has determined that a mix of professional (ie, physical therapist degree) and post-professional credentials (ie, academic doctorate) are needed by professional education program faculty.[26] In 2017, there were 2812 individuals identified as core, full-time equivalent faculty members in 1 of the 242 accredited and 25 developing professional programs, and another 1920 individuals were identified as associated faculty.[27] During that same year, there were 1180 core full-time equivalent faculty members serving in 1 of the 364 accredited and 36 developing physical therapist assitant education programs, with another 607 associated faculty.[27] Faculty of accredited clinical and non-clinical residency and fellowship education programs have an expectation of demonstrating expertise through board certification or completion of residency and fellowship education, and a specified minimum of years of specialized practice (clinical) or combination of academic, clinical, and experiential qualifications (non-clinical).[42] The number of residency and fellowship faculty continues to grow to keep pace with the development of new programs. In 2017, there were 243 accredited, 51 initial, and 20 developing residency programs, and 50 accredited, 5 initial, and 6 developing fellowship programs.[43] From 2012 to 2017 there was a 91% increase in the number of accredited residency and fellowship programs.[43] Professional education program clinical faculty are recommended to have at least 1 year of clinical experience. According to Clinical Performance Instrument data, in August 2017, individuals had served as clinical instructors (CI) within the prior 4-year period.[44] In September 2016, 29,436 individuals had served as CIs in the prior 12-month period at 1 of 17,978 clinical sites.[44] Acknowledging the increasing number of academic and clinical faculty required to support physical therapists, physical therapist assistants, and residency and fellowship education, planning for future faculty sufficiency to meet the needs of more than 1042 programs must be a priority of the profession.

Related to the need for the profession to be fully committed to diversity, equity, and inclusion is the need to develop, recruit, and retain minority faculty. In 2017, only 13.2% of core physical therapy faculty identified as non-White.[27] Intentional efforts to develop faculty who identify as a minority should also be a priority of the profession.

Readiness to Succeed in a Faculty Role

Faculty in physical therapist education programs generally assume their role with little, if any, formal training in education. Thus, most faculty have a primary professional identity as a clinician. Physical therapist educators would benefit from having a professional identity as a professional educator if that has become their primary area of practice. Professional identity development requires that one critically reflects on their professional practices. According to Elias and Merriam,[45] "true professionals know not only what they are to do, but also are aware of the principles and reasons for acting.

The person must also be able to reflect deeply upon the experience he or she has had."[(p9)] Clinical experience alone does not make a person a professional adult educator.

While some institutions have well-developed centers dedicated to teaching, learning, and assessment to support faculty development, many do not. The profession has created few development opportunities for core faculty, and those tend to be narrow in focus and limited to new or early career faculty members. Exceptions include the ABPTRFE accredited Education Leadership Institute Fellowship[46] for aspiring and current physical therapist administrators, and the Duke University Faculty Development Residency.[47]

Educational programming to support development of clinical faculty teaching skills was initiated by the APTA in 1997.[48] Since the start of that program, more than 60,000 physical therapists and physical therapist assistants (more than 50,000 physical therapists) have completed the Credentialed Clinical Instructor (level-1) course. In 2007, an advanced course was created, and more than 2000 physical therapists have earned that credential. In 2018, the advanced course was replaced by an updated level-2 course, and update courses for level-1 credentialed instructors are offered through the APTA Learning Center. These educational opportunities prepare physical therapists at an introductory level to serve as clinical preceptors, with the goal of enhancing student learning.

The profession would benefit from the creation of a developmental series of courses or experiences that prepare academic faculty who do not have a professional educational background to appreciate: (1) the roles and responsibilities of faculty in academe (eg, academic advisement, administration, clinical/faculty practice, teaching, research, service); (2) the foundations and philosophies of education, models, principles, and education theory (eg, andragogy, assessment, clinical reasoning, curriculum, experiential learning, instructional strategies, learning science, self-directed learning, situated cognition, transformative learning), leadership, and administration (eg, budget management, resource allocation, the politics of higher education); (3) educational research methods; (4) college student development; and (5) an awareness of seminal and developing literature in education. Physical therapist faculty in higher education settings must be highly regarded and respected academicians within their institutions in order to effectively advocate for the needs of their programs. Faculty who are not prepared to assume the multiple roles of faculty, especially in teaching, research/scholarship, and service, may find limited options for promotion, longevity, and success, especially at institutions that mandate a tenure track pathway. With the growth of physical therapists, physical therapist assistants, and residency and fellowship education programs, and their academic and clinical faculty needs, it is imperative that the profession support the development of faculty to maintain the physical therapist education enterprise.

CONCLUSION

The profession has a long history of promoting the evolution of physical therapist education; however, barriers to educational excellence remain. The profession is pursuing significant changes in education to achieve its vision of transforming society. The ELP is one example of how working collaboratively can propel a shared education vision forward. Aligning work across the similar interests of stakeholders will always be more sustaining than working at cross-purposes. All stakeholders have a role to play in advancing the future of physical therapist education and realizing the vision of excellence that the profession and society require. Education research, faculty sufficiency and readiness, and diversity, equity, and inclusion, and other areas adopted by the ELP are priorities for physical therapist education and addressing these issues will help the profession achieve its social mission and aims.

REFERENCES

1. Echternach JL. The political and social issues that have shaped physical therapy education over the decades. *J Phys Ther Educ*. 2003;17:26-33.
2. Moffat M. The history of physical therapy practice in the United States. *J Phys Ther Educ*. 2003;17:15-25.
3. Gwyer J, Odom C, Gandy J. The history of clinical education in physical therapy in the United States. *J Phys Ther Educ*. 2003;17:34-43.
4. Littell EH, Johnson GR. Professional entry education in physical therapy during the 20th century. *J Phys Ther Educ*. 2003;17:3-14.
5. Neiland VM, Harris MJ. History of accreditation in physical therapy education. J *Phys Ther Educ*. 2003;17:52-61.
6. American Physical Therapy Association. *Vision 2020*. http://www.apta.org/Vision2020/. Accessed January 5, 2018.
7. Hayhurst C. A vision to transform society. *PT in Motion*. 2014;6(2):20-25. http://www.apta.org/PTinMotion/2014/3/Feature/APTAVision/. Accessed January 5, 2018.
8. Education Section of the American Physical Therapy Association. About the education section. http://aptaeducation.org/about-education-section/about-us.cfm. Accessed January 20, 2018.
9. American Physical Therapy Association. Bylaws of the American Physical Therapy Association. http://www.apta.org/uploadedFiles/APTAorg/About_Us/Policies/General/Bylaws.pdf#search=%22ACAPT%22. Accessed January 20, 2018.
10. Deusinger SS, Sanders B. A new home for academic physical therapy: ACAPT's first 7 years. *J Phys Ther Educ*. 2017;31:100-104.
11. American Council on Academic Physical Therapy. Strategic initiative panels. http://acapt.org/docs/default-source/default-document-library/panel-reports---compiled-for-membership.pdf?sfvrsn=0. Accessed January 20, 2018.
12. American Physical Therapy Association House of Delegates. *Minutes*. Alexandria, VA: American Physical Therapy Association; 2013
13. American Physical Therapy Association Board of Directors. *Excellence in Physical Therapy Education Task Force Report*. Alexandria, VA: American Physical Therapy Association; 2015.
14. American Physical Therapy Association Board of Directors. *Excellence in Physical Therapy Education Task Force Report*. Alexandria, VA: American Physical Therapy Association; 2015.
15. American Physical Therapy Association. Education leadership partnership. http://www.apta.org/ELP/. Accessed January 20, 2018.
16. American Physical Therapy Association Board of Directors. *Best Practices for Physical Therapist Clinical Education Task Force Report*. Alexandria, VA: American Physical Therapy Association; 2017.
17. American Physical Therapy Association House of Delegates. Minutes. Alexandria, VA: American Physical Therapy Association; 2017.
18. American Physical Therapy Association. *Blueprint for Teaching Cultural Competence in Physical Therapy Education*. http://www.apta.org/Educators/Curriculum/APTA/CulturalCompetence/. Accessed January 20, 2018.
19. American Council of Academic Physical Therapy. Board report: diversity task force. http://acapt.org/docs/default-source/reports/diversity-task-force-final-report.pdf. Accessed January 27, 2018.
20. Cook C. 20th Pauline Cerasoli Lecture: the sunk cost fallacy. *J Phys Ther Educ*. 2017;31:10-14.
21. Urban Universities for HEALTH. Holistic Admissions in the Health Professions: findings from a national study. http://urbanuniversitiesforhealth.org/media/documents/Holistic_Admissions_in_the_Health_Professions.pdf. Accessed January 21, 2018.
22. Institute of Medicine. *In the Nation's Compelling Interest: Ensuring Diversity in the Health-Care Workplace*. Washington, DC: The National Academies Press; 2004.
23. National LGBT Health Education Center. 10 things: creating inclusive environments for LGBT people. http://www.lgbthealtheducation.org/wp-content/uploads/072315-Welcoming-Environment-Brief-WEB.pdf. Accessed January 27, 2018.
24. National Advisory Council on Nurse Education and Practice. Achieving health equity through nursing workforce Diversity. https://www.hrsa.gov/advisorycommittees/bhpradvisory/nacnep/Reports/eleventhreport.pdf. Accessed January 27, 2018.
25. The Sullivan Commission. Missing persons: minorities in the health professions. http://health-equity.lib.umd.edu/40/1/Sullivan_Final_Report_000.pdf Accessed January 27, 2018.
26. Commission on Accreditation in Physical Therapy Education. Standards and required elements for physical therapist education programs. http://www.capteonline.org/uploadedFiles/CAPTEorg/About_CAPTE/Resources/Accreditation_Handbook/CAPTE_PTStandardsEvidence.pdf. Accessed January 27, 2018.
27. Commission on Accreditation in Physical Therapy Education. Aggregate program data. http://www.capteonline.org/AggregateProgramData/?navID=47244641600. Accessed January 27, 2018.
28. Physical Therapist Centralized Application Service. *2016-2017 Applicant Data Report*. Alexandria, VA: American Physical Therapy Association; 2017.
29. Association of American Medical Colleges. Holistic admissions. https://www.aamc.org/initiatives/holisticreview/about/. Accessed January 27, 2018.

30. American Dental Education Association. Holistic admissions. http://www.adea.org/GoDental/Health_Professions_Advisors/Getting_into_Dental_School/Holistic_admissions.aspx. Accessed January 27, 2018.

31. Sedlacek WE. Why we should use noncognitive variables with graduate and professional students. *J National Assoc Advisors for the Health Prof.* 2004;24:32-39.

32. Jensen GM, Nordstrom T, Mostrom E, Hack LM, Gwyer J. National study of excellence and innovation in physical therapist education: part 1–design, method, and results. *Phys Ther.* 2017;97:857-874.

33. Jensen GM, Nordstrom T, Segal RL, McCallum C, Graham C, Greenfield B. Education research in physical therapy: visions of the possible. *Phys Ther.* 2016;96:1874-1884.

34. American Association of Medical Colleges. Core EPAs pilot participants. https://www.aamc.org/initiatives/coreepas/pilotparticipants/. Accessed January 27, 2018.

35. American Association of Medical Colleges. Education in pediatrics across the continuum. https://www.aamc.org/initiatives/epac/. Accessed January 27, 2018.

36. American Association of Colleges of Osteopathic Medicine. Osteopathic Considerations for Core Entrustable Professional Activities (EPAs) for entering residency. https://www.aacom.org/docs/default-source/med-ed-presentations/core-epas.pdf?sfvrsn=10. Accessed January 27, 2018.

37. American Association of Colleges of Pharmacy. Entrustable Professional Activities. https://www.aacp.org/resource/entrustable-professional-activities-epas. Accessed January 27, 2018.

38. Chesbro SB, Jensen GM, Boissonnault WG. Entrustable professional activities as a framework for continued professional competence: is now the time? *Phys Ther.* 2018;98:3-7.

39. American Physical Therapy Association. Education research questions in ranked priority order. http://www.apta.org/Educators/Curriculum/APTA/ResearchQuestions/. Accessed January 27, 2018.

40. Association of American Medical Colleges. Medical Education Research Certificate Program. https://www.aamc.org/members/gea/merc/. Accessed January 27, 2018.

41. Jensen GM, Hack LM, Nordstrom T, Gwyer J, Mostrom E. National study of excellence and innovation in physical therapist education: part 2–a call to reform. *Phys Ther.* 2017;97:875-888.

42. American Board of Physical Therapy Residency and Fellowship Education. *Part III: Quality Standards.* Alexandria, VA: American Physical Therapy Association; 2017. http://www.abptrfe.org/uploadedFiles/ABPTRFEorg/For_Programs/Apply/Forms/ABPTRFEClinicalQualityStandards.pdf#search=%22quality%20standards%22. Accessed July 16, 2018.

43. American Board of Physical Therapy Residency and Fellowship Education. *Annual Reports.* Alexandria, VA: American Physical Therapy Association; 2017.

44. American Physical Therapy Association. *Clinical Performance Instrument Data.* Alexandria, VA: American Physical Therapy Association; 2018.

45. Elias JL, Merriam S. *Philosophical Foundations of Adult Education.* Huntington, NY: Krieger Publishing Co.; 1980.

46. American Physical Therapy Association. Education Leadership Institute Fellowship. http://www.apta.org/ELI/. Accessed January 27, 2018.

47. Duke University. Doctor of Physical Therapy Faculty Development Residency. https://dpt.duhs.duke.edu/education/academics/residency-programs/faculty-development-residency. Accessed January 27, 2018.

48. American Physical Therapy Association. Credentialed clinical instructor program. http://www.apta.org/CCIP/. Accessed January 27, 2018.

Envisioning Our Future
The Way Forward

RE-IMAGINING THE PROFESSION
FOR THE 21ST CENTURY

As is true for all professional education, physical therapist education has the dual responsibility to prepare students for the practice of physical therapy and to also prepare them to become physical therapists; they must learn to know and do, but also to be. As we have learned in our work and as our contributors have identified, this is a challenging and complex task that requires commitment at every level of education and practice. In Part II, we identified what we learned from our academic and clinical participants about the many features of excellence to be found in today's physical therapist education, and we shared the conceptual model we built from those findings. In Part III, we used our findings and evidence from the literature to present many recommendations and collaborative actions to help transform physical therapist education; to help all physical therapist educators move toward excellence. We also identified several areas where we found gaps in today's education: interprofessional education, practice-based learning, educational research, the social contract, and collaboration across the profession. We invited several colleagues to comment on these areas, and Part IV presents their views.

In this final chapter, we hope to take this work one step further by envisioning what the physical therapist profession could be if we collectively reimagine the role of the profession, curriculum, and educational enterprise to truly prepare our students to know, do, and be physical therapists in the fullest sense.

Jensen GM, Mostrom E, Hack LM, Nordstrom T, Gwyer J.
Educating Physical Therapists (pp 237-249).
© 2019 Taylor & Francis Group.

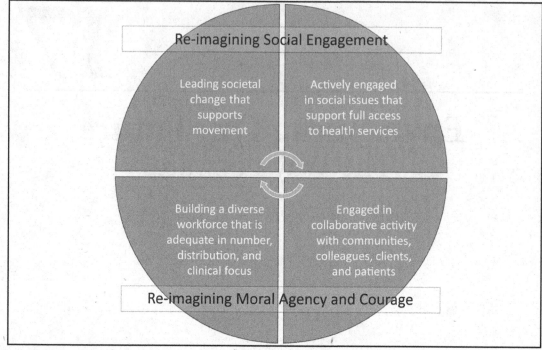

Figure 17-1. Re-imagining the profession for the 21st century.

THE PROFESSION

The American Physical Therapy Association (APTA), which serves as the primary voice of the profession, has recently adopted a new vision for the future: "Transforming society by optimizing movement to improve the human experience."[1] Such a vision demands that the members of the profession not only accept, but seek out, ways to meet the needs of society, moving beyond physical therapists' responsibilities to individual patients and clients.

The vision is supported by several principles, the first one of which states, "The physical therapy profession will define and promote the movement system as the foundation for optimizing movement to improve the health of society…The movement system is the core of physical therapist practice, education, and research."[1] As movement is the linchpin of this vision, it also behooves the profession to think as broadly as possible about society's needs to engage in movement.

The physical therapy profession must find ways to fully demonstrate social engagement. In our re-imagined future, we envision the profession will demonstrate the behaviors outlined in Figure 17-1.

1: Leading Societal Change That Supports Movement

The American health care system continues to be both expensive and ineffective compared to health care delivery around the world.[2] The Triple Aim has been proposed as a means to improve the system by improving the health of populations, improving the experience of care, and reducing the costs of care.[3,4] More recently a fourth aim has been added, to improve the work life of heath care practiitoners.[5] Concurrently, evidence continues to show the value of movement and activity to decrease mortality and morbidity and increase the quality of life.[6] Physical therapists are perfectly situated to bring this powerful intervention to bear to address all aspects of the Triple Aim, and perhaps in the process to also improve their own work life. But, this opportunity will be squandered if physical therapists do not recognize the need to address the social determinants of health. As the World Health Organization[7] states:

The social determinants of health are the conditions in which people are born, grow, live, work and age. These circumstances are shaped by the distribution of money, power and resources at global, national and local levels. The social determinants of health are mostly responsible for health inequities—the unfair and avoidable differences in health status seen within and between countries.

We cannot advise a patient to walk as a method of managing osteoarthritis if that patient has no access to safe places to walk. We cannot expect that people will make the behavioral changes that are necessary to integrate movement in their lives simply because we say so. We cannot continue to act as though treating one patient at a time, as important as that is, is sufficient to make changes for populations.

It is time that the APTA take the lead to work to effect changes in access to safe environments, in lifelong education for everyone that values movement, and in developing population-based interventions that support movement.

2: *Actively Engaged in Social Issues That Support Full Access to Health Services*

Health inequities exist when people experience the effects of poverty, unemployment and all the associated social stresses and gaps in access to important resources like education.[8] These inequities result in disparities in access to health care in the United States that exist for many different populations, including people of color and low-income groups. These groups have less access to insurance coverage, but also have less access to care itself, as well as experiencing lower quality in the care they do receive.[9] This disparity in access to health services has improved slightly since enactment of the Affordable Care Act, although disparities continue to be larger for the poor, and for people of color.[10] Yet, the susceptibility of this improvement in access to political action means that these improvements are not yet fully integrated into the US health care system. This is but one example of the need for the physical therapy profession to be actively and strongly engaged in effecting change in the health care system to reduce these disparities.

This means advocating for broader insurance coverage that provides real benefits at affordable cost and for distribution of health care services to meet the needs of these populations. It also means working to assure the best possible quality of care.

3: *Building a Diverse Workforce That Is Adequate in Number, Distribution, and Clinical Focus*

There is evidence that the needs of a diverse population are best met by a diverse health care workforce.[11,12] The aging of the US population and the growth in the number of people with chronic conditions also demand changes in the US workforce.[13] The need to think broadly about the public health of a diverse population also means that a diverse workforce with the capability to address a broad range of services is needed.[3,4] While the APTA has made statements in support of diversity in the physical therapy workforce,[14] it has been slow to act in addressing workforce issues. It has supported the development of a model to predict workforce balance for physical therapists based on several factors.[15] However, there has been no concerted effort to gather strong data that describe the current workforce. What data are available generally arise from data describing the membership in the APTA. These data show that physical therapists do not represent the diversity of the United States.[16] There is scant data on the types of sites where physical therapists practice, but much of this work is over 8 years old and there are no data that show trends.[17] There are little data on geographical distribution or on clinical practice areas. It is nearly impossible for the profession to work to develop a diverse workforce when there are minimal data to describe the current workforce.

The APTA should dedicate significant resources to understanding the current workforce and to designing incentive-based programs to build a workforce that fully meets the needs of society now and into the future.

4: Engaged in Collaborative Activity With Communities, Colleagues, Clients, and Patients

As Reeves, Fitzsimmons, and Kitto describe in Chapter 12, progress is currently being made in interprofessional education with a goal of improving collaboration across professions in direct service delivery. Currently, the primary emphasis in interprofessional education focuses on a rather narrow set of professions. Chesbro and Boissonnault, in Chapter 16, discuss the importance of collaboration within the profession. Collaboration in practice delivery is necessary, as is intraprofessional collaboration. But neither is sufficient to address the full needs of society. Rather, if physical therapists are to participate in reducing health inequalities and disparities, they must develop the skills to collaborate with anyone who can make an impact on these reductions.

The profession needs to take steps to fully engage in collaborative activities at all levels of society. This includes interactions by the APTA with other institutions and organizations. It also includes preparing physical therapists to accept advocacy roles at all levels of government and to work successfully with community groups. And it includes a new view on communication with patients that shows respect for the right of patients and clients to be in control of their own care.

Achieving the actions described here means taking full responsibility for moral agency and finding the courage to act. In Chapter 15, Purtilo and Benner describe moral agency and its importance as an obligation of the individual practitioner. Here, we refer to the moral obligation of the profession, as a moral community, and its primary agent, the APTA, to act first and primarily on behalf of society. This often means that professional leaders must display courage in helping the profession act. But if the profession is serious about transforming society through movement, there is no choice.

Re-Imagining the Curriculum
for the 21st Century

Curriculum is an essential component of professional education. While there has been continued evolution of physical therapist curricula with the move to the clinical doctoral degree,[18,19] we believe the profession must re-imagine how physical therapist curricula could produce graduates who are able to practice and lead in complex systems and fulfill our social contract with society as professionals. As Higgs suggests in Chapter 13, because the world is changing too rapidly for the content and format for learning and teaching to be based on current practice and how we teach now, curriculum frameworks need to be based on future-oriented practice. We need curriculum frameworks that are sustainable and flexible.

The profession must find ways to responsibly reframe, re-imagine and redesign curricula, and how they are delivered, that will transform physical therapist education and strengthen the profession's ability to meet societal needs. Society, including learners, will hold us accountable for meeting the ultimate desired outcome of positively contributing to health and well-being. In our re-imagined future, we envision the changes in the curriculum outlined in Figure 17-2.

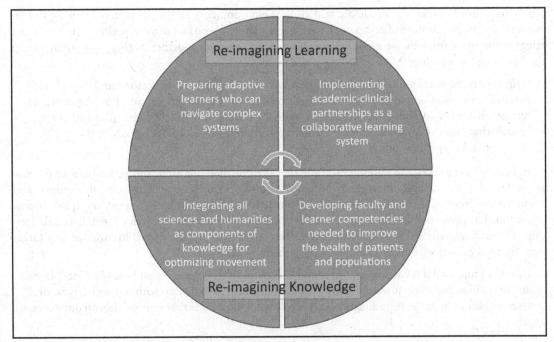

Figure 17-2. Re-imagining the curriculum for the 21st century.

1: *Preparing Adaptive Learners Who Can Navigate Complex Systems*

We must ask ourselves if our current curricula prepare our learners to meet not only current but future needs of patients, communities, and society? Health care and health care systems in the United States continue to evolve with increasing pressures to provide affordable, high-value, patient-centered care and population health.[20,21] Our learners will need the skills to engage in progressive problem solving not only for patient care but also be able to navigate complex organizations and systems as they learn and innovate in response to practice challenges. How do our curricula help learners respond creatively to situational variations or explore new ways of improving performance or developing novel solutions to problems? Learners need to have not only professional competence but capability. Christensen and Nordstrom[22] argue that the development of clinical reasoning capability is critical for the future of the profession:

> Capability…defined as the justified confidence and ability to interact effectively with other people and tasks in unknown contexts of the future as well as known contexts of today.[23(p2)]

Professional competence is foundational and learner capability is essential if we want physical therapists to be able to work effectively in unfamiliar and rapidly changing environments.

We need the Educational Leadership Partnership (ELP) to lead work that engages educators across academic and clinical organizations in identification of learner outcomes that focus on the adaptive learner who possesses both professional competence and capability.

2: *Implementing Academic-Clinical Partnerships as a Collaborative Learning System*

We found that the partnership between academic and clinical environments was a foundational element of excellence in physical therapist education. The time is now for the profession to envision our connections between our academic and clinical environments as a collaborative learning system essential for the preparation of competent, caring practitioners who can deliver quality patient care. As Higgs wrote in Chapter 13, we must bring education and practice together as these environments do the following for learning:

> Deliberately supports and challenges learners, novice practitioners, educators, and experienced practitioners, all of whom are involved in education of the next generation of practitioners, to realize what practice, good practice, means for them and to build practice identities and practice models that allow them to manifest their values and professional practice goals in the way they interpret and shape their practice.(p191)

In Chapter 12, Reeves and colleagues argue that the pressures for all health professions to prepare graduates who are "collaboration ready" require ongoing organizational engagement, support, and commitment from academic and workplace cultures that embrace and support interprofessional education. The profession is in its infancy in developing models that demonstrate formalized relationships for academic-clinical partnerships where there are mutual goals, shared knowledge that target improvement initiatives, educational needs, and quality patient care.

> Our academic and clinical communities and leaders need to put aside past held misconceptions and prejudices and move toward creating partnership models that align with our collective moral responsibilities in designing education and practice environments that improve health outcomes.

3: Integrating All Sciences and Humanities as Components of Knowledge for Optimizing Movement

Several of our past McMillan lecturers have challenged the profession to have a more integrated approach to the knowledge that undergirds physical therapist curricula,[24-30] and none more passionately than Katherine Shepard:[29]

> If every academic and clinical faculty would review just one piece of scientific evidence demonstrating the inextricable blending of mind and body and the resulting interplay of the social and biological sciences, I believe we would witness a ground swell of knowledge and insight that would enhance our ability to facilitate each patient's return to health.(p1547)

Physical therapy has focused on a biomechanical approach to movement for far too long.[31] If we are truly committed to helping society move well, then a more integrated approach to the knowledge that grounds our curricula is in order. As Purtilo and Benner remind us in Chapter 15:

> Physical therapy, like all practice disciplines, must link and translate theory of movement and assessment of problems in movement into a therapeutic action plan.(p212)

Physical therapy, as a profession of human improvement has the shared responsibility with patients in helping them manage and engage in their ability to move.[32] A more integrated knowledge base facilitates practitioners' ability to navigate uncertainty and challenge through true critical reflection and thoughtful decision making.[33,34]

> Now is the time for the ELP to lead real curricula transformation that is truly grounded in social, biomedical, and humanistic constructs that help therapists understand the human condition and its central importance in optimizing movement.

4: *Developing Faculty and Learner Competencies Needed to Improve the Health of Patients and Populations*

There continues to be overwhelming consensus that health professions education is not aligned well with what both patients and populations need.[35-38]

Professional education has not kept pace with these challenges, largely because of fragmented, outdated, and static curricula that produce ill-equipped graduates. The problems are systemic: mismatch of competences to patient and population needs; poor teamwork; persistent gender stratification of professional status; narrow technical focus without the broad understanding; episodic encounters rather than continuous care.[38(p1923)]

There is an urgent need for the profession to engage in more intentional faculty development that can facilitate transformative change in physical therapist education that is truly responsive to societal needs.[21] As Purtilo and Benner wrote in Chapter 15, academic and clinical faculty share in this responsibility.

A lag in therapy education strategies that will prepare students for rapid change may be due in part to current leadership, including faculty and practitioners who are just catching up with the fact that apparently subtle societal changes have the power to dramatically affect physical therapy practice...[(p216)]

The ELP, working across academic and clinical partnerships, needs to develop a faculty and learner competency framework that addresses content and skills necessary to improve the health of patients, populations, and delivery systems.

RE-IMAGINING THE EDUCATIONAL ENTERPRISE FOR THE 21ST CENTURY

Given the turbulence confronting the higher education and health care environments, the educational enterprise, including all 257 accredited and developing physical therapist programs,[39] with their clinical partners, and the profession's stakeholders must be considered from a systems perspective if we are to effectively image the future of the educational enterprise. As Chesbro and Boissonault described in Chapter 16, the ELP—comprised of the APTA, the American Council of Academic Physical Therapy (ACAPT), and the Academy of Physical Therapy Education—has identified several important initiatives to secure the future of physical therapist education, including diversity, education research and faculty resources. Higgs, in Chapter 13, and Purtilo and Benner, in Chapter 15, emphasized the importance of the interdependence and integration of learning across the 3 apprenticeships via experiential learning guided by expert clinician-teachers. Deepening our understanding and application of the learning sciences through theoretically grounded education research guided by the overarching, critical questions in physical therapy education is also essential if the profession is to meet its vision for the future. In our re-imagined future, we envision the behaviors in the actions of the educational enterprise outlined in Figure 17-3.

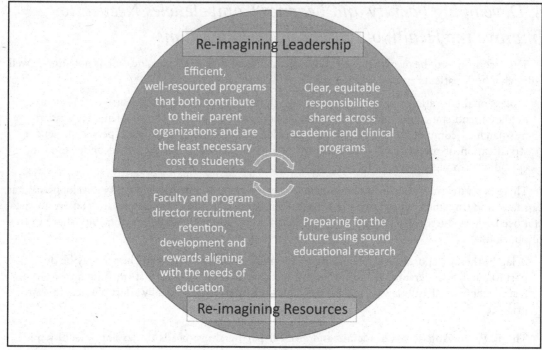

Figure 17-3. Re-imagining the educational enterprise for the 21st century.

1: Efficient, Well-Resourced Programs That Both Contribute to Their Parent Organizations and Are the Least Necessary Cost to Students

Efficient can be defined as "performing or functioning in the best possible manner with the least waste of time and effort."[40] The drive toward efficiency must be guided by a relentless pursuit of improvement through questioning everything that occurs in each program and in the system, while being attuned simultaneously to the external world of the profession in society and the internal worlds of those programs and their home institutions. We witnessed and described that relentless pursuit of improvement among our participating institutions and provide examples of it in practice in Chapter 5 and recommendations for integrating it into leadership at the institutional level and throughout physical therapy education in Chapters 9 and 11.

We are not suggesting a relentless drive toward shortening physical therapist education, but rather a considered, critical examination of the entirety of the experience of physical therapist education to ensure that we are (1) reducing unwarranted variation in learning and practice, (2) providing access to physical therapist education that is inclusive and diverse, and (3) designing student learning experiences that are the most effective possible. We must examine admission requirements, admission processes, curricular content, teaching and learning strategies, and organizational structures throughout the system of physical therapy education with these and similar criteria of quality, efficiency, and effectiveness. One of the participating academic institutions in our study recently added a hybrid Doctor of Physical Therapy program to its traditional residential program. In an interview with 2 of the leaders of the program, they identified the opportunity to question and improve their approaches to teaching and learning as a critical factor in choosing to pursue and study that model. The attitude of exploration and examination that exemplifies this approach should be taken system-wide as institutions consider the advantages and disadvantages of greater use of technology in the curriculum.

The ELP must engage the profession in a critical examination to reach consensus about required curricular content, optimal learning practices, and effective program administration for the purpose of reducing unwarranted variation in clinical practice and education and ensuring equitable access to physical therapy education to a diverse population of students.

This critical examination must include the perspective of the students who will be increasingly diverse, digital natives who are investing in their professional futures from the moment they consider applying to physical therapist programs to the time they enter practice. These students will not accept the use of ineffective teaching strategies in classrooms, labs, and clinics, nor should faculty and educational leaders. Likewise, curricular content requires a thorough, systemic analysis from the perspective of physical therapy's role in addressing the most important health problems confronting communities and individuals today. However, we need a consensus on what these priorities are and the implications for what receives less emphasis and what is eliminated from professional education. This systematic analysis must incorporate the concepts of learning we describe previously—learning to know, do, and be. We must also examine all our admission and learning practices to ensure physical therapy is a compelling profession for more diverse, digitally fluent, and socially aware students. The ACAPT and the APTA can then use the results of that consensus process to establish policies and practices that uphold these best practices, re-inforced by accreditation. Concomitant with the critical examination of the enterprise, we must have a deep understanding of the finances of physical therapist education. To these authors' knowledge, there has not been a comprehensive study of the finances of physical therapist education.

The ELP must garner resources in order to conduct systematic studies of the finances of physical therapist education.

That study must include sources of revenue, all the costs of academic education, the costs and benefits of clinical education (CE), and contribution margin to the institution, with the analysis recognizing the variability in the type of institutions that house physical therapist programs. There would be an even greater impact if there were similar studies of multiple health professions to allow meaningful comparisons of the finances of health professions education. Those studies would allow intra-institutional and interinstitutional comparisons, but more importantly, would inform health professions education and health care policy and finances at the state and national levels. Without systematic, meaningful, thorough, and accurate financial information, it is impossible to know how to best reduce the cost burden to students and operate the most efficient educational system.

That financial analysis would then provide the basis for innovation in the educational enterprise that is aimed at improving quality and efficiency. The Global Forum on Innovation in Health Professionals Education, of which the APTA and ACAPT are members, published the proceedings of a conference on financing health professions education.[41] Those proceedings can provide a foundation for meaningful change in financing physical therapist education, particularly when combined with the critical analysis of the education enterprise. As a final step:

ACAPT and the APTA should fund or promote efforts to develop innovative mechanisms and models to finance physical therapist education.

2: Clear, Equitable Responsibilities for Physical Therapist Education Shared Across Academic and Clinical Programs

As an integral component of the effort to create efficient physical therapist education programs that are the least necessary costs to students, the structural and financial relationship between the academic and clinical components of the academic physical therapy enterprise and their relationship to the physical therapy clinical environment must be scrutinized and reformed. The entire system through which CE occurs is wholly interdependent for successful outcomes among academic programs, clinical institutions, payers, governmental regulation and policy, and all the people who participate in the health care system (eg, patients and families, students, clinicians, and faculty). The viability of that interdependence was frayed by restrictions in how Medicare reimbursed services from students on clinical experiences. The interdependence is currently being frayed by several forces. While not a new phenomenon, clinic owners and health systems administrators increasingly are concerned about the cost of providing CE in an era of reduced financial margins. Students are concerned about the total cost of their education and indebtedness while valuing meaningful learning experiences, including CE, that best prepare them for practice. There are concerns over how tuition revenue is distributed in physical therapist education given that nearly 21% of the credit hours are in CE. These concerns are leading for some calls for academic institutions to pay clinical sites for student placements.[42] As we point out in Chapter 11, a thorough understanding of the costs and benefits of CE is a priority for the profession. However, a thorough understanding of the finances, including costs and benefits to all stakeholders is only the first step.

> ELP, with stakeholders in the profession, across other health professions, in health care systems, and policy, must develop sustainable structures and financing models for clinical learning in health professions education.

This effort would be integrated with efforts to understand and develop innovative approaches to finance education described previously. This effort would have a stronger impact on health policy and health systems practices if other health professions who are encountering the same issue were engaged in the discussion and solutions.

3: Faculty and Program Director Recruitment, Retention, Development, and Rewards Aligning With the Needs of Education

Shortages of qualified faculty and program directors are significant concerns in physical therapist education. In 2016 to 2017 data reported through the Commission on Accreditation in Physical Therapy Education, 8.5% of positions were vacant or projected to be vacant in the next year.[39] That report does not include data on program director vacancies, but in 2013 to 2014 there were 18 vacancies among the 225 accredited programs at the time (personal communication, Commission on Accreditation in Physical Therapy Education Staff, 2014). These vacancies threaten the viability of programs, particularly smaller programs with limited numbers of faculty members. Even though these are not new trends, there have been few studies of factors that affect faculty or program director retention in physical therapist education.[43-46]

A recent model developed for medical school faculty, with implications for physical therapy, identifies competency domains all faculty should have in today's health care environment: patient-centered care; health care processes, collaboration, and teamwork; clinical informatics, data, and tools; population and public health; policy and payment; value-based care; and health systems improvement.[21] Applying this important perspective, which is consistent with the needs to increase social engagement and strengthen the curriculum, could increase the shortage of qualified faculty.

If we are to meet the pressing needs in the profession for research in the basic sciences, clinical sciences, education and learning sciences, and health policy, and for translational research among all these areas, the future of the profession is dependent upon faculty researchers, given that the bulk of research in the profession is conducted at or under the umbrella of academic institutions. Simultaneously, one can hypothesize that with the advent of the DPT coupled with increasing interest in residency and fellowship education, the pipeline of physical therapists who pursue an advanced doctoral degree might be slowing, at least soon. Physical therapists who enter the academy through the DPT degree and residency education are not adequately prepared for the dual responsibilities of research and teaching nor are graduates of academic doctoral programs sufficiently prepared for their roles as teachers. Partnerships and shared responsibility for the education enterprise among all faculty, regardless of their route to the academy is essential.

The ELP must advance a research agenda that provides an understanding of the needs for leadership and faculty in their multiple roles, identifies institutional barriers to meeting these needs, and describes successful models for faculty selection, development, and retention. This should be coupled with immediate initiatives to support innovative demonstration projects and models for system-wide faculty appointments, teaching, and research.

Trends in how learning and instruction can be distributed over time and space via synchronous and asynchronous technologies provide potential infrastructure solutions for faculty distribution and collaboration. These technologies permit faculty to teach at more than one institution without relocating, shared curricular resources throughout the system, and open, reciprocal collaboration among members of the academy.[47] Space and time are no longer barriers to collaboration among researchers, just as they are no longer barriers for learning. The rewards that accrue to faculty members through being part of a community of researchers with shared interests and the increased productivity that the collaboration brings can be attractors for faculty given the time and motivation to pursue those partnerships.

4: *Preparing for the Future Using Sound Educational Research*

Possibilities for a re-imagined future of physical therapist education are present today, both in reality and on the near-term horizon. One of the major recommendations from the Carnegie study of medicine was a call for more student-centered flexibility towards degree attainment.[36] The Josiah Macy Jr. Foundation placed a top priority on competency-based, time-variable health education.[48] The Association of American Medical Colleges, in a recent future trend report identified on-demand learning, flipped clinics, networked discovery, high-resolution health, and rapid prototyping cycles as nonlinear, external forces that will affect medical education.[47] Two randomized-controlled trials in physical therapy that compared traditional clinical experiences with experiences in which simulation-based learning replaced a portion of the clinical experience in musculoskeletal outpatient and cardiopulmonary inpatient care provided evidence that well-planned simulation-based learning, using high-fidelity and simulated patients can play an increased role in professional education.[49,50] Current students, having been raised in a digitally-native environment, are already driving on-demand entertainment, transportation, shopping, and learning.[47] The program director where a hybrid program was initiated said in a subsequent interview, "This is the wave of the future and we want to be the leaders." Virtual reality also breaks down concepts of time and place and already provides realistic visual and auditory experiences. As haptic technology continues to improve, it is conceivable that the high-touch learning of physical therapy programs can be mediated through the virtual world as well. These technologies are not without a shadow side as they have differential effects on the 3 apprenticeships of professional education.

The ELP must expand the education research agenda to include how emerging technologies for learning and the structures for degree and credential attainment can improve access and reduce costs while achieving necessary graduate outcomes and the profession's core purpose.

These future trends will disrupt how, when, and where learning is delivered. Throughout that disruption, the challenge will be to continue our commitment to the professional formation and preparation of physical therapists who are prepared to meet the health needs of society, who are prepared to work with multiple professionals in community-based, collaborative networks, and who are master adaptive learners prepared for the uncertain—but exciting—future of health care.

CONCLUSION

We believe that action is necessary at every level of the profession—from individual academic and clinical faculty, to institutions, to the profession—if we are to meet our obligation to society to prepare physical therapists who fully integrate the 3 apprenticeships (head, hands, and heart). The recommendations proposed actions, and imagined futures presented here have emerged from our work and the work of our colleagues. It is our hope that the profession we dearly love will use these ideas to continue to transform and change in ways that truly meet the needs of society.

REFERENCES

1. American Physical Therapy Association, Vision Statement for the Physical Therapy Profession. http://www.apta.org/Vision/. Accessed September 4, 2018.
2. The Commonwealth Fund. US Health Care from a Global Perspective http://www.commonwealthfund.org/publications/issue-briefs/2015/oct/us-health-care-from-a-global-perspective. Published October, 2015. Accessed February 5, 2018.
3. Berwick DM, Nolan TW, J. The triple aim: care, health, and cost. *Health Affairs.* 2008;27(3):759-769.
4. Institute for Health Care Improvement. The triple aim. Optimizing health care and cost. *Health Care Exec.* 2009;24:64-66.
5. Bodenheimer T, Sinsky C. From triple to quadruple aim: care of the patient requires care of the provider. *Ann Fam Med.* 2014;12:573-576.
6. Haskell WL, Lee I-M, Pate RR, et al. Physical activity and public health: updated recommendation for adults from the American College of Sports Medicine and the American Heart Association. *Circulation.* 2007;116(9):1081-1093.
7. World Health Organization. About social determinants of health. http://www.who.int/social_determinants/sdh_definition/en/. Accessed February 8, 2018.
8. Weinstein JN, Geller A, Negussie Y, Baciu A, eds. *Communities in Action: Pathways to Health Equity.* Washington, DC: National Academies Press; 2017.
9. Ubri P, Artiga S. Disparities in health and health care: 5 key questions and answers. *Kaiser Family Foundation.* http://files.kff.org/attachment/Issue-Brief-Disparities-in-Health-and-Health-Care-5-Key-Questions-and-Answers. Published 2016. Accessed February 8, 2018.
10. Agency for Health Care Research and Quality. 2015 National Health Care Quality and Disparities Report and 5th Anniversary Update on the National Quality Strategy. https://www.ahrq.gov/research/findings/nhqrdr/nhqdr15/access.html. Published 2015. Accessed February 6, 2018.
11. US Department of Health and Human Services, Diversity and Inclusion Division. https://www.hhs.gov/about/agencies/asa/ohr/about-ohr/diversity-inclusion-division/index.html. Accessed February 7, 2018.
12. Cohen JJ, Gabriel BA, Terrell C. The case for diversity in the health care workforce. *Health Affairs.* 2002;21(5):90-102.
13. Dall TM, Gallo PD, Chakrabrati R, West T, Semilla AP, Storm MV. An aging population and growing disease burden will require a large and specialized health care workforce by 2025. *Health Affairs.* 2013;32(11):2013-2020.
14. ACAPT. Diversity Task Force report to the American Council of Academic Physical Therapy. https://www.acapt.org/docs/default-source/reports/diversity-task-force-final-report.pdf?sfvrsn=2. Published 2016. Accessed February 7, 2018.
15. American Physical Therapy Association. A Model to project the supply and demand of physical therapists 2010–2025, http://www.apta.org/WorkforceData/ModelDescriptionFigures/. Updated April 4, 2017. Accessed September 4, 2018
16. American Physical Therapy Association. Minutes of the APTA board of directors meeting http://www.apta.org/BOD/Meetings/Minutes/2017/12/15/. Published 2017. Accessed February 6, 2018.
17. American Physical Therapy Association. Physical therapy workforce data. http://www.apta.org/WorkforceData/. Updated May 15, 2018. Accessed February 6, 2018.
18. American Physical Therapy Association. Guide to Physical Therapist Practice. Available at: http://guidetoptpractice.apta.org/. Accessed February 7, 2018.
19. Commission on Accreditation in Physical therapy education. Standards for physical therapist education. http://www.capteonline.org/uploadedFiles/CAPTEorg/About_CAPTE/Resources/Accreditation_Handbook/CAPTE_PTStandardsEvidence.pdf. Accessed February 6, 2018.
20. Grumbach K, Lucey C, Johnston SC. Transforming from centers of learning to learning health systems: the challenge for academic health centers. *JAMA.* 2014;311(11):1109-1110.
21. Gonzalo J, Ahluwalia A, Hamilton M, Wolpaw D, Wolf H, Thompson B. Aligning education with health care transformation: identifying a shared mental model of "new" faculty competencies for academic faculty. *Acad Med.* 2018;93:256-264.

22. Christensen N, Nordstrom T. Facilitating the teaching and learning of clinical reasoning. In: Jensen GM, Mostrom E. *Handbook of Teaching and Learning for Physical Therapists.* 3rd ed. Boston, MA: Elsevier; 2013:183-199.

23. Stephenson J. The concept of capability and its importance in higher education. In: Stephenson J, Yorke M, eds. *Capability and Quality in Higher Education.* London, UK: Kogan Page; 1998:2.

24. Worthingham C. 2nd McMillan Lecture. Complementary functions and responsibilities in an emerging profession. *Phys Ther.* 1965; 45:935-939.

25. Kaiser H. 5th Mary McMillan Lecture. Today's tomorrow. *Phys Ther.* 1991;71:407-414.

26. Hislop H. 10th Mary McMillan Lecture. The not-so-impossible dream. *Phys Ther.* 1975: 1069-1080.

27. Johnson G. 20th Mary McMillan Lecture. Great expectations: a force in growth and change. *Phys Ther.* 1984;56:1690-1695.

28. Purtilo R. 31st Mary McMillan Lecture: A time to harvest, a time to sow; ethics for a shifting landscape. *Phys Ther.* 2000; 80:1112-1119.

29. Shepard KF. 38th Mary McMillan Lecture: are you waving or drowning? *Phys Ther.* 2007;87:1543-1554.

30. Jensen GM. 42nd Mary McMillan Lecture: learning: what matters most. *Phys Ther.* 2011;91:1674-1689.

31. Gibson B. *Rehabilitation: A Post-critical Approach.* Boca Raton, FL: CRC Press; 2016.

32. Cohen D. Professions of human improvement: predicaments of teaching. In: Nisan M, Schremer O, eds. *Educational Deliberations.* Jerusalem, Israel: Keter Publishers; 2005:278-294.

33. Montgomery K. *How Doctors Think: Clinical Judgment and the Practice of Medicine.* New York, NY: Oxford University Press; 2006.

34. Ofri D. Medical humanities: the RX for uncertainty? *Acad Med.* 2017;92:1657-1658.

35. Benner P, Sutphen M, Leonard C, Day L. *Educating Nurses: A Call for Radical Transformation.* San Francisco, CA: Jossey-Bass; 2010.

36. Cooke M, Irby D, O'Brien B. *Educating Physicians: A Call for Reform of Medical School and Residency.* San Francisco, CA: Jossey-Bass; 2010.

37. Colby A, Sullivan W. Formation of professionalism and purpose: perspectives from the preparation for professions program. *University of St. Thomas Law Journal.* 2008;5:404-426.

38. Frenk J, Chen L, Bhutta ZA, et al. Health professionals for a new century: transforming education to strengthen health system in an interdependent world. *Lancet.* 2010;376:1923-1958.

39. Commission on Accreditation in Physical Therapist Education. *Aggregate Program Data: 2016-2017 Physical Therapist Programs Fact Sheets.* Alexandria, VA: American Physical Therapy Association; 2017.

40. Dictionary.com. Efficient. http://www.dictionary.com/browse/efficient?s=t. Accessed February 8, 2018.

41. National Academies of Science, Engineering, and Medicine. *Future Financial Economics of Health Professional Education: Proceedings of a Workshop.* Washington, DC: National Academies Press; 2017.

42. Rucker-Hughes C, Padial C, Becker E, Becker M. Clinical site directors' perspectives on clinical education. *J Phys Ther Educ.* 2016;30(3):21-37.

43. Pagliarulo M, Lynne A. Priorities and benchmarks for new faculty in physical therapist education programs: perceptions of program directors. *J Allied Health.* 2004;33(4):271-277.

44. Pagliarulo MA, Lynna A. Needs assessment in professional-level physical therapist education programs: implications for development. *J Phys Ther Educ.* 2002;16(2):16-23.

45. Hinman MR, Brown T. Changing profile of the physical therapy professoriate—are we meeting CAPTE's expectations? *J Phys Ther Educ.* 2017;31(4):95-104.

46. Hinman M, Peel C, Price E. Leadership retention in physical therapy education programs. *J Phys Ther Educ.* 2014;18(1):39-44.

47. Association of American Medical Colleges. *Academic Medicine in 2025: Notable Trends and 5 Future Forces.* Washington, DC: Association of American Medical Colleges; 2016.

48. Josiah Macy Jr. Foundation. *Achieving Competency-Based, Time-Variable Health Professions Education.* New York, NY: Josiah Macy Jr Foundation; 2017.

49. Blackstock FC, Watson, KM, Morris NR, et al. Simulation can contribute a part of cardiorespiratory physiotherapy clinical education: two randomized trials. *Sim Health Care.* 2013;8:32-42.

50. Watson K, Wright A, Morris N, et al. Can simulation replace part of clinical time? two parallel randomized controlled trials. *Med Ed.* 2012;46:657-667.

APPENDIX A

Jensen GM, Mostrom E, Hack LM, Nordstrom T, Gwyer J.
Educating Physical Therapists (pp 251-261).
© 2019 Taylor & Francis Group.

TABLE A-1

KEY ACTIVITIES AND INITIATIVES RELATED TO PHYSICAL THERAPIST EDUCATION IN THE UNITED STATES FROM 1970 TO 2017

YEARS	ACTIVITIES/INITIATIVES	PRIMARY PURPOSE/GOAL	OUTCOMES
1974 to 1976	Project on Clinical Education in Physical Therapy; response to charge from the APTA Section for Education	Nationwide study of current status related to clinical site and faculty development and evaluation; anticipate future needs; make recommendations for standards and guidelines to be used for these activities	Final Report on Project published (1976)[a] Annotated Bibliography on Clinical Education in Health Professions (1976)[b] Handbook for Faculty Development (1977)[c]
1977 to 1978	The CAPTE approved as accrediting body for physical therapy education	Control over standards for physical therapy education in hands of the profession	Standards for the Accreditation of Physical Therapy Programs adopted by the APTA HOD (1978)
1979	The APTA HOD Motion 06-79-08-15 adopted	Advance physical therapy professional preparation to the post-baccalaureate level nationwide by 1990	

(continued)

TABLE A-1 (CONTINUED)

KEY ACTIVITIES AND INITIATIVES RELATED TO PHYSICAL THERAPIST EDUCATION IN THE UNITED STATES FROM 1970 TO 2017

YEARS	ACTIVITIES/INITIATIVES	PRIMARY PURPOSE/GOAL	OUTCOMES
1980 to 1982	Development and assessment of standards and forms for selection and evaluation of clinical centers	Address recommendations from the Project on Clinical Education in Physical Therapy	Manual published with standards, forms (1980)[d]; assessed use, reliability and validity (1982)[e]
1982	The APTA develops/sponsors workshops for educational administrators; planning for physical therapist education in the 1990s	Assist educational administrators in planning and preparing for transition to post-baccalaureate preparation of graduates	Two 5-day workshops conducted
	The APTA HOD Motion RC 83-82 adopted	Charge to study alternative models for clinical education for post-baccalaureate professional preparation	Task force on Clinical Education appointed by BOD

(continued)

TABLE A-1 (CONTINUED)

KEY ACTIVITIES AND INITIATIVES RELATED TO PHYSICAL THERAPIST EDUCATION IN THE UNITED STATES FROM 1970 TO 2017

YEARS	ACTIVITIES/INITIATIVES	PRIMARY PURPOSE/GOAL	OUTCOMES
1983	The APTA Forum—Planning for Clinical Education in 1990	Anticipate changes needed in CE as the profession moves toward graduate-level preparation	Forum proceedings published (1984)[f]
1984 to 1985	The APTA supported study of current patterns for providing CE	Describe current patterns and begin consideration of alternative models	Study findings reported, published (1985)[g]
1985	The APTA Department of Education Conference—Leadership for Change in Physical Therapy Clinical Education	Consider issues and strategies for change to advance CE for the future	Conference Proceedings published, disseminated (1986)[h]
1987	The APTA Deptartment of Education, Section for Education Conference—Pivotal Issues in Clinical Education: Present Status/Future Needs	Continue discussion about future models for CE to meet future needs	Conference Proceedings published, disseminated (1988)[i]

(continued)

TABLE A-1 (CONTINUED)

KEY ACTIVITIES AND INITIATIVES RELATED TO PHYSICAL THERAPIST EDUCATION IN THE UNITED STATES FROM 1970 TO 2017

YEARS	ACTIVITIES/INITIATIVES	PRIMARY PURPOSE/GOAL	OUTCOMES
1990 to 1994	The APTA creates 2 task forces to develop and refine voluntary guidelines for clinical education	Create voluntary guidelines/assessments for CE sites/clinical faculty (CIs, CCCEs) to enhance development and effectiveness of CE programs in sites	Guidelines for CE sites, CIs, and CCCEs published[j] first adopted by BOD (1992), HOD (1993); subsequent revision and approval (1999).[k]
1991 to 1992	The APTA forms task force on the content of post-baccalaureate entry level curricula; sponsors IMPACT conferences	Develop consensus on desired curricular content for post-baccalaureate preparation of physical therapists	Series of IMPACT conferences held around the country
1993 to 1997	The APTA creates task force to develop standardized perfomance assessment tool for CE experiences	Develop valid/reliable outcomes-based instrument that could be used for evaluation of PT and PTA student clinical performance on a voluntary basis nationwide	The APTA Physical Therapist CPI[l] is published (1997); Physical Thrapist Assistant CPI published (1998)[m]
1994 to 1997	Coalitions for Consensus Process on a Normative Model for Physical Therapist Professional Education, initiated in 1993 by the APTA Education Division, endorsed by the APTA Board of Directors; several conferences and forums conducted (1994-1997)	Create a consensus-based normative model for professional education that reflects the profession's values and vision and is responsive to changes in professional knowledge, education, and practice	A Normative Model of Physical Therapist Professional Education: Version 1997 published[n]

(continued)

TABLE A-1 (CONTINUED)

KEY ACTIVITIES AND INITIATIVES RELATED TO PHYSICAL THERAPIST EDUCATION IN THE UNITED STATES FROM 1970 TO 2017

YEARS	ACTIVITIES/INITIATIVES	PRIMARY PURPOSE/GOAL	OUTCOMES
1995 to 1996	The APTA funds grant and Department of Education, in collaboration with other stakeholders, develops training/credentialing program for clinical faculty	Develop educational program to enhance effectiveness and recognition of physical therapy clinical faculty available nationwide Develop course for credentialing trainers for the program	The APTA Clinical Instructor Education and Credentialing Program (CIECP) initiated (1996); ongoing—now known as Credentialed Clinical Instructor Program (CCIP)
1995	The APTA Consensus Conference on Professional Education at the Doctoral Level	Discuss implications of emerging doctorallevel professional preparation for physical therapists; consider strategies for consistency	
1995 to 1997	The APTA sponsors Educational Outcomes Assessment and Curriculum Development Conferences	Assist educators to develop strategies for robust outcome assessment to develop curriculum	Three conferences held annually (1995-1997)
1998	The APTA Consensus Conference on Clinical Education: *Clinical Education: Dare to Innovate*	Develop consensus on potential alternative models of clinical education for the future	Conference Proceedings published, disseminated (1998)º
1999	The APTA Conference on Post-Professional Transition to Clinical Doctorate	Develop consensus on curricular content/educational models for transition of Doctor of Physical Therapy (tDPT) degrees for baccalaureate or master's degree prepared physical therapists	The APTA Plan in support of clinical doctorate and transition doctorate (BOD 2000)

(continued)

TABLE A-1 (CONTINUED)

KEY ACTIVITIES AND INITIATIVES RELATED TO PHYSICAL THERAPIST EDUCATION IN THE UNITED STATES FROM 1970 TO 2017

YEARS	ACTIVITIES/INITIATIVES	PRIMARY PURPOSE/GOAL	OUTCOMES
1999 to 2000	First revision of *Normative Model of Physical Therapist Education*	Review/revise model to ensure consistent with current trends in education, practice, and the APTA *Guide to Physical Therapist Practice, 1st ed*.[p]	*Normative Model of Physical Therapist Professional Education: Version 2000*[q] published
2003 to 2004	Second revision of *Normative Model of Physical Therapist Education*	Review/revise model to ensure consistent with current trends in education, practice, the APTA *Guide to Physical Therapist Practice, 2nd ed*,[r] other core documents, and *Vision 2020*	*Normative Model of Physical Therapist Professional Education: Version 2004*[s] published
	Third review and revision of the APTA *Guidelines for Clinical Education*	Review/revise guidelines to ensure consistent with the APTA core documents/CAPTE evaluative criteria	
2004	Third review and revision of APTA *Guidelines for Clinical Education*	Review/revise guidelines to ensure consistent with APTA core documents and CAPTE evaluative criteria	*Guidelines and Self-Assessments for Clinical Education, 3rd ed. (2004)*[t] adopted, published
	Consensus Conference on Clinical Education: Clinical Education in a Doctoring Profession	Develop consensus on clinical education models/practices that will address the APTA's *Vision 2020* of physical therapy as a doctoring profession	Adoption of Minimum Required Skills of Physical Therapist Graduates at Entry-Level[u]
	The APTA and Education Section sponsors first national combined conference for clinical educators and academic administrators	Bring together members of academic/CE community to discuss mutual issues	First conference held 2004; became annual Educational Leadership Conference and has been held every year since

(continued)

TABLE A-1 (CONTINUED)

KEY ACTIVITIES AND INITIATIVES RELATED TO PHYSICAL THERAPIST EDUCATION IN THE UNITED STATES FROM 1970 TO 2017

YEARS	ACTIVITIES/INITIATIVES	PRIMARY PURPOSE/GOAL	OUTCOMES
2005 to 2006	Review and revision of the APTA Physical Therapist CPI	Review/revise instrument to ensure consistent with current practice, the APTA core documents, and the CAPTE evaluative criteria	Physical Therapist CPI, 2nd ed. adopted, published (2006)v
2006 to 2007	The APTA develops advanced training and credentialing program for clinical faculty to build on level-1 program	Develop an advanced educational program available nationwide to further enhance teaching effectiveness and recognition of physical therapy clinical faculty and provide a level-2 credential	Advanced Credentialed Clinical Instructor Program (ACCIP) initiated (2007), ongoing
2007 to 2008	The APTA creates Consulting Group on Uniform Outcomes Assessment	Address goals in the APTA Education Strategic Plan; suggest framework for outcomes assessment for physical therapy education programs	The APTA publication: *Outcomes Assessment in Physical Therapy Education* (2009)w
2007 to 2009	The APTA Consensus Conference Embracing Standards in Physical Therapy Clinical Education held 2007 followed by regional forums through 2009	Achieve consensus on voluntary standards/principles for clinical education for preparation of physical therapist entry-level graduates	The APTA Physical Therapist Clinical Education Principles document adopted, published (2010)x

(continued)

TABLE A-1 (CONTINUED)

KEY ACTIVITIES AND INITIATIVES RELATED TO PHYSICAL THERAPIST EDUCATION IN THE UNITED STATES FROM 1970 TO 2017

YEARS	ACTIVITIES/INITIATIVES	PRIMARY PURPOSE/GOAL	OUTCOMES
2010	The APTA issues request for proposal: *Innovation and Excellence in Physical Therapist Academic and Clinical Education*	Solicit proposals for a study to identify innovative models for academic and CE that might be replicated to meet demands of a changing society	Initial grant of $50,000 awarded for Physical Therapist Education for the 21st Century study (2011); additional funds allocated, awarded (2012, 2013)
2011	Education Leadership Institute (ELI) established	Design a fellowship program to develop education program directors with enhanced leadership skills	Competitive fellowship year-long blended learning and mentorship program initiated in 2011 with first cohort graduating in 2012; ongoing with annual cohorts of ~15 fellows.
2013	The ACAPT established and officially recognized as an APTA component by HOD	Take a leadership role in setting the direction for physical therapist academic and CE and professional development of physical therapists as leaders within the health care team	By 2018, the ACAPT had 216 member institutions initiate numerous activities to advance academic physical therapy
2013 to 2014	The APTA HOD Motions RC 12-13: *Promoting Excellence in Physical Therapist Professional Education and* RC 13-14: *Best Practice for Physical Therapist Clinical Education* both approved	These motions directed the APTA BOD to create mechanism for investigating future directions for physical therapist education	The APTA BODs appoints 2 task forces to address charges and report to BOD: EETF and BPCETF

(continued)

TABLE A-1 (CONTINUED)

KEY ACTIVITIES AND INITIATIVES RELATED TO PHYSICAL THERAPIST EDUCATION IN THE UNITED STATES FROM 1970 TO 2017

YEARS	ACTIVITIES/INITIATIVES	PRIMARY PURPOSE/GOAL	OUTCOMES
2014	The ACAPT National Clinical Education Summit held, supported by the APTA, Education Section, and Federation of State Boards of Physical Therapy	Develop a shared vision and recommendations for fostering/realizing excellence in CE in the future	Summit report and recommendations published (2015)y; several panels established to address recommendations
2014 to 2015	The EETF convenes; issues final report and recommendations	Provide info on current/emerging issues and recommendations to ensure excellence and best meet current/future health care needs	Task force report with 8 recommendations to the APTA BOD (2015); all recommendations approved
2016	Education Leadership Partnership established based on recommendation from the EETF (report to the APTA BOD, 2015)	Create entity for facilitating collaboration between the ACAPT, the Education Section, and the APTA to attain mutual goal of reducing unwarranted variation, realizing best practices, and excellence in physical therapy education	Created subgroups to address education research framework and priorities, needed infrastructure for data repository, education researcher networks; ongoing activity with several planned events in 2018 including grant writing and mentoring workshop
2016 to 2017	The BPCETF convenes; issues final report	Identify strategies and possible actions to achieve best practice in CE from professional through post-professional education	Best Practice for PT Clinical Education report presented to the APTA HOD and BOD (2017)z

APTA = American Physical Therapy Association; CAPTE = Commission on Accreditation in Physical Therapy Education; HOD = House of Delegates; CE = Clinical Education; CI = Clinical Instructor; CCCE = Center Coordinator for Clinical Education; BOD = Board of Directors; CPI = Clinical Performance Instrument; ACAPT = American Council of Academic Physical Therapy; EETF = Excellence in Physical Therapist Education Task Force; BPCETF = Best Practice in Clinical Education Task Force

References

a. Moore ML, Perry JF. *Clinical Education in Physical Therapy: Current Status/Future Needs.* Washington, DC: Section for Education, American Physical Therapy Association; 1976.

b. Moore ML, Perry JF, Clark AW, eds. *Clinical Education in the Health Professions: An Annotated Bibliography.* Washington, DC: Section for Education, American Physical Therapy Association; 1976.

c. Perry JF. *Handbook of Clinical Faculty Development.* Chapel Hill, NC: Division of Physical Therapy, University of North Carolina at Chapel Hill; 1977.

d. Barr JS, Gwyer J, Talmor Z. *Standards for Clinical Education in Physical Therapy: A Manual for Evaluation and Selection of Clinical Education Centers.* Washington, DC: American Physical Therapy Association; 1980.

e. Barr JS, Gwyer J. Evaluation of clinical education centers in physical therapy. *Phys Ther.* 1982;62(6): 850-861.

f. APTA. *Planning for Clinical Education in 1990.* Alexandria, VA: Department of Education, American Physical Therapy Association; 1984.

g. Myers RS. *Current Patterns for Providing Clinical Education in Physical Therapy.* Alexandria, VA: Department of Education, American Physical Therapy Association; 1985.

h. American Physical Therapy Association. *Leadership for Change in Physical Therapy Education.* Alexandria, VA: Department of Education, American Physical Therapy Association; 1986.

i. American Physical Therapy Association. *Pivotal Issues in Clinical Education: Present Status/Future Needs.* Alexandria, VA: Section for Education, Department of Education, American Physical Therapy Association; 1988.

j. American Physical Therapy Association. *Guidelines and Self-Assessments for Clinical Education.* Alexandria, VA: American Physical Therapy Association; 1992.

k. American Physical Therapy Association. *Guidelines and Self-Assessments for Clinical Education.* Alexandria, VA: American Physical Therapy Association; 1999.

l. American Physical Therapy Association. *Physical Therapist Clinical Performance Instrument.* Alexandria, VA: American Physical Therapy Association; 1997.

m. American Physical Therapy Association. *Physical Therapist Assistant Clinical Performance Instrument.* Alexandria, VA: American Physical Therapy Association; 1998.

n. American Physical Therapy Association. *A Normative Model of Physical Therapist Professional Education: Version 97.* Alexandria, VA: American Physical Therapy Association; 1997.

o. American Physical Therapy Association. *Clinical Education: Dare to Innovate! A Consensus Conference on Clinical Education.* Alexandria, VA: Education Division, American Physical Therapy Association; 1998.

p. American Physical Therapy Association. *Guide to Physical Therapist Practice.* Alexandria, VA: American Physical Therapy Association; 1999.

q. American Physical Therapy Association. *A Normative Model of Physical Therapist Professional Education: Version 2000.* Alexandria, VA: American Physical Therapy Association; 2000.

r. American Physical Therapy Association. *Guide to Physical Therapist Practice.* 2nd ed. Alexandria, VA: American Physical Therapy Association; 2003.

s. American Physical Therapy Association. *A Normative Model of Physical Therapist Professional Education: Version 2004.* Alexandria, VA: American Physical Therapy Association; 2004.

t. American Physical Therapy Association. *Guidelines and Self-Assessments for Clinical Education.* Alexandria, VA: American Physical Therapy Association; 2004.

u. American Physical Therapy Association. *Minimum Required Skills of Physical Therapist Graduates at Entry-Level.* Alexandria, VA: American Physical Therapy Association; 2004.

v. American Physical Therapy Association. *Physical Therapist Clinical Performance Instrument.* Alexandria, VA: American Physical Therapy Association; 2006.

w. American Physical Therapy Association. *Outcomes Assessment in Physical Therapy Education.* Alexandria, VA: American Physical Therapy Association; 2009.

x. American Physical Therapy Association. *Physical Therapist Clinical Education Principles.* Alexandria, VA: American Physical Therapy Association; 2010.

y. American Physical Therapy Association. *Clinical Education Summit Final Report and Recommendations.* Alexandria, VA: American Council of Academic Physical Therapy; 2015.

z. American Physical Therapy Association Board of Directors. *Best Practices for Physical Therapist Clinical Education Task Force Report.* Alexandria, VA: American Physical Therapy Association; 2017.

APPENDIX B

In this appendix, we supplement information found in Chapter 3 and provide additional description and detail about our study methods as follows: (1) a brief summary of the national call for participants and the site selection process; (2) an overview of the general nature and structure of the onsite visits conducted by the research team; (3) an index of data collection instruments used during site visits; and (4) selected examples of interview questions for participants at our academic and clinical sites.

SUMMARY OF NATIONAL CALL FOR PARTICIPANTS AND SITE SELECTION PROCESS

As discussed in Chapter 3, final inclusion and selection criteria for academic and clinical site participants in the study were developed based on a review of the literature on physical therapist education and the literature from the Carnegie Foundation's Preperation for the Professions Program studies and with input from a variety of stakeholders. Stakeholder input included recommendations from academic and clinical educators at the American Physical Therapy Association (APTA) Educational Leadership Conferences in addition to several rounds of review and input from our Advisory Board. The Advisory Board was comprised of leaders and representatives from the following organizations or groups: the APTA, the American Council of Academic Physical Therapy (ACAPT), the Education Section of the APTA, the Federation of State Boards of Physical Therapy, and the Foundation for Physical Therapy. Additional input was also sought from our educational research consultants and representatives from the Commission on Accreditation for Physical Therapy Education (CAPTE). Final selection criteria are provided in Chapter 3.

Following the awarding of initial funding for the study in 2011, we issued the first national call for participants and nominations in October of that year. The call was distributed using a variety of print and electronic mechanisms and went to the following individuals and groups: Program Directors of CAPTE-accredited physical therapist education programs in the United States; Directors of Clinical Education/Academic Coordinators of Clinical Education at the same accredited programs; Directors of all Residency Programs approved by the American Board of Physical Therapy Residency and Fellowship Education; members of the ACAPT; members of multiple APTA Component Sections;

Jensen GM, Mostrom E, Hack LM, Nordstrom T, Gwyer J.
Educating Physical Therapists (pp 263-271).
© 2019 Taylor & Francis Group.

and clinical education (CE) sites in the United States that had completed the APTA Clinical Site Information Form and that affiliated with 4 or more educational programs, had at least 1 APTA credentialed clinical instructor (CI) on staff, and had at least 1 clinical specialist certified by the American Board of Physical Therapy Specialties on their staff.

The review of nomination materials and selection of initial sites began early in 2012 with the goal of initiating site visits during that same year. In response to the first call for participants we received 21 nominations (11 academic sites, 10 clinical sites). With additional funding received from the APTA, we were able to select 4 sites (2 academic, 2 clinical sites) for inclusion in our initial sample. The research team reviewed, scored, and ranked all nomination materials and used a Delphi process to achieve consensus on site selection for the first round of visits.

In 2013, energized by our early site visits and recognizing the great potential an expanded sample would have for the robustness of our data and findings, we sought additional funding and were successful in receiving enough support to increase our sample size to one that was similar to those of several of the Carnegie Foundation PPP studies. We issued a second call for participants and nominations that resulted in an additional 7 sites to be considered for selection. Together, the 2 calls resulted in a final group of 15 academic institutions and 13 clinical agencies that were considered for selection. After the second call for participants, nomination materials received in both the first and second call were reviewed. In an effort to ensure geographic and institutional diversity in our sample, the team added some criteria related to these characteristics in this second round of site selections (see Chapter 4). Once again, we used a Delphi process to achieve consensus and selected 7 additional sites (4 academic, 3 clinical) for inclusion in our sample resulting in a final sample of 11 sites (6 academic, 5 clinical). Site visits to these additional sites began in 2013 and continued through 2014.

Overview of Site Visits, Data Collection Methods, and Instruments

As described previously, all 11 site visits occurred over a 2-year period from 2012 to 2014. Each site visit lasted 2 days and was preceded by an extensive review of materials and artifacts provided by the site including, but not limited to, institution/organization/program vision and mission statements, strategic plans, organizational charts, listings of faculty/staff titles, credentials and roles, curricular and assessment materials, selected course syllabi and teaching materials used in both classroom and clinical settings. During the completion of the site visits, we were also provided with additional artifacts for review relevant to interview questions or field observations.

Once onsite, data collection methods consisted of tape-recorded, semi-structured interviews with individuals and focus groups, field observations in classrooms and laboratories, and observations of selected clinical instruction or resident mentoring sessions. Field notes were written for all observations. In almost all cases, interviews and observations were conducted by 2 team members. Site visits were planned in advance to ensure that the team was able to interview and/or observe a variety of key informants including students at various points in their professional preparation, interns, residents, academic and clinical faculty, faculty outside of the discipline who had knowledge of the program/department, and academic and clinical administrators. All interviews were digitally recorded and later transcribed by a third party. We then analyzed the transcribed data and field notes and case records and case reports were prepared (see Chapter 3).

A description of the general structure of the 2-day site visits is provided in Table B-1. A specific schedule for each site visit was developed in collaboration with directors, coordinators, and participants at the sites according to the type of visit (academic institution or clinical agency). Responsibilities for data collection tasks during the visits were distributed across the team of 5 investigators.

An index of the data collection instruments (interview guides and field note forms) used during academic and clinical site visits is provided in Table B-2. We developed the interview guides based on the purpose of our study, the informants we hoped to interview during site visits (individually or in focus groups), and a review of the guides used in the Carnegie studies of medicine and nursing. Interview guides were used as applicable to the site and participants; not all interview guides were used at all sites. Field observations were completed at all sites and were usually followed by debriefing interviews with the participants observed. For example, a typical clinical teaching observation consisted of viewing an entire selected patient encounter, attending the debrief or wrap-up session between the instructor/ student or resident mentor/resident, followed by an audio-taped debriefing interview with the instructor/student or mentor/resident pair. This follow-up interview afforded a unique opportunity to ask questions of both participants and gain additional understandings about what we observed; thus, we were able to obtain both outsider and insider perspectives on what had just taken place.

As can be seen in Table B-2, there were 13 interview guides for academic site participants and 17 interview guides for clinical site participants. All interviews were semi-structured with follow-up probes to interviewees as indicated. The same field note form for observations was used at both the academic and clinical sites. Selected examples of questions included on interview guides for various participants at both types of sites are provided in Table B-3.

TABLE B-1

GENERAL STRUCTURE OF THE 2-DAY SITE VISITS CONDUCTED BY THE RESEARCH TEAM

DAY 1

Activity	Brief Description	Participants and/or Venue
Orientation and overview meeting	Introductions, overview of study background and purpose, large focus group interview	Research team and participants
Individual and focus group interviews	Description of purpose, consent procedures, interview	Academic and clinical faculty; administrators, directors, managers, coordinators, students (years 1, 2, 3), residents, resident mentors
Field observations and debriefings	Description of purpose, consent procedures with key informants, observation, debriefing interview	Classrooms: Entire lecture or laboratory sessions Clinics: Selected patient encounters—Cls/students or interns, residents, and resident mentors
Research team debriefing	Summary of Day 1, reflections, preparation and planning for Day 2	Investigators

DAY 2

Activity	Brief Description	Participants and/or Venue
Individual and focus group interviews	Description of purpose, consent procedures, interview	Academic and clinical faculty, administrators, directors, managers, coordinators, students (years 1, 2, 3), residents, resident mentors
Field observations and debriefings	Description of purpose, consent procedures with key informants, observation, debriefing interview	Classrooms: Entire lecture or laboratory sessions Clinics: Selected patient encounters—Cls/ student or interns, residents, and resident mentors
Closure meeting	Concluding remarks and questions	Research team and participants
Research team debriefing	Summary of Day 2, concluding reflections	Investigators

TABLE B-2

INDEX OF DATA COLLECTION INSTRUMENTS USED DURING SITE VISITS: INTERVIEW GUIDES AND FIELD NOTE FORMS

ACADEMIC SITES	CLINICAL SITES
Program Director	Clinical Site Manager/Physical Therapy Director
Academic Adminstrators; others ("Grand Tour Questions")	Clinical Site Administrators
Director of Clinical Education (DCE)	Clinical Site Managers (departments outside of physical therapy
Director or Research	CCCE
Director of Practice	Focus Group: CCCEs
Curriculum Chair	CI: Individual interview
Residency Director	Focus Group: CIs
Resident Mentor	Student(s): Individual interview or Focus Group
Exemplary Faculty Member	Residency Director
Focus Group: Students (years 1 to 3), Residents	Resident Mentor: Individual interview
Focus Group: Affiliated Clinical Faculty (CIs, Center Coordinators of Clinical Education [CCCEs], Mentors)	Focus Group: Resident Mentors
Focus Group: Clinical Managers of Affiliated Sites	Resident: Individual interview
Cost Questions, Multiple Participants	Focus Group: Residents
Field Note Form for observations	Focus Group: DCE, Affiliated Schools
	Director of Research
	Clinical "Grand Tour Questions," Multiple Participants
	Cost Questions, Multiple Participants
	Field Note Form for observations

Table B-3

Selected Examples of Questions From Interview Guides

ACADEMIC SITES	PARTICIPANTS
How do you view the relationship between the institutional mission/vision and your department mission/vision? How does this play out in your everyday work as Department Chair/Program Director? In your view, what is leadership? How is your leadership expressed? What distinguishes your department/program from other Physical Therapy educational programs? Can you describe 1 or 2 unique elements in your program? How do you feel your program helps your students become the physical therapists you want to see in present and future practice? What do you think are the key messages that faculty see as most important for students as they go into practice? Can you describe a major change in your program and how it occurred? Plans for future change? Describe the relationships among faculty as they teach and work together.	Program Directors, Department Chairs
Academic Grand Tour Questions This program has been identified as an exemplary program in physical therapist education. In your view, what are the elements of excellence that you attribute to this program? How is the program seen by other departments? Administrators? What distinguishes this program from other programs? Can you describe 1 or 2 unique elements? What are your plans or visions for the future?	Multiple Participants: University Administrators, Program Directors, Directors of Research, Practice and Clinical Education, Residency Directors, Curriculum Chairs, Program Faculty
Tell me about the development of the residency program. How would you describe the process to set priorities/develop curriculum for the residency program? What do you believe is the greatest value of this program for residents? What is the interaction between (entry-level) CE and residency education? How does your role as Residency Director differ from other faculty?	Residency Directors
Why do you participate in residency education? Tell me about this community as it relates to residency education and your experience as a resident mentor. Can you describe the approach, process, and activities you use for learner evaluation when you are working with residents? How and when do you provide them with information and feedback in this regard?	Resident Mentors

(continued)

TABLE B-3 (CONTINUED)

SELECTED EXAMPLES OF QUESTIONS FROM INTERVIEW GUIDES

ACADEMIC SITES	PARTICIPANTS
Can you describe a specific experience (in your educational preparation as a student/resident) that you feel has contributed to your learning and development as a physical therapist in a significant way? Tell us about how you are learning to make clinical decisions. What do you think are the key messages that your faculty think are most important as you go into practice? Which ones do you think are most important? How do you see the program (entry or residency) preparing you for practice in the future?	Students, Residents
We often talk about the integration of research and teaching/practice. What does that mean to you? Can you give me an example? What impact does the program's research activity have on the program? Faculty? Students?	Directors of Research
Why does the program have a practice? What does the practice bring to the educational program? We often talk about the integration of academic preparation and practice. What does that mean to you? Can you give me an example? How does your role as Director of Practice differ from other faculty or clinicians?	Directors of Practice
How is curriculum developed here? Who is involved? What are their roles? How do you determine if/when change is made? What changes have been made in the curriculum? Why? How are assessment, student learning and curriculum connected? What feature of the curriculum do you feel is most critical to your success (program, students)?	Curriculum Chairs
Specific follow-up questions based on field observation. What are your values and beliefs about teaching and student learning? Your overall philosophy of teaching? How has your teaching changed over time and what contributed to that change? Any change planned or anticipated for the future? Why? How? What other roles in addition to teaching do you have here? How do you manage/balance those roles?	Exemplary Faculty Members (Interview usually followed by a classroom/ laboratory observation)
Tell me about the CE component of the curriculum/program. What kind of support (is there) for this component? From faculty? From the Director/Chair? We often talk about the integration of academic preparation and practice. What does that mean to you? Can you give me an example? How does your role as DCE differ from other faculty here? What other roles in addition to the DCE do you have here? How do you manage/balance your roles? How is CE considered in setting priorities for the curriculum/program? Any change planned or anticipated (in CE) for the future? Why? What? How? What are the links between your academic faculty and clinical faculty?	DCE

(continued)

TABLE B-3 (CONTINUED)

SELECTED EXAMPLES OF QUESTIONS FROM INTERVIEW GUIDES

CLINICAL SITES	PARTICIPANTS
Why does your clinical practice/agency participate in CE? Residency education? You are here because you serve as a clinical site for (Academic Program). Why do you participate in CE for this educational program in particular? How do you select the academic institutions with whom you are willing to participate? How does the practice's relationship with the academic institution affect your clinical practice? What do you believe is the direct impact of CE on patient care (at your agency)?	Clinical Faculty: CIs and/or CCCEs, Clinical Managers/Directors affiliated with the academic program
Why does your clinical practice participate in CE? What do you believe is the direct impact of CE on patient care (at your agency)? Why does your clinic provide residency education? What is the relationship between the residency program and the entry-level CE program at your agency?	Clinical Managers/Physical Therapist Directors, Clinical Administrators, Clinical Managers (other departments), CCCEs
Tell me about this clinical community especially as it relates to clinical/residency education and your experience here as a clinical educator/residency mentor. Why do you participate in CE/residency education? How do you feel students/residents learn best in clinical settings? What do you actually do when working with students/residents to try to support and facilitate their learning? If you had one take home message or lesson that you would want students/residents to take away from their work with you as an instructor/mentor (at this site), what would that be?	CIs, CCCEs, Residency Directors, Resident Mentors
Tell me about the factors that led to the development of the residency program. How would you describe the process used to set priorities/develop curriculum for the residency program? What are the links between academic and clinical faculty? What does the residency program bring to the entry-level education program or your clinical department/agency? Specific examples?	Residency Directors

(continued)

TABLE B-3 (CONTINUED)

SELECTED EXAMPLES OF QUESTIONS FROM INTERVIEW GUIDES

CLINICAL SITES	PARTICIPANTS
Can you describe the type and level of supervision you have received from your CI/mentor during the course of your clinical experience? Can you describe the process you use to make clinical decisions with/ about your patients? What is the role of your CI/mentor in that process? An important part of any clinical experience is assessment of your performance, learning and development. Can you describe the process or activities your CI/mentor uses to evaluate your performance? How and when have they provided feedback to you? So far we have been talking primarily about the individual who helped your clinical learning. Tell us more about the environment at the clinic where you are completing this experience/residency.	Students/Residents
What are your experiences with institutional leadership relative to CE (at this agency) whether at the institutional level or within the physical therapy service? In what ways are the physical therapists or other staff at this agency involved in your program other than providing CE experiences?	DCEs at affiliated schools
Clinical Grand Tour Questions This program has been identified as an exemplary program in physical therapist education. In your view, what are the elements of excellence that you attribute to this program? How is the program seen by other departments? Administrators? What distinguishes this program from other programs? Can you describe 1 or 2 unique elements? What are your plans or visions for the future?	Multiple Participants: Clinical Managers/ Directors, Agency Administrators, CCCEs, Residency Directors, DCEs at affiliated schools, Directors of Research.
Cost Questions One of the concerns in physical therapy today is pressure from payer sources and concern over finances and payment for services. A student/ residency program introduces an additional variable into the clinical service. One of our goals is to better understand the cost/revenue balance in CE. Overall, what is your impression of the effect students/residents have on your department's finances? Is there variation based on the type of clinical experience (early vs intermediate vs terminal)? What is the relationship between the length of the clinical experience and effect on finances? What data do you collect about finances for your student/residency program? What does that data show?	Multiple Participants: Clinical Managers/ Directors, Agency Administrators, CCCEs, Residency Directors

Financial Disclosures

Dr. *Patricia Benner* has no financial or proprietary interst in the materials presented herein.

Dr. *Bill Boissonnault* has no financial or proprietary interst in the materials presented herein.

Dr. *Steven Chesbro* has no financial or proprietary interst in the materials presented herein.

Dr. *Amber Fitzsimmons* has no financial or proprietary interst in the materials presented herein.

Dr. *Jan Gwyer* has no financial or proprietary interst in the materials presented herein.

Dr. *Laurita M. Hack* has no financial or proprietary interst in the materials presented herein.

Dr. *Joy Higgs* has no financial or proprietary interst in the materials presented herein.

Dr. *Kathryn Huggett* has no financial or proprietary interst in the materials presented herein.

Dr. *Gail M. Jensen* has no financial or proprietary interst in the materials presented herein.

Dr. *Simon Kitto* has no financial or proprietary interst in the materials presented herein.

Dr. *Stephen Loftus* has no financial or proprietary interst in the materials presented herein.

Dr. *Elizabeth Mostrom* has no financial or proprietary interst in the materials presented herein.

Dr. *Terrence Nordstrom* has no financial or proprietary interst in the materials presented herein.

Dr. *Ruth Purtilo* has no financial or proprietary interst in the materials presented herein.

Index

ABPTRFE (American Board of Physical Therapy Residencies and Fellowship), 157

ABPTS (American Board of Physical Therapy Specialties), 157

academic-clinical partnerships, 5, 55-56, 107-108
   challenges and opportunities for, 9-10
   as collaborative learning system, 241-242
   cost of clinical education. *See* cost of clinical education
   as element in Culture of Excellence dimension, 35, 47-49, 73, 121-122, 131
   future for, 49, 241-242, 245-246
   paradigm case, 52-57
   recommendations for, 121-122, 131
   shared responsibilities and, 245-246
   systems-based reform, 158, 161-162

ACAPT (American Council on Academic Physical Therapy), 157, 224-225

active learning, 204-205

adaptive expertise, 85-86, 135, 163

adaptive learners, 35, 85-89
   education research on, 201-203
   evidence from academic and clinical sites, 86-87
   future for, 89, 241
   paradigm case, 87-89
   recommendations for, 133-137
   reflective questions, 137

admissions practices and policies, 206, 227-229

adult learning theory, 204

advocacy, 72, 240

aging population, 9, 140-141

American Board of Physical Therapy Residency and Fellowship Education (ABPTRFE), 157

American Board of Physical Therapy Specialties (ABPTS), 157

American Council on Academic Physical Therapy (ACAPT), 157, 224-225

Academy of Physical Therapy Education (APTE), 157, 224

American Physical Therapy Association (APTA)
   development of faculty teaching skills by, 233
   diversity and inclusion, support for, 166

funding for physical therapist education study, 27-28

historical perspectives on, 5-6, 223-224

interprofessional education and, 10, 180

leadership development programs of, 45, 118, 147-148

overview of, 223-224

partnerships and, 122, 161-162

patient-centered care, primacy of, 62

as stakeholder in physical therapist education, 157

vision statement of, 7, 118, 122, 224, 238

apprenticeship, concept of, 17

apprenticeships (or habits) of professional education, 17, 18, 20, 76-77, 127-129, 139-140, 211-221

approximations of practice, 128

APTA. See American Physical Therapy Association

APTE (Academy of Physical Therapy Education), 157, 224

autonomy, financial, 99

autonomy, professional, 217

beliefs. See shared beliefs and values

Best Practice for Physical Therapist Clinical Education Task Force (BPCETF), 161-162, 225-227

body as subject, research on, 207

CAPTE. See Commission on Accreditation in Physical Therapy Education

Carnegie Foundation, 15-22

1910 Flexner Report, 3, 15-16

Preparation for Professions Program (PPP), 16-21, 25-27

class sizes, 96, 99, 109, 148-149

clinical education, as essential part of mission, 102, 104-106, 150-151

clinical education, cost of, 10, 102, 104-107, 150-151, 161, 245-246

Clinical Education Summit, 121-122, 131, 161

clinical experiences, early authentic, 126-128

clinical imagination, 215

clinical reasoning, 86-87, 89, 136-137, 241

clinical-academic partnerships, 5, 55-56, 107-108

challenges and opportunities for, 9-10

as collaborative learning system, 241-242

cost of clinical education. See cost of clinical education

as element in Culture of Excellence dimension, 35, 47-49, 73, 121-122, 131

future for, 49, 241-242, 245-246

paradigm case, 52-57

recommendations for, 121-122, 131

shared responsibilities and, 245-246

systems-based reform, 158, 161-162

Code of Ethics for the Physical Therapist, 62

cognitive apprenticeships, 17, 20, 130-131

collaboration, in Culture of Excellence, 114, 121-122

collaboration with patient, 136-137

collaborative activities at all levels of society, 240

collaborative competencies, 176, 179-180

collaborative learning system, academic-clinical partnerships as, 241-242

Commission on Accreditation in Physical Therapy Education (CAPTE)

accreditation at doctoral degree level, 6-7

culture of excellence and, 119-120, 162

diversity, requirements related to, 228

interprofessional education and, 10, 116, 176-177, 180

requirements for control of financial resources, 158-160

communities of practice, 130-131, 207

community of education researchers, 231

Conceptual Model of Excellence in Physical Therapist Education, 23-24

Culture of Excellence, 39-57

drive for excellence, 45-47, 119-120, 203

Nexus, related to, 73

overview of, 35, 39-40

paradigm case, 49-57

partnerships, 47-49, 73, 121-122

recommendations for, 113-124

reflective questions, 114-115, 119, 120, 121

shared beliefs and values, 40-42, 73, 113-115, 122

shared leadership with a shared vision, 42-45, 96, 115-119

dimensions, overview of, 35-37

Nexus (learner- and patient-centering), 59-74

evidence from academic and clinical sites, 62-65

forms of knowledge for good clinical teaching and, 65
future for, 72
learner-centered, definition of, 60-61
lens metaphor and, 59
organizational context and, 99-100, 105
overview of, 35, 59-60
paradigm case, 66-72
patient-centered, definition of, 62
reflective questions, 73
shared beliefs and values and, 42, 73, 114-115
organizational context, 37, 95-109
academic programs, 95-102
clinical programs, 102-108
demographic data for academic sites, 97-98
demographic data for clinical sites, 103
learner- and patient-centering and, 99-100, 105
paradigm case, 100-102, 104-108
recommendations for, 147-154
reflective questions, 150, 152
Praxis of Learning, 75-93
adaptive learners, 85-89, 133-137
learner- and patient-centering and, 73, 81, 92
overview of, 35, 75-76
pardigm case, 78-79, 82-85, 87-89, 90-92
practice-based learning, 80-85, 129-132
professional formation, 89-92, 138-142
recommendations for, 125-145
reflective questions, 129, 132, 137, 142
signature pedagogy, 76-80, 126-129
research design and methods, 25-38
Carnegie studies of the professions as model for, 25-27
conceptual frameworks, evolution of, 34-37
data collection methods, 264-265, 267
data verification methods, 30, 34
demographic data for academic sites, 31-32
demographic data for clinical sites, 33

initial conceptual framework from research proposal, 28
interview questions, examples of, 268-271
national call for participants and selection process, 263-264
proposal and funding, 27-28
purpose of study, 28
qualitative case study design, 30
research team, 27, 29
selection criteria for academic and clinical sites, 29-30
site visits, structure of, 264, 266
conflict, as source of innovation and learning, 118, 122
consciousness raising, 215
continuum, learner, 128, 133-135, 163, 180-181
cost of clinical education, 10, 102, 104-107, 150-151, 245-246, 261
cost reduction, by programs, 153, 244-245
critical consciousness, 141
critical self-reflection, 86, 89, 141
critical thinking, 136-137, 201-203
cultural competence, 141
culture, organizational, 113-114
Culture of Excellence, 39-57
drive for excellence, 45-47, 119-120, 203
Nexus, related to, 73
overview of, 35, 39-40
paradgim cases
academic setting, 52-57
clinical setting, 49-52
partnerships, 47-49, 73, 121-122
recommendations for, 113-124
reflective questions, 114-115, 119, 120, 121
shared beliefs and values, 40-42, 73, 113-115, 122
shared leadership with a shared vision, 42-45, 96, 115-119
curriculum, 47, 165, 166, 204-205. *See also* specific topic
diversity of, 7, 9, 152
interprofessional education and, 10, 116, 176, 179-180
practice-based learning and, 69-72, 131, 192-198, 214
re-imagined future for, 240-243
sequential teaching and learning, 214

systematic analysis of, 245
    in workplace settings, 131-132, 179
dance metaphor for formation, 140
data catalog, creation of, 109, 133, 135, 230-231
decompositions of practice, 128
deep structure of signature pedagogies, 20, 76-77, 127-128, 204-205
demographic changes, US, 8-9, 140-141, 165-166
demographic data for academic sites, 31-32
demographic data for clinical sites, 33
dental education, 228-229
Dewey, John, 60-61
diagnostic reasoning, 136
distributed leadership, 100-102, 156, 158
diversity, commitment to, 8, 141-142, 165-166, 227-229, 239-240
doctoral degree, 6-7, 133, 138-139, 224, 246-247
doing, knowing, being, and becoming
    as framework for curricula, 193-195
    in paradigm case, 90-92
    professional practice as, 191-193
drive for excellence, 35, 45-47, 119-120, 203
early authentic clinical experiences, 126-128
Education Leadership Partnership (ELP), 11, 157, 167, 225-227
Education Leadership Institute (ELI)
    Fellowship program, 45, 118, 147-148, 156
education research, 10-11, 163, 201-209
    Education Leadership Partnership (ELP) approaches to, 229-232
    future for, 247
    learning science approach to, 133, 167, 204, 229
    practice-based education and, 206-208
    professional formation and, 205-206
    on pursuit of criticality (adaptive learning), 201-203
    on pursuit of excellence, 203
    signature pedagogy and, 203-205, 207
    systems-based reform, 167, 169
education research literacy, 231
educational enterprise, re-imagined future for, 243-247
EETF (Excellence in Physical Therapist Education Task Force), 225-227
efficiency, 153, 244-245

ELI (Education Leadership Institute)
    Fellowship program, 45, 118, 147-148, 156
ELP (Education Leadership Partnership), 11, 157, 167, 225-227
embedded mind, 212-213
embodied mind, 212-213
entrustable professional activities (EPAs), 133-134, 163, 230
episteme, 207
essential compact, 89
ethical comportment, 42, 92, 139-140, 213, 215-216
evidence-based practice, 69-72, 89, 133
excellence, concept of, 203
excellence, drive for, 35, 45-47, 119-120, 203
Excellence in Physical Therapist Education Task Force (EETF), 225-227
expertise, adaptive, 85-86, 135, 163
expertise, concept of, 85, 207
expertise, routine, 85
extended mind, 212-213
faculty, shortages of, 162, 246
faculty development, 7. *See also* learner continuum
    areas of focus for, 163
    education research and, 231
    formal training in education, 232-233
    interprofessional education and, 179, 183-184
    learning sciences as resource for, 162-163
    needs of education, alignment with, 246-247
    needs of patients and populations, alignment with, 243
    practice-based learning and, 129-130
faculty size, 149
faculty sufficiency and readiness, 162-163, 232-233
Federation of State Boards of Physical Therapy (FSBPT), 157
feedback, role of, 66-69
finances
    acquisition and management of resources, 96, 99, 109, 148-149
    clinical education costs. *See* cost of clinical education
    control of program resources, 148-149, 158-160
    education research funding, 167, 231-232

interprofessional education and, 182

leadership development related to, 147-148, 158

need for systematic study of, 245

negotiation for resources, 99, 149

principles of, 149

program efficiency and costs, 153, 244-245

revenue generation, 96, 99, 109, 148-149

financial autonomy, 99

fit for purpose, ensuring students become, 217-219

Flexner Report (1910), 3, 15-16

formation. *See* professional formation

forms of knowledge, for good clinical teaching, 65

FSBPT (Federation of State Boards of Physical Therapy), 157

funding. *See* finances

giving cultures, 114

global health system, 116-117

graduate level education, 6

habits of head, hand, heart. *See* apprenticeships

health care policies, participation in shaping, 216

health care system, trends in, 116-117

health disparities, 9, 116-117, 140-141, 164-165, 239

health professions education (HPE), financial principles of, 149

hidden (or shadow) structure of signature pedagogies, 20, 76-77, 80, 128, 137, 205

higher education, trends in, 117, 148

historical context, 3-13

  1970s to present, 5-7, 252-261

  Carnegie Foundation

    1910 Flexner Report, 3, 15-16

    Preparation for Professions Program (PPP), 16-21, 25-27

  current trends, 7-11

  origins of profession, 3-4

  Worthingham Study, 4-5

holistic review process, 228-229

human body as teacher, 20, 77-80, 126-128, 207, 212-213

humility, 219

ICE (integrated clinical education) experiences, 7

ICF (*International Classification of Functioning, Disability and Health*), 7, 62, 63-64

identity formation apprenticeship, 17, 18, 20. *See also* professional formation

implicit structure of signature pedagogies, 20, 76-77, 128, 205

innovation, 42, 119-120, 122, 162, 189-190. *See also* adaptive learners

Innovation and Excellence in Physical Therapist Academic and Clinical Education, 27-28

Institute of Healthcare Improvement, 116

integrated clinical education (ICE) experiences, 7

intellectual or cognitive apprenticeship, 17, 20

interactive learning methods, 178

interdisciplinary professional education and research, 202

International Classification of Functioning, Disability and Health (ICF), 7, 62, 63-64

interprofessional education, 167, 175-187, 202, 240

  approaches to, 178-181

  CAPTE and, 10, 116, 176-177, 180

  conceptual model for, 180-181

  evidence for, 184-186

  lessons for successful implementation of, 182-184

  resources for, 177

  spread of, 10, 176-177

  team composition for interprofessional education, 178

  Worthingham Study and, 5

Interprofessional Education Collaborative, 10, 62

interprofessional facilitators, 179

knowledge, forms of, for good clinical teaching, 65

knowledge base, integration of, for optimizing movement, 242

LAMP Institute for Leadership in Physical Therapy, 118, 156

Lancet Commission, 114-115, 116-117, 120

leadership

  control of program resources by, 148-149, 158-160

  development of, 117-119, 156, 158, 162-163

  distributed, 100-102, 156, 158

  as element in Culture of Excellence dimension, 35, 42-45, 96, 115-119

financial management. *See* finances
interprofessional education, role in, 182
needs of education, alignment with, 246-247
negotiation for resources, 99, 149
organizational context and, 96, 99, 100-102, 109, 147-150
paradigm cases, 69-72, 100-102
shortages of, 162, 246
systems-based reform, 156, 158, 162-163, 168
leading societal change that supports movement, 238-239
learner centeredness. *See* Nexus
learner competencies, aligning with patient and population needs, 243
learner continuum, 128, 133-135, 163, 180-181
learner-centered teaching, key features of, 61
learners, adaptive. *See* adaptive learners
learning outcomes for interprofessional education, 10, 180-181, 184-186
learning outcomes, performance-based, 133-135, 164-165, 229-230
learning sciences, 125-137
adaptive learners and, 133-137
education research and, 133, 167, 204, 229
for faculty development, 162-163
overview, 125-126
practice-based learning and, 85, 129-132, 212-213
signature pedagogy and, 126-129, 204
legitimate peripheral participation, 130-131
lens metaphor, 59
lifelong learners, 21
master adaptive learners, 135
mastery, 219
McMillan, Mary, 3-4
medical education, 10, 19, 133-135, 159-160, 180, 228-229, 230
mentoring
in academic sites, 64-65, 78-79
clinical reasoning skills and, 136
in clinical sites, 52, 66-69, 82-85
professional formation and, 216
metacognition, 86, 89, 135, 139, 231
mini multiple interview format, 206
mission, learner- and patient-centering in, 63, 69-72

mission, shared. *See* shared beliefs and values; shared leadership with a shared vision
mission matrix, 54
mission of clinical programs, inclusion of CE in, 102, 104-106, 150-151
Model of Excellence. *See* Conceptual Model of Excellence in Physical Therapist Education
modeling, 41, 50-51
moral (implicit) dimension of signature pedagogies, 20, 76-77, 128, 205
moral agency, 89-90, 166, 217-218
moral community, 140, 166, 240
moral courage, 142, 218-219
moral foundation, development of, 89-90, 138-142, 166
moral obligation, in patient-centered care, 62, 92
moral odyssey, 39
moral responsibility to society, 117
movement, optimizing, integration of knowledge base for, 242
movement, shared language on role of, 80, 126-128
national data set, 109, 133, 135, 230-231
National Physical Therapy Exam, 165
negotiation for resources, 99, 149
Nexus (learner- and patient-centering), 59-74
evidence from academic and clinical sites, 62-65
forms of knowledge for good clinical teaching and, 65
future for, 72
learner-centered, definition of, 60-61
lens metaphor and, 59
organizational context and, 99-100, 105
overview, 35, 59-60
paradigm cases
academic setting, 69-72
clinical setting, 66-69
patient-centered, definition of, 62
reflective questions, 73
shared beliefs and values and, 42, 73, 114-115
1910 Flexner Report, 3, 15-16
nursing education, 3, 19
organizational context, 37, 95-109
academic programs, 95-102

clinical programs, 102-108

demographic data for academic sites, 97-98

demographic data for clinical sites, 103

interprofessional education and, 182

learner- and patient-centering and, 99-100, 105

paradigm cases, 100-102, 104-108

recommendations for, 147-154

reflective questions, 150, 152

organizational culture, 113-114

outcomes, performance-based, 133-135, 229-230

outcomes for interprofessional education, 10, 180-181, 184-186

Paradgim cases

Culture of Excellence, 49-57

Nexus (learner- and patient-centering), 66-72

organizational context, 100-102, 104-108

Praxis of Learning

adaptive learners, 87-89

practice-based learning, 82-85

professional formation, 90-92

signature pedagogy, 78-79

partnerships, 5, 55-56, 107-108

challenges and opportunities for, 9-10

as collaborative learning system, 241-242

cost of clinical education. *See* cost of clinical education

as element in Culture of Excellence dimension, 35, 73

evidence from academic and clinical sites, 47-49

overview of, 47

paradigm case, 52-57

recommendations for, 121-122, 131

reflective questions, 122

future for, 49, 241-242, 245-246

shared responsibilities and, 245-246

systems-based reform, 158, 161-162, 168

patient safety and quality, 10, 116, 176

patient-centered care. *See also* Nexus (learner- and patient-centering)

definition of, 62

practice-based learning and, 81

professional formation and, 92, 138

shared beliefs and values and, 42, 73, 114-115

performance-based learning outcomes, 133-135, 163, 229-230

pharmacist education, 134, 160

phronesis, 207

physical therapist education

accreditation criteria related to financial management of, 159

future for, 109, 243-247

historical perspectives of, 3-13

1970s to present, 5-7, 252-261

current trends, 7-11

Worthingham Study, 4-5

recommendations related to, 152-153

reflective questions, 153

stakeholders in, 157

systems-based reform, 155-171

physical therapist education programs, growth in, 117, 161

positive interpersonal interaction, 122

PPP (Preparation for Professions Program), 16-21, 25-27

practice as doing, knowing, being, and becoming, 90-92, 191-193

practice wisdom, 207

practice-based evidence, in academic paradigm case, 69-72

practice-based learning

in Carnegie's PPP studies, 17, 20

education research and, 206-208

as element in Praxis of Learning dimension, 35, 80-85

evidence from academic and clinical sites, 81-82

future for, 85

overview of, 80-81

paradigm cases, 82-85

recommendations for, 129-132

reflective questions, 132

ethical comportment and, 215-216

experiential teaching and learning, 214-215

learning sciences and, 85, 129-132, 212-213

as visionary educational framework, 189-199

bringing education and practice together, 190-195

creating purposeful curricula, 192-195

model of pedagogy dimensions and practices, 195-198

pedagogical foundations of, 195
praxis, concept of, 207
Praxis of Learning, 75-93
    adaptive learners, 85-89, 133-137
    learner- and patient-centering and, 73, 81,
        92
    overview, 35, 75-76
    paradigm cases, 78-79, 82-85, 87-89, 90-92
    practice-based learning, 80-85, 129-132
    professional formation, 89-92, 138-142
    recommendations for, 125-145
    reflective questions, 129, 132, 137, 142
    signature pedagogy, 76-80, 126-129
Preparation for Professions Program (PPP),
    16-21, 25-27
productivity standards, 102, 104, 106-107,
    150-151
professional autonomy, 217
professional degree, 6-7, 133, 138-139, 224,
    246-247
professional development, arc of, 21, 133-135
professional formation, 166, 216
    in Carnegie's PPP studies, 17, 18, 20
    concept of, 89-90, 139, 205-206
    education research and, 205-206
    as element in Praxis of Learning
        dimension, 35, 89-92
        evidence from academic and clinical
            sites, 90
        paradigm cases, 90-92
        recommendations for, 138-142
        reflective questions, 142
    future for, 92, 206, 216-219
    preparing students for rapid change,
        216-217
    preparing students to be fit for purpose,
        217-219
    for readiness to succeed in faculty role,
        232-233
professional humility, 219
professional identity, 4, 8
professional identity apprenticeship, 17, 18, 20
professional preparation, 162-163, 168, 232-233
professionalism, sustainable, qualities for, 18,
    141
Professionalism in Physical Therapy: Core
    Values, 62
program efficiency and quality, 153, 244-245

program size, expansion of, 99, 148-149
Project on Clinical Education in Physical
    Therapy, 5
Quadruple Aim, 116, 175
quality improvement, 10, 45, 116
questions for reflection
    Culture of Excellence
        drive for excellence, 120
        leadership and vision, 119
        partnerships, 121
        shared beliefs and values, 115
    Nexus (learner- and patient-centering), 73
    organizational context, 150, 152
    physical therapist education, 153
    Praxis of Learning
        adaptive learners, 137
        practice-based learning, 132
        professional formation, 142
        signature pedagogy, 129
rapid change, preparing students for, 216-217
reflection on cases, 215
representations of practice, 128
residency education, participation in, by
    academic programs, 129
residency programs, growth of, 136, 232
resources, acquisition and management of, 96,
    99, 109, 148-149
respect and respectfulness, 218
respect and trust, in Culture of Excellence, 114,
    121-122
revenue generation, 96, 99, 109, 148-149
risk taking, 119-120, 162-163
role modeling, 41, 50-51
routine expertise, 85
safety and quality of care improvements, 10,
    116, 176
self-monitoring skills, 135, 139
self-reflection, critical, 86, 89, 141
sequential teaching and learning, 214
shadow (or hidden) structure of signature
pedagogies, 20, 76-77, 80, 128, 137, 205
shared beliefs and values, 35, 40-42, 73,
    113-115, 122
shared language on the role of movement, 80,
    126-128
shared leadership with a shared vision, 35,
    42-45, 69-72, 96, 115-119
shared responsibility for learning, 61, 191

Shulman, Lee S., 16-18, 20
signature pedagogy, 194. *See also* human body
    as teacher
    in Carnegie's PPP studies, 17, 18, 20-21, 80
    definition of, 18, 76
    dimensions of, 20, 76-77, 127-128, 203-205
    education research on, 203-205, 207
    as element in Praxis of Learning
        dimension, 35, 76-80
        evidence from academic and clinical
            sites, 77-78
        future for, 79-80
        overview of, 76
        paradigm cases, 78-79
        recommendations for, 126-128
        reflective questions, 129
    importance of, 20
    learning sciences and, 126-129, 204
    shadow (or hidden) structure of signature
        pedagogies, 20, 76-77, 80, 128, 137, 205
situated cognition, 129-131, 212-213, 214
social accountability, 120
social contract, 138-142
social determinants of health, 117, 140-141,
    164-165, 238-239
social justice, 141, 166
socialization, 139
societal change that supports movement,
    leadership of, 238-239
societal needs, 5, 9, 140-141
society, participation in, 92, 117, 163-166, 169,
    216, 239
stakeholders in physical therapist education,
    157
student indebtedness, 117, 246
Sullivan, William, 17
supercomplexity, 202

surface structure of signature pedagogies, 20,
    76-77, 127, 203-204
sustainable professionalism, qualities for,
    18, 141
systems-based reform, 155-171
    control of financial resources by
        professional programs, 158-160
    educational research, 167, 169
    leadership, 156, 158, 168
    overview of, 155-156
    participation in society, 163-166, 169
    partnerships, 158, 161-162, 168
    professional preparation, 162-163, 168
    stakeholders in physical therapist
        education, 157
teacher, role of, 61, 204-205
team composition for interprofessional
    education, 178
TeamSTEPPS curriculum, 116
techne, 207
technology, 117, 120, 247
thinking-in-action, 214
timeline of physical therapy education
    from 1970s to present, 252-261
transcending pedagogies, 195
transformative learning, 118, 120
Triple Aim, 116, 175, 238
uncertainty, 87-89, 135, 207
values. *See* shared beliefs and values
vision. *See* shared leadership with a shared
    vision
workforce, challenges and opportunities for,
    8-9
workforce, supply and demand of, 4, 148-149,
    164
workplace learning, 131-132, 179
World Health Organization (WHO), 62, 63-64,
    176, 238-239
Worthingham Study, 4-5

Printed in the United States
by Baker & Taylor Publisher Services